Nutrition for Special Needs in Infancy

Clinical Disorders in Pediatric Nutrition

Series Editor: Fima Lifshitz

Cornell University Medical College, New York, New York
North Shore University Hospital, Manhasset, New York

Other Volumes in Preparation

Nutrition for Special Needs in Infancy

Protein Hydrolysates

edited by

Fima Lifshitz

Cornell University Medical College
New York, New York

North Shore University Hospital
Manhasset, New York

Marcel Dekker, Inc.   New York and Basel

Library of Congress Cataloging in Publication Data

Main entry under title:

Nutrition for special needs in infancy.

(Clinical disorders in pediatric nutrition ; v. 4)
Based on a symposium held in New York on July 12,
1985, sponsored by Mead Johnson Nutritional Division.
Includes index.
1. Nutrition disorders in infants--Diet therapy--
Congresses. 2. Protein hydrolysates--Therapeutic use--
Congresses. 3. Diarrhea, Infantile--Diet therapy--
Congresses. 4. Diet therapy for infants--Congresses.
I. Lifshitz, Fima. II. Bristol-Meyers Co. Ltd. Mead
Johnson Division. Nutritional Division. III. Series.
[DNLM: 1. Infant Nutrition Disorders--diet
therapy--Congresses. 2. Protein Hydrolysates--
therapeutic use--congresses. W1 CL694 v.4 /
WS 120 N9765 1985]
RJ399.N8N874 1985 618.92'390654 85-25288
ISBN 0-8247-7517-1

MARCEL DEKKER, INC.
270 Madison Avenue, New York, New York 10016

Current printing (last digit):
10 9 8 7 6 5 4 3 2 1

Printed in the United States of America

To Jere

SERIES INTRODUCTION

Clinical Disorders in Pediatric Nutrition is a series of books designed to continuously update knowledge of the many advances in the field of pediatric nutrition. This interdisciplinary approach is intended to provide the pediatrician, neonatologist, nutritionist, gastroenterologist, and others involved with clinical disorders in pediatric nutrition, with a single-source, state-of-the-art reference work.

The first book, *Clinical Disorders in Pediatric Gastroenterology and Nutrition,* is part of the Pediatrics series published by Marcel Dekker. It focuses on four areas of great relevance to the understanding of nutritional disorders in pediatrics. Included are hepatobiliary, gastrointestinal absorption, and diarrheal disorders as well as the consequences of gastrointestinal disease. The second book (the first volume in the current series), *Carbohydrate Intolerance in Infancy,* covers, in its entirety, the subject of alterations that result from carbohydrate malabsorption. The third book, *Pediatric Nutrition: Infant Feedings Deficiencies·Diseases,* covers this subject in detail. It is divided into three major sections. The first is devoted to infant feedings, including good clinical guidelines on feeding low-birth-weight infants, design of infant formulas, and maternal and fetal nutrition. The second section discusses important nutritional deficiencies, including iron and zinc deficiencies and rickets. It also covers the area of prenatal mineral deficiencies as well as magnesium deficiency in diabetes mellitus. The final section focuses on a variety of intestinal problems in infancy, including diarrhea and malnutrition, intolerance to food proteins and necrotizing enterocolitis. The fourth book is a unique volume devoted to the subject of vitamin and mineral requirements in preterm infants.

The first four books as well as the present one, *Nutrition for Special Needs in Infancy: Protein Hydrolysates,* complement one another and together present a complete review of the most recent developments in the area of pediatric nutrition.

Fima Lifshitz, M.D.

CONTRIBUTORS

David Burston, Ph.D. Lecturer, Department of Experimental Chemical Pathology, The Vincent Square Laboratories of Westminster Hospital, London, England

David A. Cook, Ph.D. Director, Department of Nutritional Science, Mead Johnson Nutritional Division, Evansville, Indiana

Roberta A. Cooper, R.D. Pediatric Clinical Dietician, Children's Memorial Hospital, Chicago, Illinois

Angel Cordano, M.D., M.P.H., F.A.A.P. Director, Pediatric Nutrition, Mead Johnson Nutritional Division, Evansville, Indiana

Ulysses Fagundes-Neto, M.D. Associate Professor, Division of Gastroenterology, Department of Pediatrics, Escola Paulista de Medicina, São Paulo, Brazil

Brian W. C. Forsyth, M.B., Ch.B., F.R.C.P.(C) Assistant Professor, Department of Pediatrics, Yale University School of Medicine and Yale-New Haven Hospital, New Haven, Connecticut

Serem Freier, M.D. Chairman, Department of Pediatrics, Shaare Zedek Hospital, Jerusalem, Israel, and Visiting Professor, International Institute for Infant Nutrition and Gastrointestinal Disease, Children's Hospital of Buffalo, Buffalo, New York

Narmer F. Galeano, M.D. Research Fellow, Gastrointestinal Unit, Hôpital Sainte-Justine and Université de Montréal, Montréal, Québec, Canada

Harry L. Greene, M.D. Professor, Division of Gastroenterology and Nutrition, Department of Pediatrics, Vanderbilt University Medical Center, Nashville, Tennessee

Donald Hanson, Ph.D. Assistant Professor, Department of Pediatrics, Harvard Medical School, and Associate in Immunology, Children's Hospital, Boston, Massachusetts

Ralph J. Knights, Ph.D. Senior Research Scientist, Mead Johnson Nutritional Division, Evansville, Indiana

Emanuel Lebenthal, M.D. Professor, Department of Pediatrics, State University of New York at Buffalo; Chief, Division of Gastroenterology and Nutrition; and Director, International Institute for Infant Nutrition and Gastrointestinal Disease, Children's Hospital of Buffalo, Buffalo, New York

Fima Lifshitz, M.D. Professor, Department of Pediatrics, Cornell University Medical College, New York; Associate Director of Pediatrics; Chief, Pediatric Endocrinology, Metabolism, and Nutrition; and Chief, Pediatric Research, Department of Pediatrics, North Shore University Hospital, Manhasset, New York

John D. Lloyd-Still, M.D. Professor of Pediatrics, Northwestern University Medical School; Head, Division of Gastroenterology; and Director, Cystic Fibrosis Center, Children's Memorial Hospital, Chicago, Illinois

David M. Matthews, M.D. Professor, Department of Experimental Chemical Pathology, The Vincent Square Laboratories of Westminster Hospital, London, England

Nancy Moses, M.N.S., R.D. Chief Pediatric Nutritionist, Division of Pediatric Endocrinology, Metabolism, and Nutrition, Department of Pediatrics, North Shore University Hospital, Manhasset, New York

Jay A. Perman, M.D. Associate Professor, Department of Pediatrics, and Director, Pediatric Gastroenterology/Nutrition Division, Johns Hopkins University School of Medicine and Johns Hopkins Hospital, Baltimore, Maryland

Geraldine K. Powell, M.D. Associate Professor, Division of Gastroenterology, Department of Pediatrics, University of Texas Medical Branch at Galveston, Galveston, Texas

Kathy A. Powers, R.D. Pediatric Clinical Dietician, Children's Memorial Hospital, Chicago, Illinois

Claude C. Roy, M.D. Chief, Gastrointestinal Unit, Hôpital Sainte-Justine, and Professor of Pediatrics, Université de Montréal, Montréal, Québec, Canada

Alice E. Smith, M.S., R.D. Director, Clinical Dietetics, Children's Memorial Hospital, and Assistant Clinical Professor, Department of Nutrition and Medical Dietetics, University of Illinois, Chicago, Illinois

Deborah K. Sullivan, B.S. Dietetic Intern, University of Illinois, Chicago, Illinois

Saul Teichberg, Ph.D. Associate Professor of Microbiology, Department of Pediatrics, Cornell University Medical College, New York, and Chief, Electron Microscopy Section, Departments of Pediatrics and Laboratories, North Shore University Hospital, Manhasset, New York

Jon A. Vanderhoof, M.D. Professor of Pediatrics and Internal Medicine, Section of Gastroenterology and Nutrition, Department of Pediatrics, University of Nebraska, Omaha, Nebraska

W. Allan Walker, M.D. Professor of Pediatrics, Harvard Medical School, and Chief, Combined Program in Pediatric Gastroenterology and Nutrition, Children's Hospital and Massachusetts General Hospital, Boston, Massachusetts

Raul A. Wapnir, Ph.D., M.P.H. Professor of Biochemistry in Pediatrics, Cornell University Medical College, New York; Head, Laboratory of the Child Development Center, and Chief, Biochemistry Pediatric Research, Department of Pediatrics, North Shore University Hospital, Manhasset, New York

Hans U. Wessel, M.D. Professor of Pediatrics and Engineering Sciences, Northwestern University; Director of Pulmonary Function and Exercise Laboratory, Division of Cardiology, William J. Potts Children's Heart Center; and Associate Director, Cystic Fibrosis Center, Children's Memorial Hospital, Chicago, Illinois

Robert S. Zeiger, M.D., Ph.D. Chief of Allergy, Kaiser Permanente Medical Center, and Clinical Associate Professor of Pediatrics, University of California-San Diego, San Diego, California

FOREWORD

Prior to the early 1940s, allergic and postdiarrheal infants and patients with protein digestion or metabolism problems had no satisfactory dietary source of essential amino acids. In 1942, Nutramigen, the first nonantigenic source of hydrolyzed protein for enteral administration, was introduced. Use of this remarkable product is continuing to expand today, 43 years later.

Prior to the mid-1940s, only glucose, electrolytes, and vitamins were available for intravenous feeding of seriously ill patients. Not surprisingly, patients so sustained normally experienced loss of body protein during any extended illness. In 1944, Amigen, the first nonantigenic, nonpyrogenic protein hydrolysate suitable for parenteral administration, was introduced. Use of this product was effective in decreasing the loss of body protein that normally occurred during extended illnesses.

The primary ingredient for both of these pioneer products was enzymatically hydrolyzed casein, an ingredient that has been comprehensively studied, as recorded in over 400 publications.

The utility of casein hydrolysate did not end with these pioneer products, however. Rather, clinical research, experience, and observation have continued to expand the use and the indications for use of nonantigenic predigested protein:

Because enterally administered casein hydrolysate largely bypasses digestive processes, it has been useful in a wide range of conditions in which adults and infants are unable to digest or metabolize intact protein.

Because casein hydrolysate is nonantigenic, it has been useful in enteral formulas for patients—especially infants—allergic to intact protein such as milk proteins.

Because selected (aromatic) amino acids can be removed by carefully controlled processes such as charcoal treatment, highly specialized products have averted the catastrophic effect of inborn errors of protein metabolism in thousands of patients—especially phenylketonurics—to the extent that adult phenylketonurics experience a more normal life and existence, including childbearing.

Because more recent clinical observations suggest that nonantigenic "protein" sources may be useful in prophylaxis as well as management of allergy, the use of hydrolysate-based products is expanding for this indication.

Because hydrolyzed protein may be more readily reintroduced following intractable diarrhea and protein calorie malnutrition, use in such cases is enhancing the rate of recovery of infants and children from these maladies.

Because we are able to apply increasingly sophisticated basic research tools to the study of protein chemistry and metabolism, the prospect for tailoring hydrolyzed protein products to other highly specific indications appears increasingly feasible.

This book summarizes recent clinical applications for protein hydrolysates and, we hope, will suggest potential new areas of investigation for management of patients who have problems in protein nitrogen metabolism that may occur throughout the life cycle. The contributors of this book constitute an impressive assembly of experts from diverse fields of immunology, protein and nutritional biochemistry, clinical pediatrics, and enteral and parenteral nutrition. They are uniquely qualified to develop the state-of-the-art reference on protein hydrolysates, including both proven and potential areas for clinical utility and patient benefits.

On behalf of Mead Johnson Nutritional Division, I thank the authors confidently and sincerely for the good work that is assembled in this book. I also extend heartiest thanks to Dr. Lifshitz for the leadership and hard work he has invested in the organization of this volume. I trust that it will help to provide continuing benefit to thousands of patients with special protein-nitrogen needs and conditions and will provide material aid to the health care providers who will serve these patients' needs for many years to come.

Jerry L. Moore, Ph.D.
Vice President
Research and Development
Mead Johnson Nutritional Division
Evansville, Indiana

PREFACE

To be conscious that you are ignorant is a great step to knowledge.

Benjamin Disraeli

Nutrition for Special Needs in Infancy deals with the protein hydrolysates and is a much needed review that complements the vast amount of knowledge in this field of human nutrition. The theoretical considerations and the clinical use of protein hydrolysates are reviewed in a systematic fashion, representing the most current data available. Comprehensive information in this subject is thereby provided for all those interested in pediatric nutrition.

Currently, the protein hydrolysates described in this book are being used extensively to meet the special nutritional needs of many sick infants with a variety of entities. The sound principles of dietary treatment with these special formulas could not be reached until after the pathophysiology of the disease was clearly understood. The production of infant formulas to meet these needs could occur only after great advances had been made in the processing and the evaluation of cow's milk substitutes. A symposium held in New York City on July 12, 1985, sponsored by Mead Johnson Nutritional Division, brought together the contributors of this book in an attempt to integrate and disseminate current knowledge to the practicing physician and others who care for infants.

I am grateful to Dr. Angel Cordano from Mead Johnson Nutritional Division; he was instrumental in recognizing the need to gather the available information on protein hydrolysates and to organize the scientific event that led to the publication of this book. I also acknowledge the support of all other directors of Mead Johnson who sponsored this effort as well as to those who devoted long hours of work to make it happen: Messrs. Randall Alsman, Mike Lapcewich, and Lance Stalker.

As documented in this book, progress in the use of protein hydrolysates for the special nutritional needs of sick infants is impressive. However, we are only at the threshold of the acquisition of greater knowledge. Those who wish to learn may find that this volume contains substantial information that may help in the nutritional rehabilitation and care of their patients.

Fima Lifshitz, M.D.

SYMPOSIUM REFLECTIONS

The development and manufacture of casein hydrolysate in the early 1940s was pioneered by Mead Johnson. The long experience in its use taught us its value firsthand. Its early development was clearly a breakthrough in the history of pediatric nutrition. Over the years, we have learned empirically that casein hydrolysate works well in many difficult clinical situations. Many lives have been saved and made better as the result of the availability of casein hydrolysate in infant formulas and adult enteral products.

In this symposium, we had an excellent review of the modern scientific basis for the use of casein hydrolysate in the management of special nutritional needs in infancy. We have considered recent information about the digestion and assimilation, the immunologic components, and the clinical applications of this important protein source. The contents of this book will be informative to students of nutrition and pediatrics alike. We are grateful to the medical and scientific contributors who participated in the symposium and prepared the manuscripts for publication in this book.

It is exciting how much progress we have made in recent years away from empiricism and toward a better scientific understanding of the biochemical, immunological, and functional properties of casein hydrolysate. What we have known clinically for over 40 years is now definable in biochemical and physiological terms. We understand much better now the reasons that casein hydrolysate has worked so well. Moreover, this newer knowledge enables us to make important refinements in the manufacturing and quality of casein hydrolysate and to find new applications. Indeed, the future for the use of improved casein hydrolysate products to manage many special nutritional needs of infants has never looked brighter.

My congratulations to all participants for their thoughtful and informative contributions. They have brought us far but also directed us to many questions that are yet without answers.

Such is the nature of science: We move forward in small steps. I trust that the information exchanged here will stimulate further studies regarding the use of casein hydrolysate in managing the special nutrition needs of many infants and adults.

George L. Baker, M.D.
Medical Director
Mead Johnson Nutritional Division
Evansville, Indiana

CONTENTS

CLINICAL USE

Nutrition for Special Needs
in Infancy

1

Nutrition for Special Needs in Infancy

Fima Lifshitz
Cornell University Medical College, New York, and North Shore University Hospital, Manhasset, New York

I. INTRODUCTION

In the early part of this century, infants with specific reactions to milk feedings and milk sugar malabsorption were described (1,2). Since then pediatricians have recognized that there are special needs for the nutritional management of sick infants. Dextri-Maltose was introduced in 1911 for the dietary rehabilitation of patients who were not able to tolerate milk sugar and/or who were failing to thrive (3). Today, patients with carbohydrate intolerance characterized by diarrhea with excretion of acid stools and carbohydrate in feces (4) are treated with specific proprietary formulas when breast feedings are not feasible (5). These special milk formulas incorporate changes in protein and fat in addition to the substitution of other carbohydrates for lactose to meet the nutritional needs of these patients. During diarrhea there are alterations in the absorption of several nutrients which may be improved by appropriate dietary management (6).

Sound principles of dietary treatment for infants with diarrhea could only be arrived at after the pathophysiology of the disease was elucidated (7). For example, lactose which is generally considered the preferred carbohydrate in the diet of normal infants, is not desirable in infants with diarrhea. Under normal conditions, lactose enhances the absorption of minerals (8) and promotes growth of *Lactobacilli* which inhibit the establishment of pathogenic bacteria (9). However, when lactose is not absorbed, it may lead to carbohydrate intolerance which is the cause of significant alterations in infants with diarrhea

1

(10). In contrast, even though there may be malabsorption of fat in patients with gastroenteritis, (11) the fecal energy loss caused by steatorrhea in diarrheal disease is of little consequence. However, this energy loss can be critical if dietary fat is limited. Low fat formulas may be associated with a worsened nutritional state and may lead to chronic diarrhea (12). Therefore proprietary formulas for the treatment of infants with diarrhea are lactose free and provide adequate amounts of fat to meet the essential fatty acid and energy requirements with absorbable medium-chain triglycerides.

Protein sensitivity is also a factor which may lead to, or be associated with, diarrhea in infancy (13). It has long been known that intestinal permeability might be altered in gastroenteritis (14) due to a variety of factors which disrupt the intestinal epithelial barrier and allow the passage of macromolecules (15,16). Although most patients with diarrhea may generate antibody formation to dietary proteins, relatively few develop food protein sensitivity (17). In designing a formula to meet the special protein needs of sick infants, soy protein was substituted for cow's milk. However, patients who did not tolerate cow's milk protein often did not tolerate soy (17), requiring protein hydrolysates and/or other alternate sources of protein for treatment.

In this chapter some specific considerations regarding a protein hydrolysate formula are addressed. Although this formula seems to be of "ideal" composition for meeting some of the special nutritional needs of sick infants, our recommendations for special dietary formulas for non-breast-fed patients pose a number of interesting problems. Lactose-free non-cow's milk substitutes and/or protein hydrolysate formulas are generally less available and more expensive where they are most needed and least affordable. Nevertheless, this has to be viewed in relation to the possible benefit derived from early nutritional intervention. This formula may prevent life-threatening complications such as malnutrition or chronic diarrhea and/or ameliorate the morbidity of other diseases such as colic in infancy, the cause of many sleepness nights of patients and parents (18).

II. PROTEIN HYDROLYSATE FORMULA
USAGE AND IMPACT ON SEVERE
CHRONIC DIARRHEA

There are many reports in the literature of patients with severe chronic diarrhea in infancy defined in various terms. In 1968 Avery et al. (19) described patients with intractable diarrhea in whom no specific etiology could be identified. In 1970, we described malnourished infants with postinfectious chronic diarrhea in whom acquired monosaccharide intolerance was the cause of the diarrhea (20). In 1971, Hyman et al. introduced another term to define these types of patients; protracted diarrhea (21). In a comprehensive review of this subject, Sunshine et al. cited that in 48% of these patients there was a nonspecific enterocolitis which was secondary to an infectious origin (22). In the majority of these patients, there was acquired carbohydrate intolerance as described earlier (4,20). Since the pathophysiology of the disease is similar in all the above-mentioned entities, the term *chronic diarrhea with carbohydrate intolerance* seems to be more appropriate to define the syndrome. This latter term defines the principal pathophysiological alterations leading to this type of chronic diarrhea and provides a useful guide for nutritional treatment. These infants have severe chronic diarrhea and often require prolonged hospitilization for nutritional rehabilitation, generally provided in tertiary care institutions under the care of pediatric gastroenterologists (23).

In the past few years there seems to have been a general reduction in the number of patients with monosaccharide intolerance being cared for and admitted by pediatric gastroenterologists to university hospitals. This decline appeared to coincide with the increased usage by pediatricians of specific formulae for treatment of infants with diarrhea, which for many years has been recommended (24) and endorsed by the American Academy of Pediatrics (25). During the months of March and April 1985, we conducted a survey among pediatricians and pediatric gastroenterologists in the United States in order to assess the possible impact of protein hydrolysate formula usage in patients with severe chronic diarrhea. These patients were defined as patients with liquid stools for more than 2 weeks leading to dehydration and/or to "intolerance" to cow's milk formula. All relevant terms, protracted or intractable diarrhea, monosaccharide intolerance, and severe diarrhea, were used in the survey questionnaire to define the prevalence of disease regardless of the preference of the physician. However, in the majority of instances, the pediatricians surveyed preferred and identified their patients as having severe chronic diarrhea without specifying carbohydrate tolerance or other terms. Therefore, we have selected this term to define the syndrome herein. Patients with mild forms of diarrhea or with disease of short duration were not included in this survey. The survey was carried out by MARC, a market research supplier in Chicago, Illinois, and sponsored by Mead Johnson Nutritional Division.

A questionnaire was distributed to office-based pediatricians, while a second one was mailed to pediatric gastroenterologists. Of 600 office-based pediatricians randomly selected throughout the United States, 200 responded to a four-page mail questionnaire (33% response rate). Using another questionnaire, pediatric gastroenterologists were interviewed via a two-page mail questionnaire. Only pediatric gastroenterologists identified with an AMA pediatric specialty and specifically listed as gastroenterology subspecialty were included. The mailing list was 120 names long from which 81 usable questionnaires were generated (68% response rate). Approximately one week after the initial mailing a follow-up mailing of the questionnaire was issued to those who. had not responded. The follow-up letter was sent only to pediatric gastroenterologists, thus the higher response rate.

As many as 65% of pediatricians surveyed reported using protein hydrolysate formulas during the past 12 months for their infant patients under one year of age. Indications for this type of feeding as recommended by these pediatricians are listed in Table 1. The most frequently mentioned indication was chronic diarrhea. Other indications included allergy, infant colic, and miscellaneous gastrointestinal complaints.

An average of 13 patients with severe chronic diarrhea in infancy were seen by each pediatrician in one year. Therefore, it could be calculated that up to a quarter of a million U.S. infants per year may have severe chronic diarrhea. This calculation is based on the average of 13 patients per pediatrician per year found in this survey times the approximate 20,000 pediatricians who practice in the United States. We recognize that not all infants, sick or otherwise, are followed by pediatricians in this country, therefore, this number could be a conservative estimate.

In contrast, among the pediatric gastroenterologists, there was a lesser prevalence of patients with severe chronic diarrhea. Only an average of 62 patients per pediatric gastroenterologist per year were reported to have this problem in infancy. Thus, it would be calculated that a maximum of 7500 patients with this condition are being cared for in a given year by the 120 physicians practicing this subspecialty.

If the above-mentioned calculations are remotely correct, it appears that the great majority of patients with severe chronic diarrhea are cared for by pediatricians and not referred to pediatric gastroenterologists. Since specific nutritional therapy for infants with chronic diarrhea has been readily available in this country (5), it is possible that only a few of these patients require a referral to the pediatric gastroenterologist. Indeed, a protein hydrolysate formula which is now widely used by pediatricians and/or other dietary treatments may have been

Table 1 Protein Hydrolysate Use by Pediatricians in the United States in 1985

Indications	% Specifying[a]
Chronic diarrhea	59
Allergy	26
Colic	16
Miscellaneous gastrointestinal disorders	15
Upper respiratory congestion	2

[a]Sum exceeds 100% due to multiple mentions. Of 200 pediatricians, 65% used protein hydrolysate formula.

of benefit in treatment of many of these patients. Among the pediatricians who used protein hydrolysates for treatment of chronic diarrhea in the last year, 67% reported fewer referrals of their patients to specialty centers, and 61% reported fewer hospitalizations of their patients as compared with the previous three years.

On the other hand, only 41% of patients seen by pediatric gastroenterologists because of severe chronic diarrhea had already been treated with a protein hydrolysate formula. One-third of them required hospital admission. Moreover, pediatric gastroenterologists reported a 40% decline in the number of admissions of patients with severe chronic diarrhea over the past three years.

This survey suggests that aggressive nutritional treatment of the sick infant with diarrhea may result in improvement of most patients with fewer instances where deterioration of the clinical course occurs. This observation is in agreement with our report in the early 1970s that monosaccharide intolerance occurred primarily among patients who had lactose intolerance and chronic diarrhea for prolonged periods of time before nutritional treatment (4,20). In a recent prospective study (Chap. 13) we showed that most malnourished patients with postinfectious chronic diarrhea in infancy respond to a protein hydrolysate formula containing glucose polymers. In contrast, diarrhea persisted when other feedings were given and an apparent deterioration of the patient's condition occurred.

III. COST OF DIETARY TREATMENT OF SEVERE CHRONIC DIARRHEA IN INFANCY

Of all the therapeutic modalities of chronic diarrhea in infancy, nutritional treatment is the one of choice. Other forms of treatment such as antibiotics have usually not proved to be effective unless a specific infectious etiology is found. Currently we know that feedings must be offered to the infant with diarrhea unless specific complications preclude feeding or when the stool losses are massive. Breast feedings are still considered the ideal form of feeding in infancy both in health as well as in disease. However, there is controversy regarding the feeding of choice for refeeding infants with diarrhea when breast feedings are not available. Among the many considerations to ascertain the type of feedings to be recommended, there are issues that go beyond the pathophysiology of the disease. These include availability of special formulas and cost. Of course special formula preparations are more expensive and generally less available than cow's milk. In Table 2 a comparison is made of the cost of various milk formulas available; protein hydrolysate formula being the most expensive one except for human milk bought from breast milk banks.

The cost of any item can only be ascertained in terms of value. In a prospective study of the dietary treatment of malnourished infants with postinfectious

Table 2 Cost of Milk Formulas per Liter[a]

Cow's milk	$ 0.70
Enfamil and Similac	1.70
Soy protein	2.00
Nutramigen	2.90
Pregestimil	3.25
Preterm[b]	
Human-banked milk	30.00

[a]Approximate.
[b]Not commercially available.

chronic diarrhea, the use of protein hydrolysate formula was found to be very effective (Chap. 13). A rough attempt to calculate cost versus value of the treatment of such patients with protein hydrolysate formula is made below:

There were 29 patients treated for postinfectious chronic diarrhea. They had a mean of 44.5 days of diarrhea prior to admission to the hospital for treatment. During this time they were given cow's milk and/or cow's milk formula without improvement. This group of patients had a total of 1335 sick days with diarrhea before hospitalization. The cost of this is beyond our analysis. After admission to the hospital, they were treated by the usual means, which included feedings with one-half to two-thirds diluted cow's milk formula as recommended by the World Health Organization (WHO) (26) for a mean of 8.2 days of hospital treatment during which diarrhea and lactose intolerance persisted. These patients received the usual standard treatment for a total of 237 hospital days. The average cost per day is $200 in the Escola Paulista de Medicina, Matarazzo Hospital, Sao Paulo, Brazil. Therefore, the cost of this treatment for this group of patients was $47,400 for the days of diarrhea under standard usual therapy (24).

This amount of money would buy approximately 5000 liters of protein hydrolysate formula (approximately 10 dollars per liter in Brazil). This amount of formula could be sufficient for treatment (150 ml/kg per day for a 5-kg baby) for 6666 days. Since the patients fed protein hydrolysate improved diarrhea within 4 days of treatment, this amount of the "expensive formula" could treat 1666 patients for the length of time required for diarrhea to improve, or 222 patients for one month; the time required for total recovery.

This calculation of costs does not include hospitalization costs of patients while other special formulas were tried, nor does it include the deterioration which apparently took place while these were done before successful treatment with protein hydrolysate formula. Dietary treatment delays and frequent formula changes were associated with severe monosaccharide intolerance which could only be treated by total parenteral nutrition. However, it is obvious that when postinfectious chronic diarrhea occurs in malnourished infants, the usual dietary practices for the infant who is not breat fed need to be re-evaluated in the light of our current knowledge. This includes the assessment of the *value* of the various dietary therapies currently available for these patients. Of course, it would be better to prevent diarrhea through the improved sanitary conditions and encouragement of breast feedings.

IV. FINAL CONSIDERATIONS

Much has been written about human milk feedings in the past few years and its importance cannot be overemphasized. Postinfectious chronic diarrhea in infancy is a problem which occurs almost exclusively in babies who are not breast fed (27). Infants who develop diarrhea in the first few months of life need special nutritional rehabilitation when breast feeding is not available. In these patients there are multiple alterations in the absorption of several nutrients which need to be addressed in a scientific manner. Empiric and unnecessary dietary changes are often made because the disease is thought to be the result of intolerances and sensitivities, thus, delaying appropriate treatment, which could result in deterioration of the patient and aggravation of the intestinal malabsorption (Chap. 13). On the other hand, the need to meet the nutritional requirements of a child who is sick may introduce risks that may even be greater than the risk of insufficient nutrients. There is data linking feedings with the development of severe complications such as necrotizing enterocolitis (NEC) in patients whose nutritional rehabilitation is attempted (28).

The nutritional requirements of sick patients are not as simple as taking out, substituting, or changing nutrients in formula. There are other variables that determine tolerance to foodstuffs that need to be understood. Further studies need to be done to ascertain the reason for the decreased incidence of lactose intolerance despite the high lactose content of human milk (29). This is important in the development of more "humanized milk formulas" for the sick infant who has special nutritional needs. There is evidence that better processed modern cow's milk formulas have already improved "lactose tolerance" as compared with previous preparations (30). On the other hand, lactose-free soy protein formulas can also be noxious due to the lectin content (17). Additional studies are needed to understand the deterioration of the patients given several dietary trials and the development of glucose polymer intolerance (31).

Additional attempts to assess the effects of nutrients on intestinal absorption must be done to determine the optimal performance of different formulae. We recently published evidence regarding the various oral hydration solutions which may optimize jejunal absorption of water and sodium in the intestine of rats (32). This information was generally lacking, since nutrients and foodstuffs do not require the animal experimentation to prove efficacy and lack of toxicity, as required by the Food and Drug Administration (FDA) for drugs. In the case of protein hydrolysates, data is needed to provide information regarding the mode of action of these nutrients at the intestinal level. This may help explain the enhanced performance of this formula for the sick child, which has been clinically observed for many years.

REFERENCES

1. Jacobi, A. milk sugar in infant feeding. *Trans. Am. Pediatr. Soc.* 13, 150–160, 1901.
2. Lifshitz, F. Perspectives of carbohydrate intolerance in infants with diarrhea. Lifshitz, F. (ed.). Marcel Dekker, New York, 1982, pp. 3–14.
3. Cordano, A. Foreward. In: *Carbohydrate Intolerance in Infancy*. Lifshitz, F. (ed.). Marcel Dekker, New York, 1982.
4. Lifshitz, F. Secondary carbohydrate intolerance in infancy. In: *Clinical Disorders in Pediatric Gastroenterology and Nutrition*. F. Lifshitz, (ed.). Marcel Dekker, New York, 1980, pp. 327–340.
5. Cook, D. A. Infant formulas for the management of carbohydrate intolerance in infancy. In: *Carbohydrate Intolerance in Infancy*. Lifshitz, F. (ed.). Marcel Dekker, New York, 1982, pp. 237–248.
6. Lifshitz, F. Childhood diarrhea. In: *Pediatric Gastroenterology*. Silverberg, M. (ed.). Medical Examination Publishing Co., Inc., New York, 1982, pp. 286–306.
7. Lifshitz, F. Nutrition and diarrhea. In: *Manual of Clinical Nutrition*. Page, D. M. (ed.). Nutrition Publishing Co. Inc., Pleasantville, N.J., 1983, pp. 1–26.
8. Kobayashi, A., Kawai, S., Ohbe, Y., and Nagashima, Y. Effects on dietary lactose and lactase preparation on the intestinal absorption of calcium and magnesium in normal infants. *Am. J. Clin. Nutr.* 28, 681–683, 1975.
9. Barbero, G. J., Runge, G., Fischer, D., Crawford, M. N., Torres, F. E., and Gyorgy, P. Investigations on the bacterial flora, pH, and sugar content in the intestinal tract of infants. *J. Pediatr.* 40, 152–163, 1952.
10. Lifshitz, F. Perspectives of carbohydrate intolerance in infants with diarrhea. In: *Carbohydrate Intolerance in Infancy*. Lifshitz, F. (ed.). Marcel Dekker, New York, 1982, pp. 3–20.
11. Jones, A., Avigad, S., Diver-Haber, A. M. S., and Katznelson, D. Disturbed fat absorption following infectious gastroenteritis in children. *J. Pediatr.* 95, 362–366, 1979.
12. Cohen, S. A., Hendricks, K. M., Mathis, R. K., et al. Chronic nonspecific diarrhea. Dietary relationships. *Pediatrics* 64, 402–407, 1979
13. Iyngkaran, N. Intolerance to food proteins. In: *Pediatric Nutrition*: Lifshitz, F. (ed.). Marcel Dekker, New York, 1982, pp. 449–476.
14. Gruskay, F. L., and Cooke, R. E. The gastrointestinal absorption of unal-

tered protein in normal infants and in infants recovering from diarrhea. *Pediatrics,* 16, 763–769, 1955.

15. Teichberg, S., Fagundes-Neto, U., Bayne, M. A., Morton, B., and Lifshitz, F. Jejunal macromolecular absorption and bile salt deconjugation in protein-energy malnourished rats. *Am. J. Clin. Nutr.* 34, 1281–1291, 1981.

16. Teichberg, S., Lifshitz, F., Bayne, M. A., et al.: Disaccharide feedings enhance rat jejunal macromolecular absorption. *Pediatr. Res.* 17, 381–389, 1983.

17. Lifshitz, F. Food intolterance and sensitivity. In: *Advances in Pediatric Gastroenterology and Nutrition.* Lebenthal, E. (ed.). Excerpta Medica, Hong Kong, 1984, pp. 131–140.

18. Lothe, L., Lindberg, T., and Jakobsson, I. Cow's milk formula as a cause of infantile colic: A double-blind study. *Pediatrics* 70, 7, 1982.

19. Avery, G. B., Villavicencio, O., Lilly, J. R., et al.: Intractable diarrhea in early infancy. *Pediatrics* 41, 712, 1968.

20. Lifshitz, F., Coello-Ramirez, P., and Gutierrez-Topete, G. Monosaccharide intolerance and hypoglycemia in infants with diarrhea. Clinical course of 23 cases. *J. Pediatr.* 77, 595, 1970.

21. Hyman, C. J., Reiter, J., Rodnan, J., and Drash, A. L. Parenteral and oral alimentation in the treatment of the nonspecific protracted diarrheal syndrome of infancy. *J. Pediatr.* 78, 17–29, 1971.

22. Sunshine, P., Sinatra, R. R., and Mitchell, C. H. Intractable diarrhoea of infancy. *Clin. Gastroenterol.* 6, 445, 1977.

23. Lloyd-Still, J. D., Stockman, H., and Filler, R. M. Protracted diarrhea of infancy treated by intravenous elimination. *Am. J. Dis. Child.* 125, 352–364, 1973.

24. Lifshitz, F. Malabsorption syndrome and intestinal disaccharidase deficiencies. In: *Current Pediatric Therapy,* 6th ed. Gellis, S., and Kagan, B. M. (eds.). W. B. Saunders Co., Philadelphia, London, Toronto, 1973, p. 236.

25. Bartrop, R. W., and Hull, D. Transient lactose intolerance in infancy. *Arch. Dis. Child.* 48, 963–966, 1973.

26. World Health Organization. *Control of Diarrhoeal Diseases. A Manual for the Treatment of Acute Diarrhoea.* World Health Organization, Geneva, 1984, Rev. 1.

27. Auricchio, S., Della Pietra, D., and Vegnente, A. Studies on intestinal digestion of starch in man. II. Intestinal hydrolysis of amylopectin in infants and children. *Pediatrics* 39, 853–862, 1967.

28. Lifshitz, F. Necrotizing enterocolitis and feedings. In: *Pediatric Nutrition: Infant Feedings-Deficiencies-Disease.* Lifshitz, F. (ed.). Marcel Dekker, New York, pp. 513–530.

29. Okuni, M., Okinaga, K., and Baba, K. Studies on reducing sugars in stools of acute infantile diarrhea, with special reference to differences between breast fed and artificially fed babies. *Tohoku J. Exp. Med.* 107, 395–402, 1972.

30. Walker-Smith, J. A. Interrelationship between cow's milk protein intoler-

ance and lactose intolerance. In: *Carbohydrate Intolerance in Infancy*. Lifshitz, F. (ed.). Marcel Dekker, New York, 1982, pp. 155-170.

31. Fagundes Neto, U., Viarro, T., and Lifshitz, F. Tolerance to glucose polymer in malnourished infants with diarrhea and disaccharide intolerance. *Am. J. Clin. Nutr.* 41, 228-234, 1985.

32. Lifshitz, F., and Wapnir, R. A. Oral hydration solutions: Experimental optimization of water and sodium absorption. *J. Pediatr.* 106, 383-389, 1985.

THEORETICAL CONSIDERATIONS

2

Absorption of Proteins and Their Digestion Products in Early Life

David M. Matthews and David Burston
The Vincent Square Laboratories of Westminster Hospital, London, England

I. INTRODUCTION

Proteins and their digestion products—peptides and amino acids—comprise a group of compounds of greatly different molecular size and profoundly different properties. Consequently it would be useful to begin with a short account of how different types of compound are transported by the intestinal mucosa. We shall then outline, for purposes of comparison, what is known of the intestinal absorption of each class of compound in infancy and in adult life. The accounts of absorption in adults will precede with account of absorption in infancy, since, in general, so much more is known about absorption in adults.

References, which might (at least if we include digestion, the final stages of which are now known to be an integral part of the absorptive process) form an exhaustive list possibly predating Plato (1,2), will be minimized in the present account by confining them to key papers, reviews, and recent publications not dealt with in the reviews quoted herein.

II. MODES OF TRANSPORT BY THE INTESTINAL MUCOSA

A. Simple Diffusion

In the case of hydrophilic molecules, transport by simple diffusion is usually small. Uptake is believed to occur through aqueous "pores" or hydrophilic areas in the predominantly lipid cell membrane, through the "tight junctions," and also through discontinuities in the mucosa, in particular the "extrusion zones" where mucosal cells are shed at the tips of the villi. Transport of hydrophilic compounds by simple diffusion is greatest when the molecular weight is under 200, but some transport apparently by this means has been observed with substantially larger molecules; a good example is cyanocobalamin (MW $\sim$ 1300) without the aid of intrinsic factor. Lipophilic molecules diffuse readily through membrane lipid.

B. Carrier-Mediated Transport

This process depends on the substrate crossing the cell membranes by (hypothetical) carrier molecules. It is usually active (i.e., directly or indirectly dependent on metabolic energy), but in a few cases may be passive ("facilitated diffusion"). Both of these processes show saturation kinetics, in contrast to the linear rate/concentration (first-order) kinetics shown by simple diffusion. Substrates which enter the cells by carrier-mediated transport probably leave them by similar but not necessarily identical processes.

C. Pinocytosis

In this process the plasma membrane of the absorptive cells surrounds and engulfs the substrate (which may in extreme cases be particulate). The resulting vesicles traverse the absorptive cell and leave it by the reverse process of exocytosis, or they may fuse with lysosomes on the way (see Sect. III.B). Pinocytosis, like carrier-mediated active transport, is dependent on metabolic energy.

It is quite possible that more than one of the processes described above are involved in the absorption of proteins, peptides, and amino acids. A minority of peptides, especially small cyclic peptides, such as the toxin cyclochloritine, are very lipophilic and are almost certainly absorbed on a large scale by diffusion through membrane lipid (3).

III. ABSORPTION OF WHOLE PROTEINS

A. In the Adult

There was a time in the 1840s and 1850s when it was thought that all "protein" was absorbed into the body either intact or with very little modification beyond "solubilization." This view was fairly rapidly abandoned in favor of the hypothesis that "peptones" (mixtures of polypeptides) were resynthesized to plasma proteins in the wall of the small intestine (4). However, it was still believed at least 100 years ago that one protein at least must be absorbed intact, since by about 1880 it was known that ingestion of large doses of raw egg albumin led to proteinuria (later shown to be due to a mixture of egg albumin and other proteins) (5) and the observation still stands. As recently as 1949, Dent and Schilling (6) claimed that homologous serum proteins could be absorbed from the small intestine of the dog on a large scale with little or no digestion, a claim which has never been confirmed or conclusively refuted, and the validity of which Dent, a very distinguished investigator, remained convinced of for the rest of his life (C. E. Dent to D. M. Matthews, personal communication). The occurrence of food allergies, known for more than half a century, indicates that appreciable quantities of whole proteins or large protein fragments must be capable of entering the body after ingestion. While the present authors would be distressed if they were to give the impression [as some do (7)] that whole proteins were absorbed in the adult mammal on a scale sufficient to be of nutritional importance (on an immunological scale would be more correct) they feel that the idea of occurrence of the absorption of intact proteins and other macromolecules may have been dismissed too lightly by the intestinal physiologist in the recent past. Even finely particulate matter will enter the bloodstream if introduced into the intestine in sufficient dosage. The impression that absorption of whole proteins is quite negligible in the adult mammal may have been reinforced in recent years by the discovery of the phenomenon known as closure of the intestine in the neonate (see Sect. III.B). As Walker (8) puts it, "on the basis of these observations" (i.e., of *closure*) "it has been assumed that macromolecular absorption ceases entirely with epithelial cell maturation." Gardner (9) also refers to this baseless assumption.

There is now no doubt that biologically significant quantities of many proteins or large protein fragments may be absorbed into the body. Antigens to milk proteins and many other food proteins may be found in human blood. In addition, there is no reasonable doubt that a number of whole proteins including insulin, egg albumin, bovine serum albumin (BSA), bromelain (a proteolytic enzyme found in the pineapple), horseradish peroxidase (HRP), and botulinus toxin can be absorbed to some extent intact in experimental animals or humans (8). Animal investigations have shown that the major factor in intestinal uptake of whole proteins is almost certainly pinocytosis, but passage through the so-called "tight junctions" may occur, at least in certain circumstances. Entry through mucosal discontinuities such as the apical extrusion zones of the villi is another possible route of uptake. It has recently been shown that a special type of epithelial cell, the M cell or membranous epithelial cell, occurs in clusters overlying the lymphoid Peyer's patches in several species including humans. These cells, which appear to be particularly active in taking up low concentrations of protein, may provide a means for the ready access of antigens to lymphoid tissue. A large number of factors may influence whole protein absorption in health and disease, including immunological factors; but these areas are outside the scope of a compact review such as this. Walker

(8) gives the fullest account of factors influencing protein absorption, including the immunological aspect.

B. In the Infant

Neonatal mammalian small intestine has the ability to take up macromolecules, particularly γ-globulins on a massive scale by the process known as pinocytosis (endocytosis). The first hint of this came at least 80 years ago (5). The molecules are first adsorbed to the microvillous membrane, and when their concentration is sufficient the membrane invaginates to form small vesicles. Within the cell, the vesicles coalesce with lysosomes to form large vacuoles (phagolysosomes). Within these, digestion takes place, but some of the substrate escapes digestion and reaches the basolateral surface of the cell through which it passes by exocytosis, the reverse of endocytosis. After a time, from days to a few weeks, which varies between species, with cell maturation and the development of immunological defenses, the ability to take up maternal antibodies and other macromolecules is drastically reduced. This is the phenomenon known as closure. In the human infant, as opposed to the young of rodents and ruminants, passive immunity is derived almost entirely from transplacental transport of maternal antibodies before birth and not from colostrum. There is little intestinal absorption of γ-globulin, and though some protein is absorbed, closure, which may occur at about 3 months, is a less dramatic phenomenon than in some other species. There is some evidence that in the premature infant, absorptive ability for macromolecules is enhanced as it is in the neonate (8).

IV.   ABSORPTION OF PEPTIDES OF
MEDIUM SIZE

Here we are in a grey area about which little is known (3,9). From the functional point of view, a peptide of medium size is one which is too large (tetrapeptide and above) for carrier-mediated transport to polypeptides as large as insulin. Many such peptides, including small peptides unsuited for structural reasons for mediated transport, and many showing biological activity such as insulin and smaller biologically active peptides, are known to be absorbed intact on a small scale, but exactly how is another matter. Peptides of or approaching the size of insulin are probably absorbed by the same mechanisms as whole proteins. Smaller peptides may be taken up through aqueous pores, the extrusion zones, and the tight junctions, or, if lipid soluble, by diffusion through the lipid of the cell membranes of the absorptive cells. Unfortunately, nothing special is known of the absorption of peptides of medium size in infancy. This is particularly regrettable since more than one such peptide is known to occur in human milk for no apparent reason (10).

V. ABSORPTION OF SMALL PEPTIDES

A. In Adults

Until about 1970 it was generally believed that the intestinal mucosa could not take up small peptides at all or hardly at all; uptake was believed to be entirely in the form of amino acids (4). However, since the demonstration in 1968 in our laboratory and that of Siamak Adibi in Pittsburgh that di- and tripeptides could be absorbed more rapidly than the equivalent amino acids, and the demonstration of active transport of small peptides in the early 1970s, the study of the intestinal uptake of these compounds, which is clearly of major importance, has proceeded apace. As early as 1974 it was possible to write a substantial review on the subject (11). The following account is condensed from several sources (see especially Refs. 3,4,11-14). Though certain important questions remain unanswered, so much information has now accumulated that the account will have to be highly compressed.

Uptake into the absorptive cells of di- and tripeptides of normal structure such as are derived from partial hydrolysis of dietary proteins is an active process (e.g., dependent on metabolic energy). Tetra- and higher peptides are not actively transported. The process shows stereochemical specificity, peptides containing D amino acids being only slowly or very slowly transported. Substitution of the terminal amino or carboxyl group usually reduces if it does not abolish affinity for transport. This is why certain biologically active tripeptides such as thyroliberin are so poorly absorbed. Uptake of small peptides is totally independent of that of amino acids. Apparently this explains why patients with inborn inability to absorb certain groups of amino acids (Hartnup disease and cystinuria) are able to survive, because their nutritional requirements for the "affected" amino acids are met by their intact peptide uptake systems. Di- and tripeptides compete with each other for uptake, but not with free amino acids. Unlike the process of amino acid uptake, that for peptides appears to be independent of the nature of the charge on the side-chains [e.g., basic, acidic and neutral peptides all appear to be taken up by the same system(s)]. Whether there is one or more than one peptide uptake system is not yet clear (15). It is possible that more than one system exists.

Most small peptides, and here we include peptides of up to at least 6 amino acid residues, undergo a varying degree of hydrolysis in the brush border. Tripeptides, dipeptides, and free amino acids are then taken up into the absorptive cells in which, in the majority of cases, hydrolysis is completed or nearly completed by the peptidases of the cytosol. Nevertheless, there are known to be a number of di- and tripeptides which are sufficiently hydrolysis resistant to enter the blood, to some extent, intact. These include, to name but a few, glycylglycine, peptides of proline and hydroxyproline, and carnosine, the latter being a neurotransmitter peptide found in many meats, especially chicken muscle. The total extent of peptide entry into the bloodstream is in fact, after some hundred years of debate, still an unsolved question (9)! It may, in the case of some proteins such as casein or gelatin, be as high as 10% or more of the total absorption of protein digestion products.

One very important point remains to be discussed. It has long been known that the percentage absorption of amino acids from a mixture of free amino acids is very unequal. When, on the other hand, experiments were made (by intestinal perfusion in humans) on the absorption of amino acids from partial hydrolysates of proteins consisting largely of small peptides, it was found that the inequalities in percentage absorption rate were much reduced (16) and that the total absorption of amino acid nitrogen from the hydrolysates was more rapid than from the equivalent amino acid mixtures. The more even absorption of amino acids from protein hydrolysates might result in more simultaneous presentation of amino acids to the tissues and explain the numerous claims of the nutritional superiority of whole proteins over that of mixtures of free amino acids (3). This hypothesis, incidentally, seems to have passed unnoticed and untested by professional nutritionists, in spite of having been put forward on many occasions.

B. In the Infant

Little work has been done so far on peptide absorption in infancy, but what has been done is extremely exciting. It suggests that peptide uptake by the intestine, although probably already the major mode of protein absorption in adults, may be far and away more important than amino acid absorption in early infancy.

The first observations were made by Rubino and Guandalini (17) and enlarged upon by Guandalini and Rubino (18). They found that jejunal influx of glycylproline was about 10 times more rapid than that of free glycine in the perinatal period in the rabbit, declining rapidly in the first week of postnatal life and then more slowly to adult values at about 3 months (Fig. 1). The relative rapidity of peptide influx in early life was due to a high V_{max}, which might be due to an increased number of transport sites, a greater rate of translocation of carrier-substrate complex, or both. Further similar observations in the guinea pig were reported by Himukai et al. (19) who reported that influxes of glycylglycine and glycyl-leucine were much more rapid in relation to those of the constituent amino acids in animal neonates. They stressed that if it is important to replace amino acid mixtures by peptide-containing solutions in special diets for malnourished adults, as it certainly seems to be (3,16), then it may be even more so in the infant.

Auricchio (20) has reviewed the developmental aspects of intestinal peptide hydrolysis and absorption, pointing out that the high fetal and perinatal activity

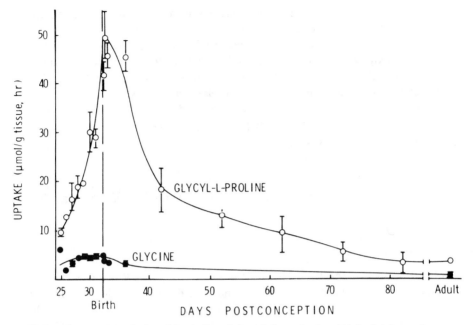

Figure 1 Uptake of glycyl-L-proline (○) and free glycine (●) in fetal, newborn, and suckling rabbits. Uptake values are means ±1 SEM. Concentrations of both substrates in the incubation medium were 0.5 mM. (From Ref. 18.)

of many intracellular peptidases in several species including the human is compatible with the importance of intestinal peptide uptake in the neonate.

VI. ABSORPTION OF AMINO ACIDS

A. In Adults

Amino acid absorption has been studied extensively for more than 30 years, since it was found to be an active process. So much is known about the process now that it cannot be properly reviewed here, especially as it is probably less important quantitatively than peptide absorption, particularly in the very young. Many good reviews are available (21-23). Amino acid uptake, like the uptake of di- and tripeptides, is a stereochemically specific active process. It is completely independent of peptide uptake, and hence amino acids do not compete with peptides for uptake, although they do so among themselves. Several distinct systems for amino acid uptake are distinguishable, dividing the amino acids into several different "transport groups." The main systems in humans are usually described as (a) for most neutral amino acids; (b) for glycine, proline, and hydroproline; (c) for the dicarboxylic (acidic) amino acids, glutamic and aspartic; and

(d) for the diamino (dibasic) amino acids, lysine, arginine, ornithine, and also cystine. The importance of exit mechanisms in amino acid and peptide absorption is well shown by the congenital defect of lysinuric protein intolerance, in which the exit mechanism for basic amino acids is defective, and such amino acids are poorly absorbed whether given in free or peptide form (see Ref. 14). This contrasts sharply with the defects of Hartnup disease and cystinuria, in which the uptake mechanisms for free amino acids are at fault and "affected" amino acids may be absorbed from peptides (see Sect. V.A) because the exit mechanisms for amino acids are intact.

B. In the Infant

Little is known about amino acid absorption in young animals, save that it is probably more rapid than later in life (18,19).

VII. CONCLUSION

In all mammalian species studied, there appear to be marked differences between intestinal absorption of proteins and their digestion products during the neonatal period and in later life. Perhaps most important is the ability of the neonate to absorb whole proteins on a massive scale, including maternal antibodies (though in the human infant, the absorption of antibodies appears to be relatively unimportant). Next, the uptake of small peptides, probably the major mode of uptake of protein digestion products in adults, is probably far more rapid in the neonate than uptake of amino acids. Finally, the absorption of amino acids themselves may be moderately more rapid in the neonate than in adult life. A last word of caution must be added. Most of the observations in the neonate have been made in experimental animals and can only be extrapolated to the human species. In this instance, such extrapolation may be fairly safe, but the possibility of species differences can never be ignored.

ACKNOWLEDGMENTS

We are deeply grateful for financial support to the Frank Odell Charity, an anonymous donor, and many other generous donors to the Children's Medical Charity which is now supporting all academic work in The Department of Experimental Chemical Pathology.

REFERENCES

1. Cary, R. J. Digestion: an historical survey. *Bull. Johns Hopkins Hosp.* 27, 142-152, 1976.

2. Rogers, Q. R., and Harper, A. E. Protein digestion: Nutritional and metabolic considerations. *World Rev. Nutr. Diet* 6, 250-291, 1966.

3. Matthews, D. M., and Payne, J. W. (eds.). *Peptide Transport in Protein Nutrition*. North Holland, Amsterdam, 1975.

4. Matthews, D. M. Memorial lecture: Protein absorption—then and now. *Gastroenterology* 73, 1267-1279, 1977.

5. Verzár, F., and McDougall, E. J. *Absorption from the Intestine* (Facsimile ed.) Hafner Publishing Co., New York, 1967, pp. 237-240.

6. Dent, C. E., and Schilling, J. A. Studies on the absorption of proteins: the amino acid pattern in the portal blood. *Biochem. J.* 44, 318-333, 1949.

7. Hemmings, W. A., and Williams, E. Q. Transport of large breakdown products of dietary protein through the gut wall. *Gut* 19, 715-725, 1978.

8. Walker, W. A. Intestinal transport of macromolecules. In *Physiology of the Gastrointestinal Tract*. Johnson, L. R. (ed.). Raven Press, New York, 1981, pp. 1271-1289.

9. Gardner, M. L. G. Intestinal assimilation of intact peptides and proteins from the diet—a neglected field? *Biol. Res.* 59, 289-331, 1984.

10. Mellander, B. In Discussion following Rubino, A. and Guandalini, S. Dipeptide transport in the intestinal mucosa of developing rabbits. In *Peptide Transport and Hydrolysis*. (Ciba Foundation Symposium 50). Elliott, K. and O'Connor, M. (eds.). Elsevier, Amsterdam, 1977, pp. 61-71.

11. Matthews, D. M. Intestinal absorption of peptides. *Physiol. Rev.* 55, 537-608, 1975.

12. Matthews, D. M., and Adibi, S. A. Peptide absorption. *Gastroenterology* 71, 151-161, 1976.

13. Matthews, D. M., and Payne, J. W. Transmembrane transport of small peptides. In *Current Topics in Membranes and Transport*, Vol. 14. Bronner, F. and Kleinzeller, A. (eds.). Academic Press, New York, 1980, pp. 331-425.

14. Matthews, D. M. Absorption of peptides, amino acids and their methylated derivatives. In *Aspartame: Physiology and Biochemistry*. Stegink, L. D. and Filer, L. J. (eds.). Dekker, New York, 1984, pp. 29-46.

15. Matthews, D. M., and Burston, D. Uptake of a series of neutral dipeptides including L-alanyl-L-alanine, glycylglycine and glycylsarcosine by hamster jejunum *in vitro*. *Clin. Sci.* 67, 541-549, 1984.

16. Silk, D. B. A., Fairclough, P. D., Clark, M. L., Hegarty, J. E., Marrs, T. C., Addison, J. M., Burston, D., Clegg, K. M., and Matthews, D. M. Use of a peptide rather than free amino acid nitrogen source in chemically defined "elemental" diets. *J. Parent. Ent. Nutr.* 4, 548-553, 1980.

17. Rubino, A., and Guandalini, S. Dipeptide transport in the intestinal mucosa of developing rabbits. In *Peptide Transport and Hydrolysis* (Ciba Foundation Symposium 50). Elliott, K. and O'Connor, M. (eds.). Elsevier, Amsterdam, 1977, pp. 61-71.

18. Guandalini, S., and Rubino, A. Development of dipeptide transport in the intestinal mucosa of rabbits. *Pediatr. Res.* 16, 99-103, 1982.

19. Himukai, M., Konno, T., and Hoshi, T. Age-dependent changes in intes-

tinal absorption of dipeptides and their constituent amino acids in the
guinea pig. *Pediatr. Res.* 1271-1275, 1980.

20. Auricchio, S. Developmental aspects of brush border hydrolysis and absorp-
    tion of peptides. In *Textbook of Gastroenterology and Nutrition in In-
    fancy*. Lebenthal, E. (ed.). Raven Press, New York, 1981, pp. 375-384.

21. Wiseman, G. Absorption of protein digestion products. In *Biomembranes*,
    Vol. 4A, *Intestinal Absorption*. Smyth, D. H. (ed.). Plenum Press, London-
    New York, 1974, pp. 363-481.

22. Lerner, J. *A Review of Amino Acid Transport Processes in Animal Cells and
    Tissues*. University of Maine Press, Orono, Maine, 1978.

23. Munck, B. G. Intestinal absorption of amino acids. In *Physiology of the
    Gastrointestinal Tract*. Johnson, L. R. (ed.). Raven Press, New York, 1981,
    pp. 1097-1122.

3

The Effects of Sodium Replacement on Peptide Uptake by the Small Intestine

David Burston and David M. Matthews
The Vincent Square Laboratories of Westminster Hospital, London, England

I. INTRODUCTION

It has been shown (1,2) that peptide absorption plays a large part in perinatal nutrition in animals and it is almost certain that a similar situation exists in humans. Although the general requirements for peptide transport are now well known (3) there are still some areas in which more basic research is needed, one such area is whether or not peptide transport is sodium-dependent. Many small molecules, including monosaccharides and amino acids, are transported together with sodium, the sodium entering the cell via its electrochemical gradient and providing the driving force for the transport of the cotransported substrate. With the demonstration by Craft et al. (4) and Adibi and Phillips (5), that uptake of amino acids from peptides was more rapid than from their constituent amino acids, implying uptake of intact peptide, investigators wondered whether peptide uptake, like the uptake of amino acids was sodium-dependent. The first experiments in this area (6) gave negative results, but this is not surprising as they were carried out in isolated loops of intestine in vivo, so that even though the lumen was sodium free, as the intestine had an intact blood supply the mucosal surface was unlikely to have been free of sodium. The first demonstration that peptide transport was sodium-dependent was reported by Rubino et al. (7) who showed that sodium replacement by choline reduced Gly-Pro uptake under conditions of influx. From 1972 to 1974 our group (8,9) using everted rings of hamster jejunum showed that 20 min uptake of two hydrolysis-resistant

Table 1 Sodium Dependence of Peptide Uptake by Small Intestine

Reference	Technique	Peptide(s)	Substituent(s)	Na^+ dependent
Matthews et al. (6)	Rat jejunum in vivo	Gly-Gly	Mannitol	No
Rubino et al. (7)	Rabbit ileum in vitro	Gly-Pro	Choline	Yes
Addison et al. (8)	Hamster jejunum in vitro	Gly-Sar	K^+, Li^+	Yes
Matthews et al. (9)	Hamster jejunum in vitro	Carnosine	K^+, choline, Tris	Yes
Cheeseman and Smyth (10)	Rat small gut in vitro	D-Leu-Gly	Choline	Yes
Sigrist-Nelson (11)	Rat brush-border vesicles	Gly-Leu	K^+	Yes
Cheesman and Parsons (12)	Frog small gut in vitro	Gly-Leu Leu-Gly	K^+	No
Heading et al. (13)	Rat small gut in vitro	L-Tyr-D-Ala L-Tyr-Gly	K^+	Yes
Himukai and Hoshi (14)	G. pig ileum in vitro	Gly-Leu	Mannitol	No
Ganapathy et al. (15)	Rabbit small gut brush-border vesicles	Gly-Pro	K^+	No
Berteloot et al. (16)	Mouse brush-border vesicles	Gly-Leu	Mannitol	No
Ganapathy et al. (17)	Rabbit brush-border vesicles	Gly-Sar	K^+, Li^+, Rb^+, Cs^+, Choline, tetraethylammonium, mannitol	No

dipeptides, glycylsarcosine and carnosine (β-alanyl-L-histidine) was considerably reduced in the absence of sodium and the rings were unable to concentrate the peptides. In these experiments sodium was replaced by KCl, LiCl, choline, and Tris but only a single (5 mmol/liter) substrate concentration was used. As a result of these experiments it was thought that peptide transport was indeed sodium-dependent. Since 1974, however, a number of papers have appeared sugggesting that peptide transport is not sodium-dependent. Table 1 shows a selection from a list of about 20 papers, half of which suggest that peptide transport is sodium-dependent and half of which suggest it is not. There are two papers on the list which are of special interest. Cheeseman and Parsons (12) reported that peptide transport was not sodium-dependent when not accumulative, inferring it was only sodium-dependent when concentrative. Secondly, Ganapathy and co-workers (17), using brush-border membrane vesicles, suggested that peptide transport was not sodium-dependent but was proton-dependent and that the effects seen in sodium replacement experiments in intact tissue were due to the removal of sodium from the sodium/hydrogen ion antiport system.

The literature is now very confused and is made more difficult by the fact that many investigations have been carried out as a minor part of some larger investigation and have involved only one set of experimental conditions and one concentration of peptide. Also, most workers have studied the transport of peptides which are readily susceptible to brush-border and intracellular hydrolysis which further complicates the issue.

We have now carried out a more thorough investigation of the problem using a wide range of substrate concentrations and studying uptake both with and against an apparent electrochemical gradient. The peptide used was glycylsarcosine which is sufficiently resistant to hydrolysis to accumulate intact in the tissue.

II. METHODS

A full description of the methods used in this investigation can be found in Matthews and co-workers' studies (9,18), but briefly, the methods used were as follows: In the experiments under influx conditions, rings of everted hamster jejunum weighing 10–20 mg were incubated in a range of concentrations of $[^{14}C]$ Gly-Sar in 0.5 ml Tris-phosphate sodium chloride buffer pH 5 or in a similar buffer in which the sodium chloride was replaced by various substituents. A pH of 5 was used since it minimizes extracellular hydrolysis without causing a reduction in uptake. The rings were incubated in glass tubes at 37°C under oxygen for 2 min with shaking. After removal from the incubation medium the rings were rinsed in cold NaCl or an appropriate solution of the replacing substituent, blotted on filter paper, and placed in 1 ml of 6% sulfosalicylic acid. The rings were then extracted by heating the capped tubes in a boiling water bath for 5 min at 100°C. After centrifugation 0.5 ml of supernatant was added to 15 ml of xylene-based scintillation fluid and radioactivity was counted in a liquid scintillation counter. In the experiments in which uptake was measured against a concentration gradient, rings of everted hamster jejunum weighing 10-20 mg were placed in 25-ml conical flasks containing various concentrations of unlabelled glycylsarcosine in 3 ml Tris-phosphate sodium chloride buffer or a similar buffer in which the sodium chloride was replaced by various substituents. The flasks were gassed with oxygen and incubated at 37°C for 20 min with shaking. At the end of this time the rings were removed, rinsed in the appropriate cold washing solution, blotted, and weighed. The rings were extracted with 1 ml of 6% sulfosalicylic acid as described earlier and analyzed on a Locarte amino acid analyzer.

Uptake under influx conditions was expressed as μmol g initial wet wt.$^{-1}$ min^{-1} and the total uptake curves were analyzed by nonlinear regression analysis having first obtained an approximate estimate of K_d by the method of self-inhibition. The parameter K_d in these experiments represents total nonmediated influx and is a combination of nonsaturable uptake into the cells plus uptake into the extracellular space. From the nonlinear regression analysis, the kinetic constants V_{max}, K_t, and K_d were obtained and the mediated uptake curves were plotted. In the experiments against a concentration gradient, uptake was expressed as μmol g final wet wt. for 20 min.

III. RESULTS

A. Effects of Sodium Replacement on Peptide Transport Under Influx Conditions

When sodium was replaced by other members of Periodic group 1a there was either, as seen with potassium and cesium (Fig. 1), a small reduction in total uncorrected uptake (that is uptake containing both a nonmediated component and uptake into the extracellular space) over the whole concentration range, or in the case of sodium replacement by lithium (not shown), uptake was reduced up to a concentration of about 45 mmol/liter and above this concentration the uptake curve was slightly higher. Correction of the uptake curves for the nonmediated component of transport resulted in mediated uptake curves that were in all cases substantially reduced compared with the controls (Fig. 2).

Replacement of sodium by the nonmetallic compounds choline and mannitol resulted in a small reduction in total influx at concentrations above 10 mmol/ liter but below this uptakes were similar to, or lower than, the controls (Fig. 3).

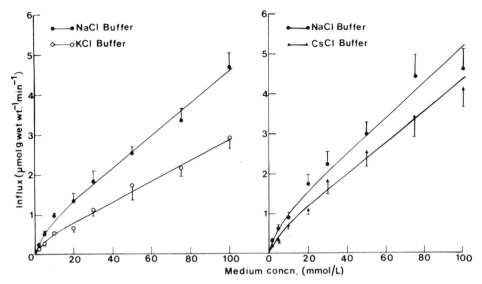

Figure 1 Plot of total influx ±SEM of $[^{14}C]$ Gly-Sar in NaCl, KCl, and CsCl buffers into rings of everted hamster jejunum over the concentration range 1–100 mmol/L. The lines for Gly-Sar influx are calculated from K_t, V_{max}, and K_d.

In contrast to the replacement by the metallic ions, correction of the total uptake curves for the nonmediated component of transport resulted in curves for mediated uptake which were actually increased at the higher concentrations compared with the controls. In the case of choline there was a "cross-over" at 8 mmol/liter and at the lower concentrations influx was slightly lower than in the sodium buffer (Fig. 4).

The values obtained for the kinetic constants with the various sodium replacements are summarized in Table 2. The kinetic constants obtained with the sodium buffer controls, at the same time as those in the substitute buffer, are shown in brackets. The control values vary somewhat because the different sets of experiments were carried out over a period of time. The changes in K_t values were not consistent, both lithium and cesium giving a reduction in K_t, but there was an increase with potassium. Replacement of sodium by choline and mannitol, on the other hand, gave an increase in K_t. The changes in V_{max} were more consistent, replacement by the metallic ions giving a considerable reduction in V_{max} compared with the controls, whereas choline and mannitol gave an increase. With regard to K_d, all values, with the exception of that in lithium were reduced compared to the control values.

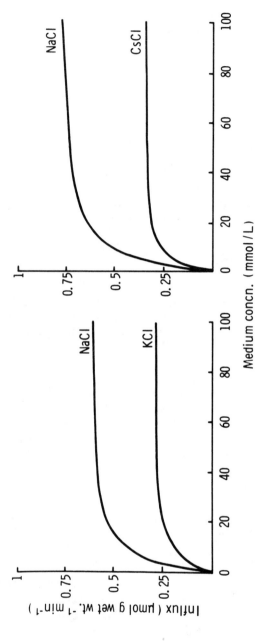

Figure 2 Calculated mediated influx of Gly-Sar in NaCl, KCl, and CsCl buffers into rings of everted hamster jejunum. The lines were calculated from K_t and V_{max}.

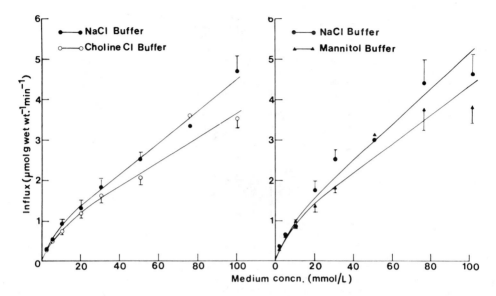

Figure 3 Plot of total influx ±SEM of $[^{14}C]$ Gly-Sar in NaCl, choline, and mannitol buffers into rings of everted hamster jejunum. The lines were calculated from K_t, V_{max}, and K_d.

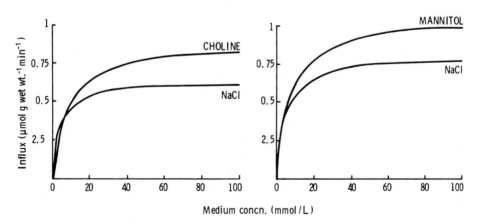

Figure 4 Calculated mediated influx of Gly-Sar in NaCl, choline, and mannitol buffers into rings of everted hamster jejunum. The lines were calculated from K_t and V_{max}.

Table 2 Effects of Substituting Medium Na on Kinetic Parameters of Uptake of Gly-Sar by Rings of Everted Hamster Jejunum[a]

Na Replaced by	K_t mmol/l	V_{max} μmol/g/min	K_d[c] μmol/g/min mmol
LiCl	3.0 ± 0.68[b] (5.6 ± 0.83)	0.32 ± 0.064 (0.85 ± 0.118)	0.041 ± 0.0020 (0.030 ± 0.0022)
KCl	5.2 ± 1.70 (3.9 ± 0.73)	0.30 ± 0.097 (0.64 ± 0.102)	0.025 ± 0.0021 (0.039 ± 0.0025)
CsCl	3.2 ± 1.05 (5.0 ± 1.26)	0.36 ± 0.098 (0.81 ± 0.188)	0.040 ± 0.0032 (0.044 ± 0.0047)
Choline	7.9 ± 1.67 (3.9 ± 0.73)	0.89 ± 0.175 (0.64 ± 0.102)	0.028 ± 0.0027 (0.039 ± 0.0025)
Mannitol	7.2 ± 2.15 (5.0 ± 1.26)	1.07 ± 0.311 (0.81 ± 0.118)	0.033 ± 0.0127 (0.044 ± 0.0047)

[a]Figures in brackets represent values obtained in sodium buffers.
[b]S.E.
[c]Total nonmediated uptake including uptake into inulin space.

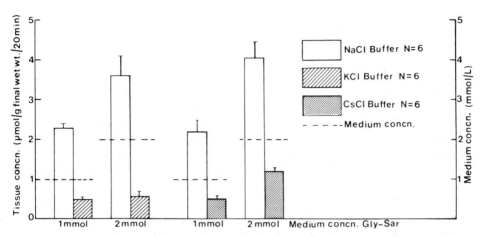

Figure 5 Graph of 20-min uptake ±SEM of Gly-Sar 1 and 2 mmol/L in NaCl, KCl, and CsCl buffers into rings of everted hamster jejunum.

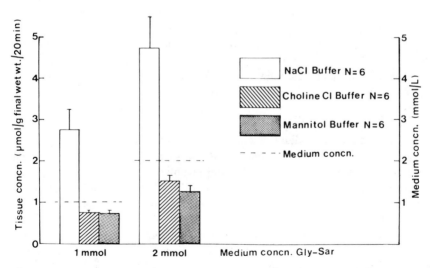

Figure 6 Graph of 20-min uptake ±SEM of Gly-Sar 1 and 2 mmol/L in NaCl, choline, and mannitol buffers into rings of everted hamster jejunum.

A. Effects of Sodium Replacement on Peptide Transport Against an Apparent Electrochemical Gradient

A 20 min uptake from substrate concentrations of 1 and 2 mmol/liter resulted in significant tissue concentration of Gly-Sar in the sodium buffer (Figs. 5 and 6). The effects of replacing sodium by the other metallic ions and by choline and mannitol was similar in all cases. Concentration was abolished and uptake was reduced to 20–30% of the control values (Figs. 5 and 6). The greater reductions were seen when sodium was replaced by the other metallic ions.

IV. DISCUSSION

In attempting to explain all the conflicting results in the literature, a number of variables must be considered. As shown in Table 1 these include the peptides studied, the substituents for sodium used, the species of animal employed, whether jejunum, ileum, or whole small intestine was used, the experimental conditions, and the nature of the preparations employed. The conflict in the literature is not surprising when you consider that even with the relatively simple experiments reported here the results are conflicting, influx being considerably reduced but not abolished when the metallic ions, lithium (Li), potassium (K), and cesium (Cs) are substituted for sodium but sodium-independent when choine and mannitol are used, under concentrative conditions sodium-dependent in all cases. In view of these findings we can no longer maintain that peptide uptake is sodium-dependent in that the presence of sodium is always essential for maximal rate of uptake—though the large reduction in the presence of metallic ions and under concentrative conditions remains to be explained. Our results with the metallic ions resemble those of Rubino et al. (7) who found that replacement of sodium by choline inhibited Gly-Pro influx into rabbit ileum by reducing V_{max}, in contrast to the effect on glycine where V_{max} was unchanged and K_t was increased. As a result of these experiments Rubino et al. suggested that peptide transport can take place in the absence of sodium but that it is more rapid in the presence of sodium, as sodium facilitates translocation of the peptide-carrier complex. However, the situation must be more complex than this because the substitution of sodium by choline and mannitol in our experiments caused an increase rather than a reduction in mediated influx. A possible explanation is that, peptide transport is not sodium-dependent, but that potassium, cesium, and lithium in some way complex with the carrier thereby causing a reduction in the rate of translocation, whereas choline and mannitol do not complex. This hypothesis should be testable by inhibition experiments with varying concentrations of replacing substituent.

The reduction in uptake and failure to concentrate when sodium is replaced by choline and mannitol in the 20 min uptake experiments, as opposed to the absence of any effect in the influx experiments, might be explained by the work of Ganapathy et al. (17), who believe that intestinal uptake of peptide is the result of cotransport with protons and, that while replacement of sodium may have no effect on peptide uptake by brush border vesicles, it might inhibit peptide uptake by intact intestine owing to the inactivation of the sodium-hydrogen ion antiport system. The existence of a jejunal sodium-hydrogen antiport system has recently been shown in humans (19). In the present work, under influx conditions at pH 5 there will be an inwardly directed proton gradient and in the absence of sodium, hydrogen ions will enter the cell but will not be pumped out again. Therefore, although in the presence of choline and mannitol there is no inhibition of uptake over the first few minutes, probably because the endogenous sodium is being utilized, as the peptide and hydrogen ion concentrations in the cell increase, and in the absence of a blood supply, and thus the normal homeostatic mechanisms, the cell will become more and more acidotic, thus inhibiting metabolism and, in turn, in the experiments under concentrative conditions, mediated uptake. In the 20 min uptake experiments in which sodium is replaced by the metallic ions there will be inhibition of initial uptake superimposed on the inhibition caused by the inactivation of the sodium-hydrogen antiport. This is supported by the greater reduction in 20-min uptake when sodium is replaced by the other metallic ions.

In summary, the results show that under influx conditions, peptide transport appears to be largely sodium-dependent when sodium is replaced by other metallic ions, but sodium-independent when replaced by choline and mannitol. Under concentrative conditions all the replacements caused a reduction in uptake and abolished the ability to concentrate.

ACKNOWLEDGMENTS

We are grateful to Dr. M. L. G. Gardner, Department of Biochemistry, University of Edinburgh, for carrying out the nonlinear regression analysis of the kinetic curves. We are also grateful, for financial support, to the Frank Odell Charity, an Anonymous Donor, and many other generous donors to the Children's Medical Charity, which is now supporting all academic work in the Department of Experimental Chemical Pathology.

REFERENCES

1. Rubino, A., and Guandalini, S. Dipeptide transport in the intestinal mucosa of developing rabbits. In *Peptide Transport and Hydrolysis. Ciba Foundation Symposium 50.* Elsevier Excerpta Medica, New York, 1977, pp. 61–71.
2. Himukai, M., Konno, T., and Hoshi, T. Age-dependent change in intestinal absorption of dipeptides and their constituent amino acids in the guinea pig. *Pediatr. Res.* 14, 1272–1275, 1980.

3. Matthews, D. M. Intestinal absorption of peptides. *Physiol. Rev.* 55, 537–608, 1975.

4. Craft, I. L., Geddes, D., Hyde, C. W., Wise, I. J., and Matthews, D. M. Absorption and malabsorption of glycine and glycine peptides in man. *Gut* 9, 425–437, 1968.

5. Adibi, S. A., and Phillips, E. Evidence for greater absorption of amino acid from peptide than from freeform by human intestine. *Clin. Res.* 16, 446, 1968.

6. Matthews, D. M., Lis, M. T., Cheng, B., and Crampton, R. F. Observations on the intestinal absorption of some oligopeptides of methionine and glycine in the rat. *Clin. Sci.* 37, 751–764, 1969.

7. Rubino, A., Field, M., and Shwachman, H. Intestinal transport of amino acid residues of dipeptides. 1. Influx of the glycine residue of glycyl-proline across the mucosal border. *J. Biol. Chem.* 246, 3542–3548, 1971.

8. Addison, J. M., Burston, D., and Matthews, J. M. Evidence for active transport of the dipeptide carnosine (β-alanyl-L-histidine) by hamster jejunum in *Sci.* 43, 907–991, 1972.

9. Matthews, D. M., Addison, J. M., and Burston, D. Evidence for active transport of the dipeptide carnosine (β-alanyl-L-histidine) by hamster jejunum in vitro. *Clin. Sci. Mol. Med.* 46, 693–705, 1974.

10. Cheeseman, C. I., and Smyth, D. H. Interaction of amino acids, peptides and peptidases in the small intestine. *Proc. R. Soc. London Ser. B.* 190, 149–163, 1975.

11. Sigrist-Nelson, K. Dipeptide transport in isolated intestinal brush-border membrane. *Biochim. Biophys. Acta* 394, 220–226, 1975.

12. Cheeseman, C. I., and Parsons, D. S. The role of some small peptides in the transfer of amino nitrogen across the wall of vascularly perfused intestine. *J. Physiol.* 262, 459–476, 1976.

13. Heading, C. E., Rogers, C. S., and Wilkinson, S. Absorption of two tyrosine containing dipeptides from the small intestine and rectum of the rat. *J. Physiol.* 278, 21P, 1978.

14. Himukai, M., and Hoshi, T. Mechanisms of glycyl-L-leucine uptake by guinea pig small intestine: Relative importance of intact-peptide transport. *J. Physiol.* 302, 155–169, 1980.

15. Ganapathy, V., Mendicino, J. F., and Leibach, F. H. Transport of glycyl-L-proline into intestinal and renal brush border vesicles from rabbit. *J. Biol. Chem.* 256, 118–124, 1981.

16. Berteloot, A., Khan, A. H., and Ramaswamy, K. Characteristics of dipeptide transport in normal and papain-treated brush border membrane vesicles from mouse intestine. II Uptake of Gly-Leu. *Biochim. Biophys. Acta* 686, 47–54, 1982.

17. Ganapathy, V., Burckhardt, G., and Leibach, F. H. Characteristics of glycylsarcosine transport in rabbit brush-border membrane vesicles. *J. Biol. Chem.* 259, 8954–8959, 1984.

18. Matthews, D. M., and Burston, D. Uptake of a series of neutral dipeptides including L-alanyl-L-alanine, glycylglycine and glycylsarcosine by hamster jejunum in vitro. *Clin. Sci.* 67, 541–549, 1984.
19. Booth, I. W., Strange, G., Murer, H., Fenton, T. R., and Milla, P. J. Defective jejunal brush-border Na/H exchange: A cause of congenital secretory diarrhoea. *Lancet* 2, 1066–1069, 1985.

4

The Role of Protein Breakdown Products in the Absorption of Essential Trace Elements

Raul A. Wapnir

Cornell University Medical College, New York, and North Shore University Hospital, Manhasset, New York

I. INTRODUCTION

Essential trace elements are necessary dietary requirements and key participants in a variety of biological functions. Many natural products of animal or plant origin satisfy the daily needs of humans once the lactation period has been completed. For the purpose of this review, we will focus on the luminal phase of intestinal absorption, since this stage in the assimilation of trace elements is directly linked to the composition of the diet and other exogenous variables, and has received the least attention from the investigators in the field. In addition, our interest will center on the role that another key dietary element, protein, and its breakdown products, especially small peptides and amino acids, will play in the absorptive process.

This chapter will be concerned with elements normally required in amounts below 0.5 mmol/day (1), and among those, the transition elements which have elicited the greatest interest in recent years: iron, zinc, manganese, and copper. We have also included specific sections on calcium and magnesium, for which the recommended dietary allowances in humans exceed 1 mmol/day. However, since these two elements are divalent, as the remaining trace elements to be considered, their inclusion is supported by chemical analogy and physiological behavior.

A number of contributing factors have demonstrated effect on the intestinal absorption of nutritionally important minerals. Table 1 enumerates these variables, some of which will be individually discussed later in this chapter.

Table 1   Intraluminal Factors Capable of Altering the Intestinal Absorption of Trace Elements

---

Oxidation status of the metal
Chemical nature of the metallic compound
  Inorganic substances
  Organic forms of the element
Interactions in the luminal space with

Dietary substances	Proteins and breakdown products
	Carbohydrates (simple and complex)
	Fats and hydrolysis products
	Fiber and sequestering substances
	Other metals and cations
	Anions
Secretions	Salivary
	Gastric
	Pancreatic
	Biliary
	Intestinal
	Water fluxes, pH

Interactions at the intestinal membrane with
  Glycocalyx
  Unstirred layer
  Membrane transporters
  Membrane pores
  Membrane turnover products
  Foreign substances

Essential metals capable of existing at more than one level of oxidation, such as iron, manganese, and copper, may be absorbed by different mechanisms depending on the valence of the cation, which can change its interactions with other components of the diet. Such elements could be available to the gut as inorganic salts, rarely in unsupplemented diets, and occasionally in semisynthetic formulations provided to humans or used for animal experimentation. However, a well-balanced diet of natural products would contain mostly organic forms of trace metals.

Once ingested, and absorbed into the intestinal tract, minerals will be subjected to interactions with all types of dietary products and their hydrolytic products; with fiber or other naturally occurring sequestering substances, with other cations, and with available anions. The absorptive process, in turn, will be regulated, in part, by the contents of secretions appearing in the gastrointestinal tract, the bidirectional exchanges of water continuously occurring in the gut, and the pH changes at different points of the lumen.

Beyond the alterations in the molecular configuration of the products containing trace elements up to their point of absorption, there are possible interactions at the intestinal mucosal levels with the glycocalyx and its surrounding unstirred layer; specific membrane transporters capable of actively translocating those elements; membrane pores open to bulk flow of dissolved solutes of low-molecular weight (LMW); membrane turnover products which may be similar to dietary substances, but may be present at significant concentration only in the immediate vicinity of the brush border; and foreign substances which may be minor constituents or contaminants of the diet, bacteria, cellulose, and so on.

II. IRON

The intestinal absorption of iron probably has been more extensively studied than any other mineral of nutritional significance (2). Most investigators have differentiated the origin of dietary sources of iron as heme or nonheme type. In heme, iron is bivalent, and it is at this lower oxidation state at which it is normally absorbed. Humans take up ferrous more effectively than they do ferric iron. Stomach acidity may play a role in extracting iron from foodstuffs, especially those low in protein and heme. Iron in heme is taken up by the intestinal mucosa by an endocytotic process, and once in the enterocyte, the metal follows a similar path to that followed by iron from other sources. Nonheme iron binds to specific high-affinity receptors in the small intestine and the transport process across the mucosa is an energy-dependent, mediated mechanism.

For our purposes we will omit questions related to iron sufficiency status and absorption, although there is little doubt that animal protein intake and iron repletion are closely linked. The earliest association of protein-derived products and iron absorption stems from the clearly demonstrated inverse relationship between meat consumption and iron deficiency (3). Although hemoglobin and myoglobin rarely supply more than one tenth of the iron ingestion in developed countries, this fraction is highly bioavailable, and provides one third of adult requirements (4). However, it has been shown that hemoglobin ingested in the absence of meat is not so well absorbed (5). Such findings support the implication that other protein derivatives which are present in various types of meat, or which can be generated during the processing or cooking of meat may play a substantial role in the bioavailability of iron. Among these products, amino acids or polypeptides have drawn logical attention. This notion had been advanced many years ago (6). More recently, the focus has centered on cysteine as an important adjuvant of iron absorption (4,7). Increased availability had also been observed where amino acids were added to a staple vegetable food (8).

Since it has been noted that human milk is capable of preventing anemia, even when it is the sole source of food for up to 12–18 months, iron absorption promoters have been proposed to be present in fresh human mammary gland secretions. Cysteine and taurine, which are found in high concentrations in human breast milk, may be likely candidates for that role (9). Nevertheless, additional intrinsic factors which may be present in breast milk may be no less important.

These findings have theoretical and practical interest since it has been previously shown that nutritionally superior proteins, such as those derived from eggs, negatively affected iron absorption due to the presence of phosphoproteins with great affinity for iron (10,11). Binding of iron was equally observed in soy protein isolates, which reduced nonheme iron absorption in humans (12).

Another condition in which iron from a high-molecular weight protein such as ferritin (MW = 500,000) is better absorbed was demonstrated when a serving of veal added to ferritin increased iron absorption from 1.7% to 6.6%. Since veal alone was enough to assure a 13.2% iron absorption, it was assumed that amino acids or small peptides liberated during veal digestion were the putative agents responsible for the increased iron absorption (13).

In in vitro experiments, iron salts mixed with animal protein obtained from fish meal increased iron uptake fourfold, as compared with the sulfate. The uptake of the element was improved only 67% by a soy protein isolate, while the addition of whey had no effect (14).

III. ZINC

The interrrelationships between zinc, protein, and amino acids are probably those that have been most intensively studied. The knowledge that many metalloproteins have one or several zinc atoms tightly bound in their molecules, and that zinc easily binds to serum proteins and amino acids in vitro and in vivo (15–18), became an indicator of the possible role that proteins and/or their products of hydrolysis may have in the luminal phase of zinc absorption.

Brush-border binding agents have been proposed as the gap step in the internalization of zinc (19). Since the 1970s, a variety of molecular species have been favored as the most likely candidates. Many of them were further analyzed and found to have a peptidelike structure. Reports from Evans' laboratory (20,21) presented evidence of zinc:LMW ligand complexes. A polypeptide capable of binding zinc was later described in rat intestinal mucosa (22).

A different view was opened when, instead of mucosal-binding proteins or polypeptides, the focus shifted to luminal factors or substances which could enhance the absorptive process. In particular, there has been increasing evidence to support the view that the transfer of zinc across the mammalian small intestinal mucosa is mediated, at least, in part, by an LMW ligand. This contention is supported by the fact that free zinc ions can only be present at negligible concentrations at the pH of the small intestine, and also because of the high affinity of zinc for proteins and semidigested peptide fragments (17). Therefore, it appears likely that zinc should be chelated with LMW ligands and cross the brush border by passive or active transport mechanisms. This would be synthesized in what has been generically defined as "a more absorbable form" of the metal (14,23–25).

The proven therapeutic value of human breast milk in the treatment of acrodermatitis enteropathica (26), a condition known to be due to zinc malabsorption, prompted attempts to elucidate the nature of the LMW agents present in maternal milk which made zinc more available than when provided from processed milk. In addition to the postulated positive effects on zinc absorption of citrate and picolinate (27–29), which elicited a lively debate a few years ago, several investigators noted that certain amino acids greatly enhance zinc intestinal absorption. The addition of lysine, cysteine, and glycine plus histidine to zinc sulfate produced higher serum zinc levels than the ingestion of the inorganic salt by itself (30). Also, cysteine added to chicken feed increased the absorption of zinc as compared with formulations without the free amino acids (31). This confirmed earlier studies which showed increased zinc absorption and therapeutic effect in the zinc-deficiency syndrome elicited in the chick (32). Schwarz and Kirchgessner (33) remarked that protein nutritional levels were an important factor in efficient zinc absorption. But when they added large amounts of histidine, in proportions ranging from 250:1 to 2000:1 in relation to zinc, no improvement in absorption was observed.

The need to maintain LMW:zinc ratios within well-defined limits appears to be a prerequisite as important as the presence of an effective chelator and the dissociation constants of the ligand:metal complexes. In studies using ileal perfusion techniques we showed that certain organic acids and amino acids were effective for allowing a considerable rate of zinc absorption with little or no change in the velocity of transport, even at ligand:zinc ratios exceeding 65:1 (25). Among these were glucuronic and galacturonic acids, and the natural amino acids, glutamate, glycine, tryptophan, as well as glycylglycine. However, other LMW substances, such as citrate, picolinate, histidine, and DL-histidine-L-histidine showed zinc absorption rates which were progressively lower with higher ratios. For actively transported substances, this suggested transport (K_t) competition. Appropriate kinetic analysis, also conducted under in vivo conditions, showed that there was competitive inhibition (K_i) between histidine and the 2 histidine:zinc complex. The K_t of the complex increased from 0.54 to 1.46 mM in the presence of a 20 mM excess of the AA. The K_i could be estimated to be approximately 4 mM. This phenomenon was also stereospecific, since the unnatural D stereoisomer allowed for only minimal mediated transport. The report concerning the effectiveness of the dipeptide glycylleucine, in an approximate proportion of 67:1 in enhancing zinc absorption, although not so of the individual amino acid, underlines the specificity of the LMW:zinc complexes transporters, even under conditions of ligand excess (34).

Also, if the proportion between the amino acid and zinc is maintained under isotonic perfusion conditions, the absorption of zinc in the presence of tryptophan, histidine, proline, and cysteine is greater than in the absence of AA, both through the jejunum and the ileum (Figs. 1 and 2). Preceding experiments have shown that the colonic mucosa is capable of dissociating zinc from LMW ligands such as amino acids or a nonhydrolyzable dipeptide, and absorbing the metal without taking up the ligand (35).

Further support to the identity and size of LMW ligands was obtained from experiments in which zinc was perfused through the jejunum and ileum of rats in the presence of a protein hydrolysate (mean MW = 165). No stimulation of zinc

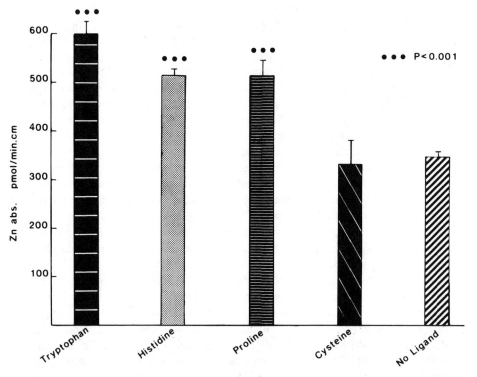

Figure 1   Absorption of zinc from a 0.153 mM solution, by rat jejunum in vivo, in the presence of 0.306 mM of the indicated amino acids, in an isotonic, nonelectrolyte solution. The bars denote the means ± SEM of 48 determinations. The significance between means as shown in the chart compare with perfusions in the absence of ligands (one-way analysis of variance).

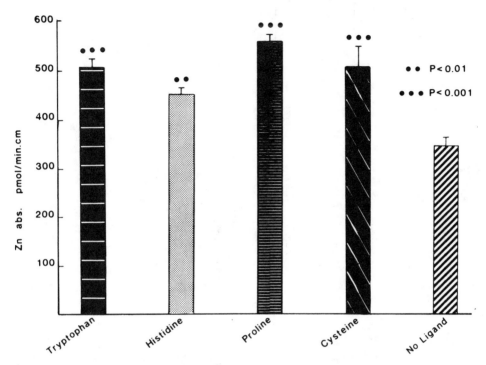

Figure 2 Absorption of zinc by rat ileum in vivo, in the presence of twice the concentration of an amino acid, under the conditions described in the legend of Figure 1.

absorption was noted in either area of the gut, although net water influx was much higher in the presence of the protein hydrolysate (Table 2). These results can be interpreted as if the large excess of protein breakdown products (± 400:1) was inhibitory of a mediated transport, since bulk transport should have favored a greater absorption of zinc. However, the excessive ligand:zinc ratio may be closer to physiologic conditions than a more favorable proportion of LMW ligands to the metal.

Another insight on the chemical specificity of LMW compounds has been obtained from comparisons of the effectiveness of amino acids and some of the non-amino acid homologs as ligands for the absorption of zinc. Preliminary studies have shown that tryptophan is superior to tryptophol, histidine is more effective than imidazole, and cysteine surpasses acetyl-N-cysteine in the translocation of zinc across the jejunum and ileum of the rat (36).

It has been known for some time that zinc, which is a constitutive part of, or is ingested with proteins of animal origin, such as casein, is more available than equivalent amounts from a high-quality protein of vegetable origin such as soy-

Table 2 Rat Jejunal and Ileal Absorption of Zinc and Copper, and Water Absorption in the Presence of Protein Hydrolysate

Protein hydrolysate	Zinc absorption (pmol/min × cm)		Water absorption (µl/min × cm)		Copper absorption (pmol/min × cm)		Water absorption (µl/min × cm)	
	Jejunum	Ileum	Jejunum	Ileum	Jejunum	Ileum	Jejunum	Ileum
+	149.6 ± 23.3 (48) (NS)	181.7 ± 13.7 (48) (NS)	0.917 ± 0.097	0.909 ± 0.073	15.3 ± 2.1 (42)	33.6 ± 2.8 (43)	1.904 ± 0.58	1.412 ± 0.051
−	166.8 ± 19.1 (48)	135.4 ± 20.6 (48)	0.087 ± 0.092 [a]	0.167 ± 0.081 [a]	54.2 ± 10.4 [a] (48)	79.4 ± 7.4 [a] (48)	−0.944 ± 0.143 [a]	−0.468 ± 0.100 [a]

[a]$p < 0.001$ (Student's t-test).
The perfusates initially contained either 0.153 mM zinc, or 0.031 mM copper, in an isotonic, buffered NaCl solution.
The protein hydrolysate consisted of a 1% proteose-peptone No. 3 (Difco) solution contributing 60 mOsm/kg.
(N) = number of determinations.

bean (37,38). This will eventually reflect on the zinc nutritional status of the whole organism (39). The presence of organic phosphates such as phytate (inositol hexaphosphate) in foods of vegetable origin is a key factor in the bioavailability of zinc. Phytate has been shown to bind zinc very tightly. Diets very rich in phytate, such as those based in cereals, can even lead to zinc nutritional deficiency (40). In animal experiments, using body weight gain and femur zinc content as indicators, it has been shown that a phytate:zinc ratio not exceeding 10 is tolerable, but if the proportion exceeds 20 it becomes unacceptable. That is why the bioavailability of zinc from a product free from phytate, such as beef, is 7 to 8 times greater than that of soy protein concentrate and about twice as high that of rapeseed protein concentrate (41). Significant results have also been obtained from work done on rats fed infant formulas containing protein derived from whey which proved to be superior to casein-based sources, since this bypasses phosphoproteins which tend to bind zinc very tightly and reduce its bioavailability (42,43).

There is evidence to postulate that large proteins bind zinc with very low dissociation constants (14). This generalization was substantiated by the total suppression of ileal zinc absorption observed when an intact protein was added to a perfusion solution under otherwise optimal conditions (25). This binding of zinc to the proteins may become looser with the release of smaller peptides from the larger molecule. Actual information in this regard is still limited, since only dissociation constants for some amino acids and a few dipeptides have been determined (16). The LMW ligand:zinc complexes may then be translocated into the enterocyte both by mediated and nonmediated routes. The general concept outlined above was supported by the findings of enhanced zinc absorption by the simple addition of amino acids to a low-protein animal feed. Such enrichment improved zinc nutritional status to an extent even greater than the addition of zinc to the diet (44).

IV. MANGANESE

The luminal phase of manganese absorption has received even less extensive probing than that of other trace elements. Since this metal can be toxic when ingested in large amounts, the nature of the diet may play a role in regulating excessive absorption of manganese. Thus, if a low-protein (10%) diet is fed to rats, they will become more susceptible to the toxic effects of the metal than animals fed an appropriate concentration (21%) (45).

The considerable interaction between manganese and other trace elements, particularly iron, leads to variable absorption of the former (46). This may explain the inverse relationship in the absorption of the two metals from formulas supplemented with iron, rather than the nature of the high-protein diet (47).

Cow's milk contains both more casein and three to eight times more manganese than human breast milk (6 μg/liter). The role of lactose in manganese absorption in unknown, although it may contribute to its facilitated absorption from cow's milk. There is a substantial difference in how manganese is bound to ligands in milk from different species. Extrinsically labeled manganese was found to be totally bound to LMW fractions, presumably polypeptides of MW < 1000, in an infant formula, and up to 85% bound in cow's milk (48). In contrast, none of the tagged manganese was found bound to LMW fractions of human breast milk, with the totality of the metal distributed between a 407,300-dalton fraction (90%) and a 128,000-dalton protein. The high availability of manganese from infant formulas became a source of concern when this element was added as a supplement in bottled feedings, thus prompting a reduction of the overall levels of the trace element in many manufactured preparations (49).

Animal experiments have also shown that the LMW ligands present in bovine milk and derived infant formulas are responsible for the greater absorption of manganese, as compared to human breast milk (50). More recently, externally tagged manganese served to demonstrate a similar (80%) whole body elemental uptake from cow's milk or a formula prepared from it, against a 60% uptake from a soy protein formula (51).

Kinetic studies conducted in vivo revealed that the presence of LMW ligands, such as citrate or histidine, enhanced the initial manganese transport rates fourfold. In the ileum, the active translocation of the metal in the presence of twice the amino acid concentration had a K_t = 0.056 mM and a V_{max} equal to 158 pmol/min $\times$ cm. These data are in agreement with the concept of enhanced manganese absorption from dietary sources rich in LMW putative ligands (52).

V. COPPER

Absorption of this element has been studied in many species, from cattle to humans. In a standard American diet, vegetables, particularly potatoes, and to a lesser extent animal proteins are the best sources of copper. The general view of copper metabolism is now well understood (53). Absorption of copper across the small intestinal mucosa can occur by mediated and nonmediated processes (54,55). Most inorganic salts of this element are well absorbed, the acidity of the stomach being a possible explanation for its release from insoluble forms (56). Copper present in vegetables or plants occurs as neutral or anionic complexes, probably related to organic acids or lectins, and has a better bioavailability than the sulfate (57). This is so in spite of the strong binding that phytate exerts on copper, which can result in a decreased body retention of this element, as has also been demonstrated in the case of zinc (58).

The extraction process required to transfer copper bound to large molecules makes processed foods, or those containing smaller breakdown products more readily available sources of copper. This may explain why cooked meat has been shown to reverse a copper deficiency developed in rats fed raw meat (59). In other studies carried out with rats in vitro, it was shown that copper added to either fish or soybean meals produced a fourfold increase of uptake in relation to the sulfate, supporting the view that protein-derived products has a positive influence in the mucosal phase of copper absorption (60). From a different standpoint, it has been argued that dietary protein may reduce bioavailability of copper, as determined by its liver content. However, an opposite view could be held, regarding protein deficiency as a factor impairing copper mobilization from the liver (53).

It has been proposed that since copper forms well characterized, and tightly bound complexes with amino acids, these chelates could be the most important vehicles for the translocation of the element (61). These postulates derive from earlier studies on the uptake of copper by body tissues, in particular liver slices in vitro (62,63). However, later studies have shown that when ^{64}Cu is used to follow the intestinal absorption of the element in the rat, whether the form is ionic, or copper is presented with histidine or with protein, no differences could be detected (56). However, even if most of the copper could be released by the acidity of the stomach, a variety of potential ligands present in the intestinal secretion can again bind the metal. The copper complexes prepared with saliva, gastric, and duodenal secretions of rats can easily be dialyzed, while preparations made with bile retain copper very tightly (64,65).

Nutritional studies in adult males have demonstrated an improvement in copper absorption from 36 to 52% when the subjects were shifted from a low- to a high-protein diet (66). Although milk and other dairy products rich in protein are poor sources of copper, there are large discrepancies in the distribution of this element among different fractions. In cow's milk, almost all copper is equally bound to the casein and the LMW fractions. However, in human breast milk, more than half the amount of copper present is retained by whey and a far smaller proportion is bound to LMW ligands (67).

Although at physiological concentrations of free amino acids, such as those present in serum, the transmembrane passage of copper is stimulated (62,63), a large excess of an amino acid with great affinity for copper, such as histidine, can both enhance its absorption as well as accelerate its urinary elimination (68). In this case, the absorption enhancement of copper, when offered to rats in a diet with 8% histidine, was enough to compensate a copper depletion that could be elicited by a high intake of histidine alone. However, in a study done on adolescent girls, this positive effect of amino acids could not be demonstrated, since copper balance was not altered by the addition to the diet of threonine, methionine, or lysine (69).

Similar inhibitory results were obtained in our laboratory with intestinal perfusions of a 0.031 mM solution containing copper and a physiologic excess of a protein hydrolysate, approximately in a 2000:1 proportion to the metal. A sharp depression of copper absorption was noted, in spite of a high net influx of water (Table 1). The solution perfused as control, containing an equivalent osmotic contribution of choline, failed to elicit water absorption, although copper transport was considerable, and proportionately greater than that of other trace elements. These data suggest that the small intestinal absorption of copper occurs via LMW:copper complexes, whose uptake may be partially inhibited by an excess of high-affinity ligands competing with the same active sites of the brush border.

The nature and MW of the putative ligands that could be involved in the transport of copper and zinc across the small intestinal mucosal membrane could be different or similar. Since zinc and copper often behave as antagonistic in many mammalian systems, this may be suggestive of parallel transport routes, and high-affinity sites for these two elements. Although the antagonism at the nutritional level has been repeatedly reported (70-72), more specific details remain to be clarified.

VI. CALCIUM AND MAGNESIUM

These two elements actually fall outside the category of trace minerals by virtue of their considerable daily dietary requirements. Moreover, due to their chemical properties and biological considerations, they may be less influenced by protein breakdown products of LMW such as amino acids, or small peptides, as well as by organic acids, all of which may still play a role in the luminal phase of their absorption.

A key factor in the absorption of calcium by the mammalian small intestine is the vitamin D-induced calcium-binding protein, first described in the chick intestinal mucosa (73). These findings were later extended to human small intestine (74). The role of the active form of vitamin D, 1,25-dihydroxycholecalciferol, synthesized in the kidney, but capable of binding to a specific cytosolic receptor in the intestinal epithelial cell and stimulating calcium absorption through the synthesis of transport protein, has been well documented (75,76).

Although some high-protein-containing foods, such as dairy products, are rich in calcium and an excellent source of this element and of protein, the magnitude of the calcium:phosphorus ratio appears to be more important than other nutritional factors in maintaining calcium balance (77). There are several reports indicating that an excess of protein in the diet results in losses of calcium through the urine (78). If the protein intake leads to a negative calcium balance of 40 mg/day, menopausal women may suffer a loss of as much as 1% of their skeletal tissue per year (79). A similar effect, but relating hypercalciuria to the free amino acids provided in total parenteral nutritional solutions, has also been reported. In this situation, the amino acid-associated calcium losses may be linked to renal effects of increased permeability of amino acid:calcium complexes and impaired renal tubular resorption of the chelated element (80).

There have been several reports linking some amino acids to calcium absorption and excretion. Lysine and arginine have been shown to enhance calcium absorption in experimental animals (81). No difference between D- and L-lysine was noted. However, the solubility of the amino acid:calcium complex was not a factor, since glycine:calcium was very soluble, but was not effective in enhancing calcium absorption.

Stimulation of water absorption may be a key factor in the enhancement of calcium transport. Although most natural amino acids are known to promote water influx, this effect has only been well documented with absorbable sugars, which also increase calcium uptake (82,83). In general, permeability of the small intestinal mucosa may be a significant factor in transmembrane passage of this element, since juvenile rats undergoing intestinal perfusion showed net calcium efflux into the lumen (84).

Using an in vivo jejunal perfusion procedure, we investigated the effect that a protein hydrolysate may have on the absorption of calcium and magnesium (Table 3). In spite of a stimulation of water influx and net water absorption, due to the presence of a mixture of amino acids and small peptides, calcium absorption was not affected, confirming that a preponderant fraction of calcium absorption is accomplished by a mediated process (82).

Metabolic and nutritional studies have yielded controversial results on the interrelationship between calcium and magnesium intestinal absorption. At the luminal level there may be a variety of factors which can affect the uptake of both elements in a similar way. In humans, recent studies suggest that the observed relationship between both elements may be related to their competitive binding to macromolecules, proteins, or undigestible matter in the intestinal lumen, which may provide a differential availability of either calcium or magnesium in various nutritional situations (85).

The absorption of magnesium at the intestinal brush border has only been explored to a limited extent. Luminal pH appears to have a negligible effect, as well as biliary secretion. Water fluxes may have a preponderant role in determining effectiveness of magnesium absorption (85).

The role of protein in the intestinal absorption of magnesium has not been well clarified. Early reports stated that the intestinal absorption of this element was increased by a higher protein intake (86,87). Since these studies included calcium as well, their later rebuttal (88,89) casts doubt about absorption enhancement of either of these two cations.

Only incidental information has offered a possible role to amino acids as enhancers of magnesium absorption. Magnesium aspartate has been considered to be a more effective vehicle for that element than an inorganic salt in the treatment of experimental cardiopathy in animals (90).

Ashmead et al. have reported a substantial stimulation of magnesium uptake from rat jejunum in vitro by casein or soy protein. When compared to the

Table 3 Absorption by Rat Jejunum, in vivo, of Magnesium and Calcium, and Water Fluxes in the Presence of Protein Hydrolysate

Protein hydrolysate	Magnesium absorption (nmol/min × cm)	Calcium absorption (nmol/min × cm)	Net water absorption (µl/min × cm)	^3H_2O Influx (µl/min × cm)	Water secretion (µl/min × cm)	r Water/Mg	r Water/Ca
+	2.235 ± 0.229 a	5.925 ± 0.250 (NS)	1.336 ± 0.053 b	5.87 ± 0.15 b	4.54 ± 0.14 NS	0.598[c]	0.126
−	0.948 ± 0.439	6.300 ± 1.286	0.925 ± 0.122	5.27 ± 0.13	4.35 ± 0.19	0.964[c]	0.908[c]

[a] $p < 0.025$;
[b] $p < 0.005$;
[c] $p < 0.001$ (intergroup comparisons by Student's t-test. r = Pearson's correlation coefficient).
The perfusates initially contained 1.18 mM magnesium, and 2.54 mM calcium, at a pH 7.4, in an isotonic solution. The protein hydrolysate was the same described in Table 2, and in the text.
N = 48 determinations in each group.

soluble magnesium sulfate (= 100), the mucosal uptake from the carbonate was 214; from whey, 144; from soy protein, 158; and from whole fish meal, 261 (14). The undefined nature of the transport substrates leaves still other questions unanswered.

Experimental conditions similar to those used for calcium absorption studies in the presence of a protein hydrolysate showed a very marked increase of magnesium jejunal absorption in the presence of a protein hydrolysate which contributed 60 mOsm/kg to an isotonic electrolyte solution (Table 3). Magnesium absorption more than doubled and this improvement of the element uptake was much greater than the stimulation of net water absorption. The latter effect was to be expected from the presence of a protein hydrolysate containing breakdown products with a mean molecular weight of 165, which signifies the presence of mostly free amino acids and dipeptides. The lower correlation in the absorption of calcium and magnesium with water uptake, when absorbed in the presence of the protein hydrolysate, supports the view that amino acid or dipeptide:magnesium or calcium complexes may be formed which can be translocated independently of bulk flow by mediated mechanisms, possibly the same mechanisms that can effect amino acid passage, a situation which has been shown to occur in the case of zinc (25).

VII. CONCLUSIONS

The preceding information suggests a tentative unified view for the possible involvement of LMW ligands, especially protein breakdown products, in the absorptive process of essential trace elements of nutritional significance. This synthesis is diagrammatically shown in Figure 3.

In a normal diet, most metallic (divalent or trivalent) components will be ingested as covalently bound to large molecules, generally proteins of variable charge and quaternary conformation. Cations such as calcium and magnesium may appear as well as organic salts. Initial protein hydrolysis may yield large polypeptides with or without metals. These large breakdown products will be progressively split by proteolytic enzymes yielding LMW peptides, some of which will again contain one or several atoms of the essential elements.

A key parameter of such a sequence is related to the affinity of the proteins for the metal. Larger proteins bind metals most tightly, thus exhibiting the lowest affinity constant K_{mP}. The bonds between small protein fragments and the metal will tend to become progressively weaker with the release of smaller peptides. This translates into affinity constants of increasing magnitude (Fig. 3).

At the absorption site, the trace element will be solubilized due to its chelation by LMW ligands derived not only from the native dietary proteins, but also from luminal secretions and brush-border mucosal turnover which will add to the exogenous pool. These endogenous ligands may also be peptides, amino

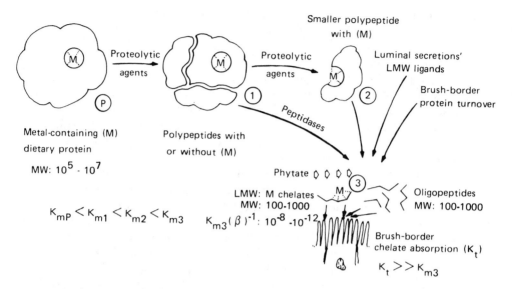

Figure 3 Schematic representation of digestion and absorption of a metal-containing dietary protein (P). Luminal proteolytic agents break down the protein to polypeptides with or without the metallic element (M) (1), and to smaller polypeptides (2) containing M. Further hydrolysis, plus other protein breakdown products from the brush-border mucosal turnover and luminal secretions with potential ligands produce relatively low-molecular-weight chelates (LMW: M) and other oligopeptides and free amino acids (3). Phytate, if present, will compete with the formation of LMW:M complexes. The affinity constants binding M to fragments of decreasing MW increases from K_{mP} through K_{m3}, representing the LMW:M chelate, which is generally of the order of $10^{-8}-10^{-12}$ M. Active absorption at the brush border may occur by transporters with an affinity K_t far greater than the dissociation constant K_{m3} of the LMW:M complex. Absorption may also take place by diffusion.

acids, or organic acids capable of forming chelates with the metals. These complexes will be available for uptake by the small intestinal mucosa, by paracellular flow following the movement of fluid, or by energy-requiring transporters capable of translocating the LMW:metal complexes. The presence of amino acids, sodium, and monosaccharides can enhance trace-metal absorption by fluid uptake stimulation, a well-known resultant of the active cotransport of these nutrients with sodium. This mediated route may be shared by one or several amino acids or small peptides, which may compete or indirectly regulate the absorption of the element. This phenomenon, added to the secretory passage of some of these elements into the lumen and eventual loss in the stools may constitute an important phase of trace-element homeostasis.

REFERENCES

1. Mertz, W. The essential trace elements. *Science* 213, 1332–1338, 1981.
2. Lynch, S. R. Iron. In *Absorption and Malabsorption of Mineral Nutrients.* Solomons, N. W. and Rosenberg, I. H. (eds.). Alan R. Liss, New York, 1984, pp. 89–124.
3. Takkunen, H., and Seppanen, R. Iron deficiency and dietary factors in Finland. *Am. J. Clin. Nutr.* 28, 1141–1148, 1975.
4. Bjorn-Rassmussen, E., and Hallberg, L. Effect of animal proteins on the absorption of food iron in man. *Nutr. Metab.* 23, 192–198, 1979.
5. Bothwell, T. H., Charlton, R. W., Cook, J. D., and Finch, C. A. *Iron Metabolism in Man.* Blackwell, Oxford, 1979.
6. Kroe, D., Kinney, T. D., Kaufman, N., and Klavins, J. V. The influence of amino acids on iron absorption. *Blood* 21, 546–551, 1963.
7. Martinez-Torres, C., Romano, E., and Layrisse, M. Effect of cysteine on iron absorption in man. *Am. J. Clin. Nutr.* 34, 322–327, 1981.
8. Martinez-Torres, C., and Layrisse, M. Effect of amino acids on iron absorption from a staple vegetable food. *Blood* 35, 669–675, 1970.
9. McMillan, J. A., Landaw, S. A., and Oski, F. Iron sufficiency in breast fed infants and the availability of iron from human milk. *Pediatrics* 38, 686–693, 1976.
10. Callender, S. T., Marney, S. R., and Warner, G. T. Eggs and iron absorption. *Br. J. Haematol.* 19, 657–663, 1970.
11. Monsen, E. R., and Cook, J. D. Food iron absorption in human subjects. V. Effects on the major dietary constituents of a semisynthetic meal. *Am. J. Clin. Nutr.* 32, 804–810, 1979.
12. Cook, J. D., Morck, T. A., and Lynch, S. R. The inhibitory effects of soy products on nonheme iron absorption in man. *Am. J. Clin. Nutr.* 34, 2622–2629, 1981.
13. Layrisse, M., Martinez-Torres, C., Renzi, M., and Leets, I. Ferritin iron absorption in man. *Blood* 45, 688–696, 1975.
14. Ashmead, H. D., Graff, D. J., and Ashmead, H. A. *Intestinal Absorption of Metal Ions and Chelates.* Charles C Thomas, Springfield, 1985, p. 121.
15. Prasad, A. S., and Oberleas, D. Binding of zinc to amino acids and serum proteins in vitro. *J. Lab. Clin. Med.* 3, 416–425, 1970.
16. Hallman, P. S., Perrin, D. D., and Watt, A. E. Computed distribution of copper (II) and zinc (II) ions among seventeen amino acids present in human plasma. *Biochem. J.* 121, 549–555, 1971.
17. Giroux, E. L., and Henkin, R. I. Competition for zinc among serum albumin and amino acids. *Biochim. Biophys. Acta* 273, 64–74, 1972.
18. Henkin, R. I. Metal-albumin-amino acid interactions: chemical and physiological interrelationships. *Adv. Exp. Med. Biol.* 48, 297–327, 1974.
19. Cousins, R. J. Regulation of zinc absorption: Role of intracellular ligands. *Am. J. Clin. Nutr.* 32, 339–345, 1979.
20. Hahn, C., and Evans, G. W. Identification of a low molecular weight 65-Zn complex in rat intestine. *Proc. Soc. Exptl. Biol. Med.* 144, 793–795, 1973.

21. Evans, G. W., Grace, C. I., and Votava, H. J. A proposed mechanism for zinc absorption in the rat. *Am. J. Physiol.* 228, 501–505, 1975.

22. Schricker, B. R., and Forbes, R. M. Studies on the chemical nature of a low molecular weight zinc binding ligand in rat intestine. *Nutr. Rep. Intl.* 18, 159–165, 1978.

23. Duncan, J. R., and Hurley, L. S. Intestinal absorption of zinc: A role for a zinc-binding ligand in milk. *Am. J. Physiol.* 235, E556–E559, 1978.

24. Bonewitz, R. F., Voner, C., and Foulkes, E. C. Uptake and absorption of zinc in perfused rat jejunum: The role of endogenous factors in the lumen. *Nutr. Res.* 2, 301–307, 1982.

25. Wapnir, R. A., Khani, D. E., Bayne, M. A., Lifshitz, F. Absorption of zinc by the rat ileum: Effects of histidine and other low molecular weight ligands. *J. Nutr.* 113, 1346–1354, 1983.

26. Hurley, L. S., Lonnerdal, B., and Stanislowski, A. G. Zinc citrate, human milk and acrodermatitis enteropathica. *Lancet* 1, 677–678, 1979.

27. Evans, G. W. Normal and abnormal zinc absorption in man and animals. The tryptophan connexion. *Nutr. Revs.* 38, 137–141, 1980.

28. Evans, G. W., and Johnson, E. C. Zinc absorption in rats fed a low-protein diet and a low-protein diet supplemented with tryptophan or picolinic acid. *J. Nutr.* 110, 1076–1080, 1980.

29. Lonnerdal, B., Stanislowski, A. G., and Hurley, L. S. Isolation of a low molecular weight zinc binding ligand from human milk. *J. Inorg. Biochem.* 12, 71–78, 1980.

30. Giroux, E., and Prakash, N. K. Influence of zinc-ligand mixtures on serum zinc levels in rats. *J. Pharm. Sci.* 66, 391–395, 1977.

31. Shah, B. G. Chelating agents and bioavailability of minerals. *Nutr. Res.* 1, 617–622, 1981.

32. Nielson, F. H., Sunde, M. L., and Hoekstra, W. G. Effect of some dietary synthetic and natural chelating agents on the zinc deficiency syndrome in the chick. *J. Nutr.* 89, 35–42, 1966.

33. Schwarz, F. J., and Kirchgessner, M. Tierexperimentelle Untersuchungen zur Zn-Absorption bei verschiedenen Dunndarmabschnitten und Zn-Verbindugen. *Nutr. Metab.* 18, 157–166, 1975.

34. Steinhardt, H. G., and Adibi, S. A. Interaction between transport of zinc and other solutes in human intestine. *Am. J. Physiol.* 247, G176–G182, 1984.

35. Wapnir, R. A., Garcia-Aranda, J. A., and Mevorach, D. E. K. Differential absorption of zinc in protein-energy malnutrition. *J. Am. Coll. Nutr.* 3, 275, 1984.

36. Wapnir, R. A., and Stiel, L. Zinc intestinal absorption: Specificity of amino acids as ligands. *Fed. Proc.* 44, 994, 1985.

37. O'Dell, B. L. Effect of dietary components upon zinc availability. A review with original data. *Am. J. Clin. Nutr.* 22, 1315–1322, 1969.

38. Sandstrom, B., and Cederblad, A. Zinc absorption from composite meals. II. Influence of the main protein source. *Am. J. Clin. Nutr.* 33, 1778–1783, 1980.

39. Pedersen, B., and Eggum, B. O. Interrelations between protein and zinc utilization in rats. *Nutr. Rep. Intl.* 27, 441–453, 1983.
40. Prasad, A. S., Miale, A., Farid, Z., Schulert, A., and Sandstead, H. H. Zinc metabolism in patients with the syndrome of iron deficiency anemia, hypogonadism and dwarfism. *J. Lab. Clin. Med.* 61, 537–549, 1963.
41. Shah, B. G., and Belonje, B. Bioavailability of zinc in beef with and without plant protein concentrates. *Nutr. Res.* 4, 71–77, 1984.
42. Harzer, G., and Kauer, H. Binding of zinc to casein. *Am. J. Clin. Nutr.* 35, 981–987, 1982.
43. Knauff, K. H. Influence of protein source on zinc bioavailability from infant formulas. *Fed. Proc.* 44, 1506, 1985.
44. Magee, A. C., and Lugeye, K. K. Effect of zinc on growth and trace mineral status of rats fed low protein diets supplemented with amino acids. *Fed. Proc.* 44, 543, 1985.
45. Murthy, R. C., Lal, S., Saxena, D. K., Shukla, G. S., Ali, M. M., and Chandra, S. V. Effect of manganese and copper interaction on behavior and biogenic amines in rats fed a 10% casein diet. *Chem. Biol. Inter.* 37, 299–304, 1981.
46. Thompson, A. B. R., Olatunbosum, D., and Valberg, L. S. Interrelation of intestinal transport system for manganese and iron. *J. Lab. Clin. Med.* 78, 643–655, 1971.
47. Gruden, N. Suppression of transduodenal manganese transport by milk diet supplemented with iron. *Nutr. Metab.* 21, 305–309, 1977.
48. Chan, W. Y., Bates, J. M., Jr., and Rennert, O. M. Comparative studies of manganese binding in human breast milk, bovine milk and infant formula. *J. Nutr.* 112, 642–648, 1982.
49. Lonnerdal, B., Keen, C. L., Ohtake, M., and Tamura, T. Iron, zinc, copper and manganese in infant formula. *Am. J. Dis. Child.* 137, 433–439, 1983.
50. Bates, J., Chan, W., Mahood, A., and Rennert, O. M. Human milk, bovine milk and infant formula ligand-bound manganese transport in the rat. *Fed. Proc.* 42, 817, 1983.
51. Keen, C. L., Bell, J. G., and Lonnerdal, B. Manganese uptake and retention from human milk, cow's milk and infant formulas in the suckling rat. *Fed. Proc.* 44, 1850, 1985.
52. Garcia-Aranda, J. A., Wapnir, R. A., and Lifshitz, F. In vivo intestinal absorption of manganese in the rat. *J. Nutr.* 113, 2601–2607, 1983.
53. Solomons, N. W. Biochemical, metabolic, and clinical role of copper in human nutrition. *J. Am. Coll. Nutr.* 4, 83–105, 1985.
54. Crampton, R. F., Matthews, D. M., and Poisner, R. Observations on the mechanism of absorption of copper by the small intestine. *J. Physiol.* 178, 111–119, 1965.
55. Evans, G. W. Copper homeostasis in the mammalian system. *Physiol. Revs.* 53, 535–570, 1973.
56. Marceau, N., Aspin, N., and Sass-Kortsak, A. Absorption of copper 64 from gastrointestinal tract of the rat. *Am. J. Physiol.* 218, 377–384, 1970.

57. Mills, C. F. The dietary availability of copper in the form of naturally oc-curring organic complexes. *Biochem. J.* 63, 190–193, 1956.

58. Davis, N. T., and Nightingale, R. The effects of phytate on intestinal absorp-tion and secretion of zinc, and whole body retention of zinc, copper, iron and manganese in rats. *Br. J. Nutr.* 34, 243–250, 1975.

59. Moore, T., Constable, B. J., Day, K. C., Impey, S. G., and Symonds, K. R. Copper deficiency in rats fed upon raw meat. *Br. J. Nutr.* 18, 135–142, 1964.

60. Ashmead, H. Tissue transportation of organic trace minerals. *J. Appl. Nutr.* 22, 42–51, 1970.

61. Kirchgessner, M., and Grassman, E. The dynamics of copper absorption. In *Proceedings of WAAP/IBP International Symposium on Trace Element Metabolism in Animals*. Mills, C. F. (ed.). E. & S. Livingstone, Edinburgh, 1970, pp. 277–287.

62. Neumann, P. Z., and Silverberg, M. Active copper transport in mammalian tissues—a possible role in Wilson's disease. *Nature* 210, 414–416, 1966.

63. Harris, D. I. M., and Sass-Kortsak, A. The influence of amino acids on cop-per uptake by rat liver slices. *J. Clin. Invest.* 46, 659–667, 1967.

64. Gollan, J. L., Davis, P. S., and Deller, D. J. Binding of copper by human alimentary secretions. *Am. J. Clin. Nutr.* 24, 1925–1935, 1971.

65. Gollan, J. L. Studies on the nature of complexes formed by copper with hu-man alimentary secretions and their influence on copper absorption. *Clin. Sci.* 49, 237–244, 1973.

66. Greger, J. L., and Snedeken, S. M. Effect of dietary protein and phosphorus levels on the utilization of zinc, copper and manganese by adult males. *J. Nutr.* 110, 2243–2251, 1980.

67. Fransson, G. B., and Lonnerdal, B. Distribution of trace elements and min-erals in human and cow's milk. *Pediatr. Res.* 17, 912–915, 1983.

68. Harvey, P. W., Hunsaker, H. A., and Allen, K. G. D. Dietary L-histidine in-duced hypercholesterolemia and hypocupremia in the rat. *J. Nutr.* 111, 639–647, 1981.

69. Price, N. O., and Bunce, G. E., Effect of nitrogen and calcium on balance of copper, manganese and zinc in pre-adolescent girls. *Nutr. Rep. Intl.* 5, 275–284, 1972.

70. Van Campen, D. R. Copper interference with the intestinal absorption of zinc-65 by rats. *J. Nutr.* 97, 104–108, 1969.

71. Greger, J. L., Zaikis, S. C., Abernathy, R. P., Bennett, O. A., and Huffman, J. Zinc, nitrogen, copper, iron and manganese balance in adolescent females fed two levels of zinc. *J. Nutr.* 108, 1449–1456, 1978.

72. Burke, D. M., DeMicco, F. J., Tapper, L. J., and Ritchey, S. J. Copper and zinc utilization in elderly adults. *J. Gerontol.* 36, 558–563, 1981.

73. Wasserman, R. H., and Taylor, A. N. Vitamin D-induced calcium binding protein in chick intestinal mucosa. *Science* 152, 791–793, 1966.

74. Alpers, D. H., Lee, S. W., and Avioli, L. V. Identification of two calcium-binding proteins in human small intestine. *Gastroenterology* 62, 559–565, 1972.

75. DeLuca, H. F., and Schones, H. K. Metabolism and mechanism of action of vitamin D. *Ann. Rev. Biochem.* 45, 631–675, 1976.
76. Weiser, M. M. Calcium. In *Absorption and Malabsorption of Mineral Nutrients*. Solomons, N. W., and Rosenberg, I. H. (eds.). Alan R. Liss, New York, 1984, pp. 15–68.
77. Allen, L. H. Calcium bioavailability and absorption: A review. *Am. J. Clin. Nutr.* 35, 783–789, 1982.
78. Margen, S., Chu, J. Y., Kaufman, N. A., and Calloway, D. H. Studies in calcium metabolism. I. The calciuretic effect of dietary protein. *Am. J. Clin. Nutr.* 27, 584–589, 1974.
79. Heaney, R. P., and Recker, R. R. Effects of nitrogen, phosphorus, and caffeine on calcium balance in women. *J. Lab. Clin. Med.* 99, 46–57, 1982.
80. Bengoa, J. M., Sitrin, M. D., Wood, R. J., and Rosenberg, I. H. Amino acid induced hypercalciuria in patients on total parenteral nutrition. *Am. J. Clin. Nutr.* 38, 264–270, 1983.
81. Irving, J. T. *Calcium and Phosphorus Metabolism*. Academic Press, New York, 1973, pp. 25–26.
82. Pansu, D., Chapuy, M. C., Milani, M., and Bellaton, C. Transepithelial calcium transport enhanced by xylose and glucose in the rat jejunal ligated loop. *Calcif. Tissue Res.* 21, 45–56, 1976.
83. Norman, D. A., Morawski, S. G., and Fordtran, J. S. Influence of glucose, fructose and water movement on calcium absorption in the jejunum. *Gastroenterology* 78, 27–35, 1980.
84. Ghishan, F. K., Jenkins, J. T., and Younoszai, M. K. Intestinal calcium loss in infant rats. *Proc. Soc. Exptl. Biol. Med.* 161, 70–73, 1979.
85. Bengoa, J. M., and Wood, R. J. Magnesium. In *Absorption and Malabsorption of Mineral Nutrients*. Solomons, N. W., and Rosenberg, I. H. (eds.). Alan R. Liss, New York, 1984, pp. 69–88.
86. McCance, R. A., Widdowson, E. M., and Lehmann, H. The effect of protein intake on the absorption of calcium and magnesium. *Biochem. J.* 36, 686–691, 1942.
87. Hunt, S. M., and Schofield, F. A. Magnesium balance and protein intake level in adult human female. *Am. J. Clin. Nutr.* 22, 367–376, 1969.
88. Toothill, J. The effect of certain dietary factors on the apparent absorption of magnesium by the rat. *Br. J. Nutr.* 17, 125–131, 1963.
89. Allen, L. H., Oddoye, E. A., and Margen, S. Protein-induced hypercalciuria: A longer term study. *Am. J. Clin. Nutr.* 32, 741–749, 1979.
90. Seelig, M. S. *Magnesium Deficiency in the Pathogenesis of Disease*. Plenum Medical Books, New York, 1980, p. 263.

5

Morphological Alterations in Small Intestinal Epithelial Surfaces During Nutrient Transport

Saul Teichberg
Cornell University Medical College, New York, and North Shore University Hospital, Manhasset, New York

I. INTRODUCTION

The absorptive epithelial cells of the small intestine are polarized columnar cells specialized for digestive and nutrient transport functions. A significant factor in the efficiency of the absorptive and transport functions of these cells concerns their two major surface macrodomains; the luminal-facing microvillar brush border and basolateral surface plasma membrane. The mucosal microvillar surface amplifies the absorptive-digestive surface 25–30-fold, and this zone is further complicated by a "fuzzy" coat of acidic mucopolysaccharide complexed with oligosaccharidases and other digestive enzymes. The basolateral surface of the absorptive epithelial cell is much less well characterized and has been referred to as the "dark side" of the epithelium (1). The basolateral surface of the absorptive epithelial cell is also amplified in area by means of a large folded plasma membrane that interdigitates with the membrane of adjacent cells. This basolateral surface contains many key transport proteins; for example, the Na^+-K^+ ATPase (1-3), that drives sodium and water absorption from lumen to plasma and adenylcyclase, the key enzyme of cyclic adenosine monophosphate (cAMP)-mediated secretion (4,5). In addition, there are less well characterized transport carriers on the basolateral surface that mediate the translocation of nutrients such as amino acids from epithelial cell interior to extracellular space (6).

The two major absorptive epithelial surface macrodomains, microvilli and basolateral, are functionally and structurally separated by a zona occludens or tight junction, which prevents lateral membrane fluidity, resulting in a general segregation of transport proteins to either the mucosal or basolateral surface (3). Interchange of membrane between the two major surface domains appears to occur only during vesicular bulk transport in membrane-delimited vesicles such as that involved in secretory IgA translocation from basolateral to mucosal surface (7) or the translocation of immunoglobulin (8) trophic factors (9), or other proteins (10) by endocytosis from the intestinal lumen. Although there is a lack of membrane fluidity across the tight junction, in low resistance, "leaky" epithelia such as the small intestine and gallbladder, fluid and sodium absorption is largely paracellular; that is, between the epithelial cells and through the tight junctional zone (11,12). Because the intestinal epithelium absorbs and secretes fluid simultaneously, the division of bidirectional fluxes between cells of different zones along the villus tip to crypt axis has been under investigation. While absorptive, fluid influx is generally thought to be restricted to cells on the upper portion of villi, questions of overlapping function and bidirectional fluxes in the same cells have not been fully resolved (3,13). Although perceived in electron micrographs as static structures, the plasma membranes of both the mucosal and basolateral surfaces of absorptive epithelial cells are dynamic changing structures. These surfaces turn over their components and undergo a variety of translocations both within the fluid lateral plane of the membrane and between the cell interior and surface.

This chapter focuses on some of the dynamic movements and changes in the mucosal and basolateral surface membranes of small intestinal epithelia during feeding and exposure to nutrients, including proteins and their digestive products such as amino acids. A large body of evidence indicates that both the microvillous surface as well as the basolateral cell membrane undergo dramatic alterations during the changing physiological conditions seen during nutrient and fluid absorption. The possible role of vesicle-mediated membrane transport in the regulation of nutrient absorption is also discussed.

A. The Microvillar Surface

Microvilli of the small intestinal epithelium can modify their membrane surface in a variety of ways. These include a contraction-associated process and by membrane addition and shedding.

1. Contractile-Associated Microvillar Motion

The ability of microvilli to undergo contraction-associated movements can be related to their underlying structural organization. Microvilli contain a polarized core of 20–30 thin parallel actin filaments linked by other proteins such as villin and fimbrin and associated with the calcium regulatory protein calmod-

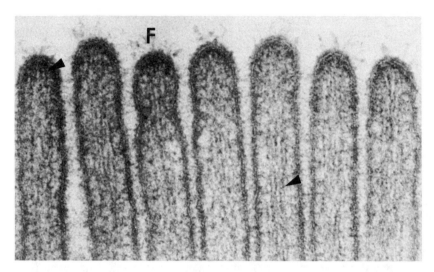

Figure 1 Electron micrograph of the microvillar surface showing the "fuzzy" coat (F) and slender microvilli. Note the core of thin filaments (arrowheads) that run parallel to the microvillar axis and appear to insert into the plasma membrane at the tip. (X90,000.)

ulin (14). The filamentous actin core inserts into the apex of the microvillar plasma membrane (Fig. 1), while the base of the filament core extends into the terminal web and intertwines with a variety of terminal web, nonactin filaments and myosin. The terminal web filaments are associated with actin, myosin, and other proteins at belt desmosome (zonula adherens) sites at the basolateral cell margin. Addition of adenosine triphosphatase (ATP) to isolated brush borders results in contraction, that is calcium dependent, involves movements of the filament systems relative to the basolateral desmosmal anchorage (14,15), and is mediated by desmosomal (zonula adherens) myosin. The motion observed in vitro during this contraction consists of a fanning out (14) of the microvilli. Such a phenomenon during feeding would have an appreciable effect on the movement, circulation, and contact of nutrients with the absorptive surface. This could in effect, "stir" the unstirred layer adjacent to the microvillar membrane, bringing disaccharides, peptides, amino acids, fatty acids, and monoglycerides into more frequent contact with surface digestive enzymes and carrier proteins. It has been hypothesized that this contraction could also modify the permeability of the tight junction or zona occludens (14). Observing microvillar movements in vivo is clearly more difficult; some in vivo studies suggest that there may be rapid shortening and microvillar extension during hypertonic feedings (16). Such contraction of the microvilli themselves could be mediated by core actin and terminal web myosin, but remains to be more fully documented (14). The localized "motility" produced by microvillar movements mediated by intracellular filamentous contractile proteins could have a significant effect on the physiology of intestinal absorption and transport.

2. Microvillar Elongation and Shedding

The microvillar surface of intestinal absorptive cells also shows dramatic morphological changes in the extent and turnover of microvillar surface membranes during feeding and nutrient absorption. This process involves microvillar elongation and membrane shedding (14,17).

Studies on experimental animals indicated that microvilli elongate during feeding; microvilli of fasted rats are significantly shorter than those of fed animals (17). Tall microvilli from fed animals also show a microvesicular shedding from their tips, as if membrane were continually released into the gut lumen (Fig. 2). The simplest interpretation of these observations is that feeding, either by a neuroendocrine pathway or directly, induces metabolic changes in absorptive epithelial cells leading to rapid addition of mucosal surface membrane (possibly with new digestive and transport proteins) resulting in microvillar elongation. Simultaneously, there appears to be a continual shedding from the microvillar tip of membranous microvesicles into the gut lumen in a manner that superficially resembles the production turnover and shedding of membrane from rod photoreceptors (18). Thus, the morphological aspects of this process are compatible with a stimulation of the synthesis and turnover of microvillar components.

Our recent observations indicate that when an infant formula is infused into the intestine of young experimental rats, a similar process of microvesicular shedding can be induced (Fig. 2). Perhaps this is a normal process that also occurs during feeding of human infants.

However, many aspects of this interesting process of microvesicular elongation and shedding remain to be clarified. For example, is elongation due to added membrane fragments with newly synthesized digestive enzymes produced on the endoplasmic reticulum (19,20)? Do the fragments, presumably added by exocytosis to the surface, gradually migrate up the microvilli intact where they are used and eventually turned over by microvesicular shedding? Or, alternatively, are membrane components randomized within the microvillar membrane? If there is a sequence of addition and turnover of the same proteins, there should be some stoichiometric relation between shed enzyme and transport molecules and newly added molecules. Are protein components as well as lipids shed and, if so, do shed proteins function enzymatically in the intestinal lumen? How specific is the shedding phenomena; nonabsorptive cells such as mucus-producing cells may also show evidence of this process (17). Furthermore, we need to know whether there are specific classes of nutrients that induce this

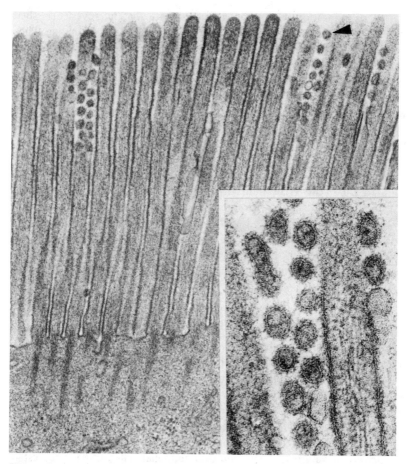

Figure 2 Electron micrograph of a portion of the microvillar brush border from the jejunum of a rat infused with infant formula. At focal sites in the jejunum, microvilli appear unusually long and show evidence of microvesicular shedding of membrane at their apices (arrowhead). (X30,000.) The inset, at a higher magnification, shows that the small microvesicles retain the fuzzy coat and characteristic double membrane of the microvilli, further indicating that they derive from the microvilli themselves. (Inset X100,000.)

sequence. Evidence from in vivo pathophysiological studies suggest that lectins present in the diet produce a similar, but even more dramatic effect on microvilli (21), leading to enough microvesicular shedding to damage the epithelial cell surface. Although such an effect of lectins might explain microvesicular shedding during pathophysiological conditions, they provide no data on the stimulation of elongation. Our observations indicate that microvesicular shedding can also be induced by a simple nutrient like glycerol, a triglyceride. Thus, lipids or their digestive products might well play a role in normal microvesicular shedding. In our experience, the presence of luminal amino acids such as glycine, phenylalanine, and tryptophan, dipeptides, or potential metabolic products of tryptophan such as 5-hydroxytryptophan and serotonin do not induce microvesicular shedding or elongation when they are present in the intestinal lumen for up to 60 minutes in isotonic-buffered saline. However, when glycerol is present along with the amino acids, microvesicular shedding is initiated.

Overall, microvillar elongation and shedding appears to be a normal phenomenon associated with feeding. This process is likely to reflect a stimulation of the addition and turnover of transport proteins during feeding, although this remains to be further clarified. The precise nutrients or classes of nutrients that induce this process and its possible physiological mediators remain to be better defined. The degree of specificity, the physiological role in digestion and absorption, and the effect of certain pathophysiological agents on this process also remain to be detailed.

3. Microvillar Membrane Retrieval and Endocytosis

Another significant aspect of the movement of membrane to an from the microvillar surface of absorptive epithelial cells concerns endocytosis, exocytosis, and related vesicular transport phenomena. In preweaning neonatal animals, endocytosis mediates the transport of immunoglobulins and possible trophic factors (8-10). In postweaning mammals, the possible physiological role of vesicle-mediated movements of microvillar plasma membrane between the surface and intracellular endosomal compartments remains to be better defined.

In neonatal preweaning animals, the role of endocytosis in absorption of immunoglobulins, IgG in proximal jejunum (15), and in the absorption of trophic factors such as nerve growth factor by ileal epithelial cells (9), has been established. These endocytic processes involve mucosal surface receptor-mediated mechanisms (22) that are able to sort the specific proteins, avoid lysosomal degratory mechanisms, and transport the molecules transcellularly to the basolateral intracellular space. In addition, a nonspecific ileal endocytosis of macromolecules into large digestive vacuoles may be nutritionally important in neonatal animals, where other digestive processes are not yet as fully developed (22,23).

In postweaning intestine, endocytosis of intact proteins also occurs in small quantities across absorptive epithelia (10,24-26), across specialized "M" microfold cells (27), or across epithelia in which normal barrier integrity is compromised either by malabsorbed nutrients (28) or by bacterial products (29-32). The normal quantitatively small, transport of intact protein across the absorptive intestinal epithelium has been associated with antigen sampling by the local immune system (33,34), and the possible evolution of food protein sensitivities such as in cow's milk protein sensitivity (35) is discussed elsewhere in this volume.

However, the possible role of the low levels of normal endocytosis at the mucosal surface of absorptive epithelial in mature animals remains a relatively unexplored process. Unfortunately, the glycoprotein marker usually used to detect this process, horseradish peroxidase, does not discriminate well in the gut between specific receptor-mediated and fluid-phase endocytosis.

An attractive hypothesis concerns the possibility that plasma membrane internalization, reflected by endocytosis of tracer at the microvillar mucosal surface is related to the regulation of nutrient and electrolyte absorption. Such a process could involve addition of transport carriers or specialized plasma membrane with permeability characteristics to the surface by exocytosis and retrieval of these or other membrane fragment components by endocytosis. In a variety of other epithelia, the regulation of fluid transport (36,37), hydrogen ion transport (36), and sodium transport (37) can be regulated by membrane exchange. Several indirect but suggestive observations hint that this process may be involved in small intestinal epithelia. During longer-term horseradish peroxidase exposure, the tracer continues to gradually accumulate in terminal web multivesicular bodies (MVB), tubules, and vesicles, and remains restricted to that zone; the tubular extensions from MVBs in the intestine resemble those shown to mediate dissociation of ligand and receptor (38) in other epithelial systems (Fig. 3). This longer term endocytosis is markedly inhibited by chloroquine (39), a lysosomotropic agent that raises lysosomal and endosomal pH (40), interfering with traffic to and from these compartments and eventually inhibiting receptor-associated endocytosis in other cellular systems. The inhibition of endocytosis is thought to be due to failure of receptor-recycling to the surface. Since chloroquine has also been shown to alter intestinal transport functions (42), the possibility exists that vesicle-mediated membrane translocation is linked to regulation of fluid and electrolyte transport regulation. Clearly, the possibility that circulation of membrane-carrying key transport proteins to and from the microvillar mucosal membrane in the form of vesicles and tubules that also fuse with intracellular endosomal or lysosomal compartments remains to be more fully detailed.

As a potential general mechanism, a vesicle-mediated shuttling of transport-related proteins to and from the surface and endocytic compartments may operate at either the microvillar or basolateral cell surface.

C. The Basolateral Surface

1. Plasticity of the Basolateral Surface During Fluid Absorption

The other major plasma membrane macrodomain of the absorptive epithelium of the small intestine, the basolateral surface, may also undergo significant trans-

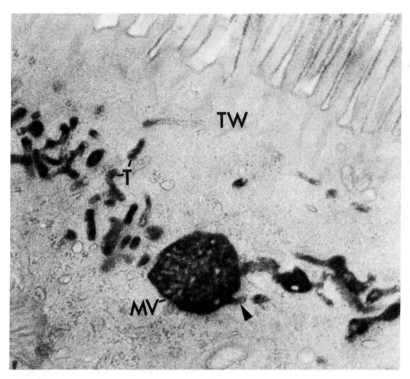

Figure 3 Portion of a rat jejunal epithelial cell from an intestinal loop, continually exposed to a macromolecular tracer, horseradish peroxidase, for over 60 min. In some villi, the epithelial cells show extensive tracer uptake into tubules (T) and multivesicular bodies (MV) in the region beneath the terminal web (TW). Note the tubular extension (arrowhead) from the multivesicular body. (X37,000.)

formation during nutrient transport. Electron microscopic evidence from small intestinal epithelia taken together with studies on living gallbladder epithelium indicate that net fluid absorption results in an expansion of the lateral intercellular spaces between absorptive epithelial cells (43,44). In the intestinal villi, this effect is graded, dilation being most striking in the upper villus zone. The intercellular fluid expansion is believed to be due to the two-membrane, standing osmotic gradient mechanism of fluid absorption (11,12) involving a neutral NaCl transport from intestinal lumen to cell interior, driven by an electrochemical sodium gradient, and a pumping of sodium against a gradient from cell interior to the intercellular space in exchange for potassium by an energy-dependent Na^+-K^+ ATPase. The result is an elevation of intercellular sodium

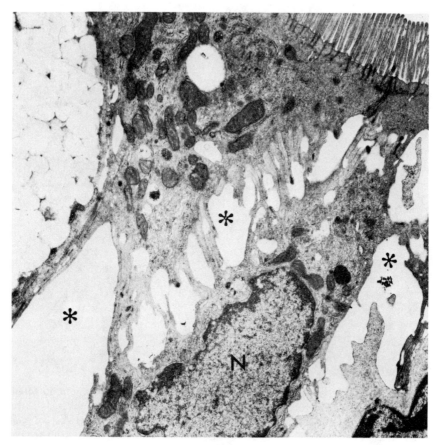

Figure 4 Ileal epithelium from an intestinal loop exposed to buffered isotonic NaCl and 20 mM glycine, where water and sodium absorption are enhanced. Note the dilated intercellular spaces (asterisks) between adjacent absorptive cells. Nucleus, N. (X4800.)

sufficient to pull water in osmotically and largely by a paracellular route. The result is a fluid-induced expansion of the intercellular space (Fig. 4). During nonabsorptive or secretory states, the epithelial intercellular space is collapsed (always in the crypt zone). In the upper portions of villi, during nonabsorptive or secretory states, the interdigitations and contact of basolateral plasma membranes appear maximal. By contrast, fluid expansion decreases contact and also appears to decrease basolateral plasma membrane folding. In other epithelia, such as the mammalian bladder (37), expansion by volume can lead to new

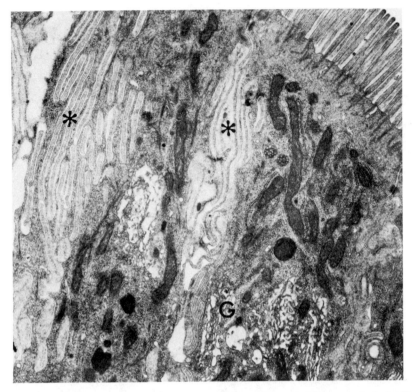

Figure 5 Ileal epithelium from a loop exposed to 20 mM serotonin in buffered isotonic NaCl. With serotonin, fluid absorption is markedly suppressed. Note the extensive interdigitated basolateral plasma membranes (asterisks) of adjacent cells. The intercellular space appears collapsed as compared with the glycine-treated loops. Golgi apparatus, G. (×6600.)

surface membrane addition to accommodate swelling; this has also been associated with the turnover of amiloride-sensitive sodium transport (37). This appears relatively unlikely to occur in small intestinal epithelium because of the extensive basolateral surface amplification that would allow sufficient expansion of fluid space. However, this process remains to be more fully defined in the small intestine. In this expansion/collapse process during fluid transport, leaky epithelia have been described as having the property of a thin-walled elastic tube (44).

Because organic nonelectrolytes such as amino acids and possibly dipeptides are absorbed by Na^+-dependent processes (6,45), the absorption of these nu-

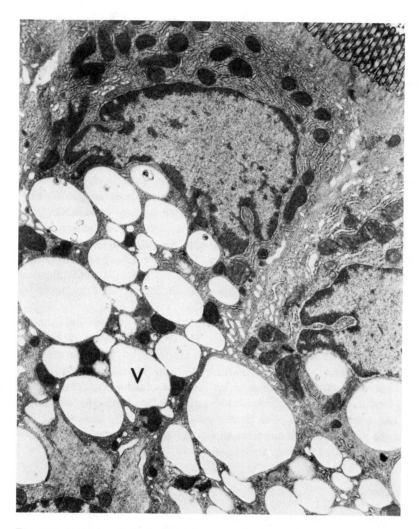

Figure 6 In the early stage of inhibition of fluid and sodium absorption associated with luminal 20 mM L-tryptophan there is a striking formation of clear, apparently swollen, vacuoles (V) in the serosal side of the cytoplasm of ileal absorptive epithelial cells. The mucosal side of the cell appears relatively unaffected. The intercellular space appears relatively collapsed. (X6600.)

trients can also be linked to alterations in the basolateral surface of intestinal epithelial cells. For example, in experimental animals there is a striking expansion in the lateral intercellular space between intestinal epithelial cells when glycine or L-phenylalanine, amino acids that enhance fluid absorption, are present in the gut lumen. On the other hand, the inhibition of fluid absorption by serotonin (Fig. 5) or L-tryptophan (46-50) is associated with collapse of the intercellular space with tightly apposed epithelial cells.

Studies with L-tryptophan (L-Trp) suggest that the inhibition of water influx from lumen to plasma may be mediated by changes in the organization of the epithelium. Thus, early suppression of water influx with L-Trp is associated with swollen vacuoles in the serosal epithelial cytoplasm, particularly in the ileum (Fig. 6). Over longer periods, this evolves into clear mucosal damage. The early vacuoles may be derived from the basolateral membrane and contain Na^+ pump sites. The swollen vacuoles are reminiscent of cation-dependent fluid-filled vacuoles found in other secretory epithelia (51). Similar changes also occur with the dipeptides, tryp-glycine or glycine-tryp. This may be due in part to luminal cleavage of the dipeptides to amino acids. A further potential mechanism concerns the possibility that the fluid absorption suppression of L-tryptophan is partly due to local conversion to serotonin (52).

It is clear that much remains to be learned about the regulatory phenomena at the basolateral surface of the epithelium. The evidence of transport inhibition by tryptophan lends support to the view that nutrients such as amino acids may exert important regulatory effects on the balances of fluid and electrolyte transport. Thus, when nutrients such as amino acids are added as supplements, as in infant formulae, the consequences to intestinal mucosal integrity and to net water and electrolyte absorptive process should be carefully investigated. The role of the spectrum of amino acids, dipeptides and tripeptides on fluid transport processes needs to be fully elaborated.

II. SUMMARY

The major plasma membrane macrodomains of absorptive epithelial cells (mucosal microvillar and basolateral) appear to be dynamic and changing surfaces that may be structurally altered in a variety of ways during nutrient and fluid absorption and transport. These include (a) contractile-related microvillar movements that may serve a role in increasing contact of substrate for digestion and absorption with the microvillar surface; (b) the elongation of brush-border microvilli and microvesicular shedding from the tips of microvilli during feeding that indicates a transient increase in absorptive surface and may also reflect an important mechanism of digestive enzyme and carrier protein turnover; and (c) the plastic characteristics of the basolateral membranes during water and electrolyte absorption that relates to their ability to permit large variations in intercellular space during fluid absorptive or secretory phases. A mechanism is hypothesized for the regulation of numbers of transport proteins that involves vesicle-mediated addition and retrieval of plasma membrane to either mucosal or basolateral surface. Finally, the role of protein-digestive products, principally amino acids, in the regulation of absorptive–secretory processes of the intestinal epithelium is briefly discussed.

REFERENCES

1. Wright, E. M., Mircheff, A. K., Hanna, S. D., Harms, V., van Os, C. H. Walling, M. W., and Sachs, G. The dark side of the intestinal epithelium: The isolation and characterization of basolateral membranes. In: *Mechanism of Intestinal Secretion*. Binder, H. (ed.). Alan Liss, New York, 1979, pp. 117–130.

2. Stirling, C. E. Radioautographic localization of sodium pump sites in rabbit intestine. *J. Cell Biol.* 53, 704–714, 1972.

3. Trier, J. S., and Madara, J. L. Functional morphology of the mucosa of the small intestine. In: *Physiology of the Gastrointestinal Tract*, vol. 2. Johnson, L. R. (ed.). Raven Press, New York, 1981, pp. 925–962.

4. Field, M. Intracellular mediators of secretion in the small intestine. In: *Mechanism of Intestinal Secretion*. Binder, H. (ed.). Alan Liss, New York, 1979, pp. 83–91.

5. Field, M. Secretion by the small intestine. In: *Physiology of the Gastrointestinal Tract*, vol. 2. Johnson, L. R. (ed.) Raven Press, New York, 1981, pp. 963–982.

6. Munck, M. G. Intestinal absorption of amino acids. In: *Physiology of the Gastrointestinal Tract*, vol. 2. Johnson, L. R. (ed.). Raven Press, New York, 1981, pp. 1097–1122.

7. Kagnoff, M. E. Immunology of the digestive system. In: *Physiology of the Gastrointestinal Tract*. Johnson, L. R. (ed.). Raven Press, New York, 1981, pp. 1337–1359.

8. Rodewald, R. Intestinal transport of antibodies in the newborn rat. *J. Cell Biol.* 58, 189–211, 1973.

9. Gonnella, P. A., Siminowski, K., Owen, L., Bernanke, J., Neutra, M. R., and Murphy, R. A. Transepithelial transport of nerve growth factor (NGF) across the ileal epithelium of sucking rats. *Fed. Proc.* 44, 810, 1985.

10. Walker, N. A. Intestinal transport of macromolecular. In: *Physiology of the Gastrointestinal Tract*. Johnson, L. R. (ed.). Raven Press, New York, 1981, pp. 1271–1290.

11. Shultz, S. G., Frizzell, R. A., and Nellans, H. N. Low transport by mammalian small intestine. *Ann. Rev. Physiol.* 36, 51–91, 1974.

12. Munck, B. G., and Schultz, S. G. Properties of the passive conductance pathway across in vitro rat jejunum. *J. Membr. Biol.* 16, 163–174, 1974.

13. Madara, J. L. Increases in guinea pig small intestinal transepithelial resistance induced by osmotic loads are accompanied by rapid alterations in absorptive cell tight-junction structure, *J. Cell Biol.* 97, 126–136, 1983.

14. Mooseker, M. A., Border, E. M., Conzelman, K. A., Fishkind, D. J. Howe, C. L., and Keller, T. C. S. Brush border cytoskeleton and integration of cellular functions. *J. Cell Biol.* 99, PE2, 104s–112s, 1984.

15. Rodewald, R., Newman, S. B., and Karnovsky, M. J. Contraction of isolated brush borders from the intestinal epithelium, *J. Cell Biol.* 70, 541–554, 1976.

16. Teichberg, S., Lifshitz, F. L., Pergolizzi, R., and Wapnir, R. A. Response of rat intestine to a hyperosmotic feeding. *Pediatr. Res.* 12, 720–725, 1978.

17. Misch, D. W., Giebel, P. E., and Faust, R. G. Intestinal microvilli responses to feeding and fasting. *Eur. J. Cell Biol.* 21, 269–279, 1980.

18. Young, R. N. The renewal of rod and cone outer segments in the rhesus monkey. *J. Cell Biol.* 49, 303–318, 1971.

19. Grand, R. J., Montgomery, R. K., and Perey, A. Synthesis and intracellular processing of sucrase-isomaltase in rat jejunum. *Gastroenterology* 88, 531–538, 1985.

20. Weiser, M. M., Neumeier, M. M., A. Quaroni, and Kirsch, K. Synthesis of plasmalemmal glycoproteins in intestinal epithelial cells. Separation of Golgi membranes from villus and crypt cell surface membranes; glycosyltransferase activity of surface membrane. *J. Cell Biol.* 77, 722–734, 1978.

21. Lorenzsonn, V., and Olsen, W. A. In vivo responses of rat intestinal epithelium to intraluminal dietary lectins. *Gastroenterology* 82, 838–848, 1982.

22. Gonnella, P. A., and Neutra, M. R. Membrane bound and fluid phase macromolecules enter separate prelysosomal compartments in absorptive cells of suckling rat ileum. *J. Cell Biol.* 99, 909–917, 1984.

23. Cornell, R., and Padykula, H. A. A cytological study of intestinal absorption in the suckling rat *Am. J. Anat.* 125, 291–316, 1969.

24. Cornell, R., W. A. Walker, and Isselbacher, K. J. Small intestinal absorption of horseradish peroxidase: A cytochemical study. *Lab. Invest.* 25, 42, 1977.

25. Walker, W. A., and Isselbacher, K. J. Uptake and transport of macromolecules by the intestine: A possible role in clinical disorders. *Gastroenterology* 67, 531–547, 1974.

26. Fagundes-Neto, U., Teichberg, S., Bayne, M. A., Morton, B., and Lifshitz, F. Bile salt enhanced rat jejunal absorption of a macromolecular tracer. *Lab. Invest.* 44, 18–26, 1981.

27. Owen, R. L. Sequential uptake of horseradish peroxidase by lymphoid follicle epithelium of Peyer's patches in the normal unabstracted mouse intestine: An ultrastructural study. *Gastroenterology* 72, 440–451, 1977.

28. Teichberg, S., Lifshitz, F., Bayne, M. A., Fagundes-Neto, U., Wapnir, R. A. and McGarvey, E. Disaccharide feedings enhance rat jejunal macromolecular absorption. *Pediatr. Res.* 17, 381–389, 1983.

29. Gullikson, G. W., Cline, W. S., Lorenzson, V., Benz, L., Olsen, W. A., and Bass, P. Effects of anionic surfactants on hamster small intestinal membrane structure and function: Relationship to surface activity. *Gastroenterology* 73, 501–511, 1977.

30. Cline, W. S., Lorenzson, V., Benz, L., Bass, P., and Olsen, W. The effect of sodium ricinoleate on small intestinal function and structure. *J. Clin. Invest.* 58, 380–390, 1976.

31. Teichberg, S., McGarvey, E., Bayne, M. A., and Lifshitz, F. Altered jejunal macromolecular barrier induced by alpha-dihydroxy deconjugated bile salts. *Am. J. Physiol.* 245, G122–G132, 1983.

32. Teichberg, S., Fagundes-Neto, U., Bayne, M. A., and Lifshitz, F. Jejunal macromolecular absorption and bile salt deconjugation in protein-energy malnourished rats *Am. J. Clin. Nutr.* 34, 1281–1291, 1981.

33. Walker, W. A., and Isselbacher, K. J. Intestinal antibodies. *N. Engl. J. Med.* 297, 767–773, 1977.

34. Walker, W. A., Isslebacher, K. J. and Bloch, K. J. Intestinal uptake of macromolecules: Effect of oral immunization. *Science* 177, 608–610, 1972.

35. Walker-Smith, J. A., Harrison, M., Kilby, A., Phillips, A., and France, N. E. Cow's milk sensitive enteropathy. *Arch. Dis. Child.* 53, 375–380, 1978.

36. Gluck, S., Cannon, C., and Al-Awqati, Q. Exocytosis regulation urinary acidification in turtle bladder by rapid insertion of H^+ pumps into the luminal membrane. *Proc. Natl. Acad. Sci.* (U.S.A.) 79, 4327–4331, 1982.

37. Loo, D. D. F., Lewis, S. A., Ifshin, M. A., and Diamond, J. M. Turnover membrane insertion and degradation of sodium channels in rabbit urinary bladders. *Science* 221, 1288–1290, 1984.

38. Geuze, H. J., Slot, J. W., Strous, G. J. A. M. Lodish, H. F., and Schwartz, A. L. Intracellular site of asialglucoprotein receptor-ligand uncoupling: Double label immuno electron microscopy during receptor-mediated endocytosis. *Cell* 32, 277–287, 1983.

39. Teichberg, S., Bayne, M. A., Roberts, B., Lifshitz, F. Inhibition of endocytosis in rat ileal epithelium by chloroquine. *Fed. Proc.* 43, 728, 1984.

40. Steinmann, R. M., Mellman, I. S., Muller, W. A., and Cohn, Z. A. Endocytosis and the recycling of plasma membrane. *J. Cell Biol.* 96, 1–27, 1983.

41. Gonzalez-Noriega, A., Grubb, J. H., Talkad, V., and Sly, W. Chloroquine inhibits lysosomal enzyme secretion by impairing receptor recycling *J. Cell Biol.* 85, 839–852, 1980.

42. Fogel, R., Sharp, G. W.G., and Donowitz, M. Chloroquine stimulates absorption and inhibits secretion of ileal water and electrolytes. *Am. J. Physiol.* 243, G117–G126, 1982.

43. Tomasini, J. T., and Dobbins, W. O. Intestinal morphology during water and electrolyte absorption. A light and electron microscopy study. *Digest. Dis.* 15, 226–238, 1970.

44. Spring, K. R., and Hope, A. Size and shape of the lateral intercellular spaces in a living epithelium. *Science* 200, 54–58, 1978.

45. Addison, J. M., Burston, D., and Matthews, D. M. Evidence for active transport of the dipeptide glycylsarcosine by hamster jejunum in vitro. *Clin. Sci.* 43, 907–911, 1972.

46. Teichberg, S., Wapnir, R. A., Zdanowicz, M., Roberts, B., and Lifshitz, F. Morphological alterations in L-tryptophan treated ileum. *Fed. Proc.* 44, 812, 1985.

47. Munck, B. G., and Rasmussen, S. N. Characteristics of rat jejunal transport of tryptophan. *Biochem. Biophys. Acta* 389, 261–280, 1975.

48. Cooke, H. J., and Cooke, A. R. Effect of tryptophan on transport properties of newborn rabbit jejunum. *Am. J. Physiol.* 242, G308–G312, 1982.

49. Markowitz, J., Wapnir, R. A., and Fisher, S. E. Effect of intraluminal L-tryptophan (TP) on water flux in the perfused rat jejunum. *Gastroenterology* 84, 1240, 1983.
50. Wapnir, R. A. Intestinal osmotic effects of carbohydrate malabsorption. In: *Carbohydrate Intolerance in Infancy*. Lifshitz, F. (ed.). Marcel Dekker, New York, 1982, pp. 121–135.
51. Leslie, B. A., and Putney, J. W. Ionic mechanism in sevretatogogue-induced morphological change in rat parotid gland *J. Cell Biol.* 97, 1119–1130, 1983.
52. Kisloff, B., and Moore, E. W. Effect of serotonin on water and electrolyte transport in the in vivo rabbit small intestine. *Gastroenterology* 71, 1033–1038, 1976.

6

The Mechanisms of Allergic Reactions and Local Antibody Production in Infancy

W. Allan Walker
Harvard Medical School, Children's Hospital, and Massachusetts General Hospital, Boston, Massachusetts

Donald Hanson
Harvard Medical School and Children's Hospital, Boston, Massachusetts

I. INTRODUCTION

An important adaptation of the gastrointestinal tract to the extrauterine environment is its development of a mucosal barrier against the penetration of antigens and antigenic fragments present in the intestinal lumen. At birth, the newborn must be prepared to deal with bacterial colonization of the gut, with formation of toxic byproducts of bacteria and viruses (enterotoxins and endotoxins) and with the ingestion of antigens (milk and soy proteins) and their fragments. The potentially immunologic active substances, if permitted to penetrate the mucosal epithelial barrier under adverse circumstances (increased absorption of antigens or abnormal immune responsiveness) can cause inflammatory and allergic reactions, which may result in gastrointestinal and systemic disease states (1).

To protect against the potential danger of invasion across the mucosal barrier, the infant must develop an extensive system of defense mechanisms within the lumen and on the luminal surface; these mechanisms act to control and maintain the epithelial surface as an impermeable barrier to the uptake of antigens and large antigenic fragments. These defenses include a unique immunologic response (dimeric IgA antibody) to controlled penetration of luminal antigens including production of local antibodies uniquely suited to protection in the luminal environment (secretory component attached to dimeric IgA) and the control of a systemic response (immune tolerance). The result of this physiologic immune response to luminal antigens is the absence of adverse immune reactions.

The purpose of this review is to summarize the evidence for an altered mucosal barrier to proteins and protein fragments in human newborns, to consider factors contributing to mature mucosal barrier function in the human, and finally to stress the consequences (intestinal allergic reactions, etc.) of antigen penetration across an immature intestinal mucosa during infancy.

II. CONCEPT OF THE MUCOSAL BARRIER

As a result of a variety of recent observations (2) it is now apparent that nonimmunological processes working independently and in concert with the local mucosal immune system collectively comprise an effective barrier, "the mucosal barrier," to the attachment and penetration of antigens and fragments present in the intraluminal environment. Table 1 lists some of the processes which comprise the mucosal barrier. Of particular importance is our greater appreciation for the mucus coat overlying the microvillous membrane surface in this defense process. These aspects of intestinal host defense will be stressed. Other aspects have been reviewed previously (3).

A. Mucus Coat

The thickness and composition of the mucus coat overlying the microvillous surface contributes to the defense of mucosal surface against antigens and antigen

Table 1 Representative Components of the Mucosal Barrier to Antigens/Fragments

Nonimmunologic
Intraluminal
Gastric barrier
Proteolysis
Peristalsis
Mucosal surface
Mucus coat
Microvillous membrane
Immunologic
Secretory IgA system
Combination of immunologic and nonimmunologic
Immune complex-mediated mucus release from goblet cells
Immune complex-facilitated mucosal surface proteolysis
Kupffer cell phagocytosis of immune complexes

fragment attachment and penetration. With increase of mucus discharge from goblet cells onto the mucosal surface, the physical thickness of the mucus coat can expand, providing a more extensive physical barrier to the diffusion of antigens from the lumen to the microvillous surface. This enhanced thickness of the mucus coat may be a contributing factor in the expulsion phenomenon for parasites and microbial antigens described by Miller and Nawa (4). Another protective property of mucus relates to the observation that microorganisms can attach to carbohydrate moieties (receptors) of glycoprotein components of the microvillous surface. Examples of this phenomenon are the mannose receptor (5) for *Escherichia coli* and the fucose receptor for *Vibrio cholera* (6). Recent studies from our laboratories (J. Snyder and W. A. Walker, unpublished observations) and others (7) suggest that mucus may contain similar carbohydrate moieties which can actually act as receptor inhibitors, thereby specifically interfering with the attachment of microorganisms and antigens to the microvillous surface. Interference with bacterial attachment by carbohydrate mucus inhibitors provides evidence for a specific protection against antigen penetration. Figure 1 depicts this concept with antigen antibody complexes. Additional studies in this area are needed to further delineate this process.

PHYSICAL BARRIER   LECTIN BINDING   ANTIGEN ALONE

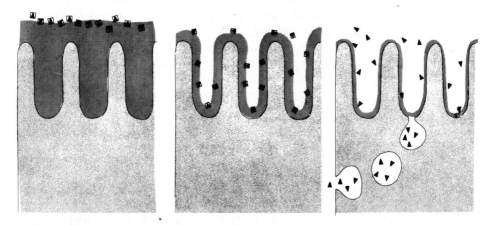

Figure 1 Mechanism of mucus protection in small intestine (IgG complexes). Diagrammatic representation of intestinal secretions coating the intestinal surface as a mucosal barrier to intestinal allergens. Formation of antigen-antibody complexes results in increased release of mucus to form a physical barrier to allergen diffusion. These allergen-antibody complexes also bind to the mucus coat in lectin-like fashion to prevent penetration of the enterocyte. (From Stern and Walker, 1985, with permission of *Pediatr. Clin. North Am.*)

B. Membrane Composition

The composition of the intestinal cell membrane changes as the epithelial cell migrates up the villus (8-10) and as the animal ages (11-13). Changes in membrane composition may determine whether antigen or fragments bind to the cell. Bresson et al. (14) have studies isolated microvillous membranes from the intestine of newborn and adult rabbits. They have shown that the membrane protein/phospholipid ratio is dramatically decreased in membranes of newborns compared to those of adults. In addition, they noted increased cholera enterotoxin binding to microvillous membranes of newborns compared to those of adults. These studies of the development of the intestinal surface may help us to better understand why antigen transport is greater early in life and why newborns have a high incidence of allergic diseases. In recent studies, a direct association between maturity of the microvillous membrane and antigen attachment has been demonstrated (Fig. 2) (15).

C. Immunologic Components of the Mucosal Barrier

The adequacy of local immune function in the gastrointestinal tract affects the attachment and penetration of ingested antigen and fragments. IgA is the immunoglobulin present in highest concentration in intestinal secretions (16,17). It has been postulated that this immunoglobulin prevents the transport of antigen and antigen fragments by complexing with them in the lumen or within the mucus coat, thereby impeding adsorption (1,18). The concentration of IgA in saliva, stool, and serum of newborn animals and humans (19-22) is decreased, and it has been hypothesized that this transient deficiency can in part account for the increased attachment of antigens to the intestinal surface and as noted, in newborn animals. This hypothesis is supported by studies of patients with selective IgA deficiency. These patients have circulating immune complexes and precipitating antibodies to absorbed bovine milk proteins (23). Again, when the sera of IgA-deficient individuals were studied for the appearance of complexes after the ingestion of milk, 3-7 subjects had increases in antibody-antigen complexes, which peaked at 120-150 min (24). In another three subjects there was a tendency toward the formation of two peak concentrations of complexes, the first at 30-60 min and the second 120-150 min after drinking milk. Additionally, the circulating immune complexes found in some patients contained bovine milk proteins. Presumably the same process occurs in the transient IgA deficiency of the newborn as a contributing factor in the increased incidence of intestinal allergy, a common gastrointestinal disease occurring during infancy, and in the increased incidence of immune complex disease (nephritis, rheumatoid arthritis) in selective IgA-deficient patients.

Another important component of mucosal immunity is the access of intestinal antigens to lymphoid elements in Peyer's patches, a necessary first step in the

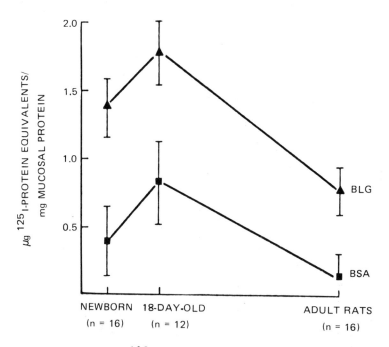

Figure 2 Binding of ^{125}I-labelled bovine serum albumin (BSA) and beta-lacto-globulin (BLG) by the jejunal microvillous membrane in the rat, showing the effect of maturity. Numbers of animals (n) are given in parentheses. Means ± 1 SD are shown. Protein concentration of BSA and BLG, 0.1 mg/ml; microvillous membrane protein concentration, 1.5 mg/ml. Differences in binding between 18-day-old and adult groups are statistically highly significant (p < 0.001) for both proteins. (From Stern et al., 1984, with permission of *Pediatr. Res.*)

secretory IgA cycle (18). Several investigators (25,26) have demonstrated that protein antigens can also traverse the epithelial barrier of the intestine. This occurs in the distal small intestine via specialized M (microfold) cells overlying Peyer's patches. Electron microscopic studies of these cells indicate that they have few microvilli, a poorly developed glycocalyx, and an absence of lysosomal organelles. Using electron microscopy, Owen has observed the uptake and processing of horseradish peroxidase by M cells (25,26). This marker is first taken up by these specialized cells and then extruded into an extracellular space, where it is phagocytosed by lymphoid cells circulating through Peyer's patches (25,26). This type of antigen absorption in the gut has not yet been shown to occur via receptors, but nonetheless appears to represent an important access route for ingested antigens and fragments and viruses (27) to reach lymphoid tissues and thereby stimulate the local and distant immune system. Figure 3 depicts our current concept of the IgA cycle in the gut (28). More research is needed to de-

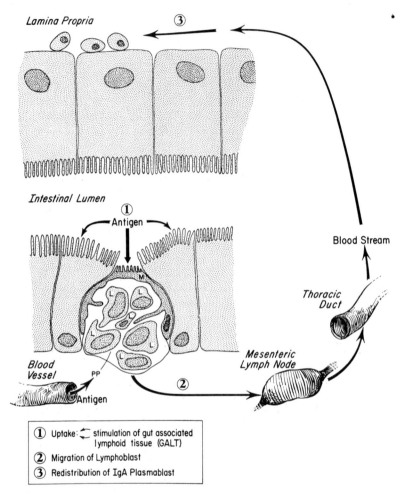

Figure 3 IgA plasma cell cycle. Schematic representation of the cell cycle for IgA-producing plasma cells populating the intestinal mucosa. Lymphocytes (L) within gut-associated lymphoid tissues (GALT), primarily Peyer's patches (PP) of the ileum, are stimulated by antigens entering from the intestinal lumen (1) via specialized epithelium (M cells), across conventional absorptive cells, or from the systemic circulation. Lymphoblasts migrate to mesenteric nodes for further maturation (2) and then enter the systemic circulation as plasmablasts to redistribute along intestinal mucosal surfaces (3) and produce secretory IgA antibodies in response to intestinally absorbed antigens. Symbols in figure: (1) uptake of luminal and systemic antigen by gut-associated lymphoid tissue (GALT); (2) migration of lymphoblast; and (3) redistribution of IgA plasmablast to submucosal sites. (From Walker and Isselbacher, 1977.)

fine the composition of the M-cell membrane surface and to determine whether its composition is important in antigen/fragment attachment.

In summary, one can state that lymphoid elements in the gastrointestinal tract respond uniquely to lumenal antigens which are geared to optimize handling of these antigens. A physiologic immune responsiveness to mucusal antigens entails a two-part response, including the IgA response as discussed above and a preferential inhibition of systemic (IgE, IgG) responsiveness through the stimulus of T suppressor cell clones which act to modulate the conversion of lymphoblasts to plasma cells predisposed to producing systemic antibodies. This phenomenon known as "tolerance" seems to be uniquely the property of antigens or fragments crossing the mucosal surface (29). Figure 4 diagrammatically depicts this two-part response of intestinal lymphoid elements to luminal antigens.

D. Combined Effect of Immunologic and Nonimmunologic Components of the Mucosal Barrier

Several recent observations have suggested that the local immune process in addition to its inherent protective properties can also augment the protective capacity of the previously mentioned nonimmunologic components of the mucosal barrier (Table 1). Representative examples illustrate this phenomenon. In previous work (30) we reported that the proteolysis of intestinal antigens was considerably greater in immunized animals than in nonimmunized controls, and that enhanced proteolysis most likely resulted from the interaction of immune complexes present in the mucus coat with pancreatic enzymes adsorbed onto the surface of the intestine after secretion into the lumen. Another example of combined protection is the enhanced discharge of goblet cell mucin occurring in intestinal anaphylaxis, as reported by Lake et al. (31). Using radiolabelled goblet cell mucus to quantify release, Lake showed that IgE-mediated mast cell discharge of histamine resulted in enhanced release of goblet cell mucus into the intestinal tract. This observation probably explains the expulsion of parasites associated with an increased mucus coat, described by Miller and Nawa (4), and may represent an important factor in host protection against parasitic infestation of the intestine.

A final example of the combined effect of immunologic and nonimmunologic processes in controlling host defense at the mucosal surface is the role of Kupffer cells in clearing immune complexes absorbed from the gastrointestinal tract. Several years ago in an animal model, we demonstrated that immune complexes to intestinal antigens formed on the intestinal surface or within the intestinal interstitium were cleared more readily by Kupffer cells in the liver than were antigens alone (32). This second line of mucosal defense may be important in preventing Gram-negative microorganisms gaining access to the portal

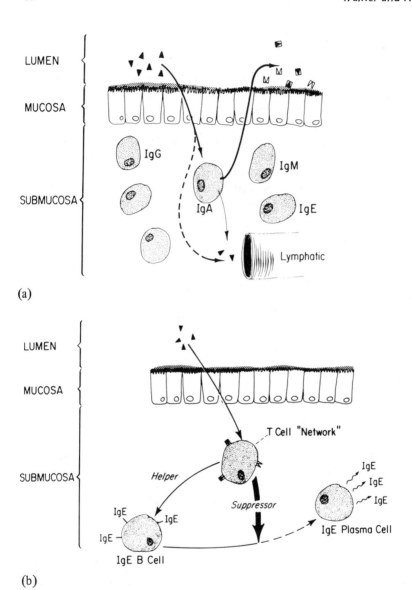

Figure 4 Physiologic immune response to intestinal antigen. Intestinal antigens evoke a local IgA response after crossing mucosal surfaces (a) and interacting with IgA-producing plasma cells previously primed by the IgA cycle. In addition, antigens and antigenic fragments can trigger a T-cell suppressor activity which presumably contributes to a tolergenic IgE/IgG systemic response (b).

circulation and in the clearance of endotoxins and food antigens known to be taken up into the portal circulation.

III. DEFICIENCIES OF THE MUCOSAL BARRIER TO ANTIGENS AND THEIR FRAGMENTS

If the complex process of mucosal barrier defense is disrupted, or if specific deficiencies in components of barrier function exist, an increased incidence of antigen-induced intestinal diseases may ensue. Table 2 lists examples of circumstances that have resulted in disruption of mucosal barrier function and an increased incidence of gastrointestinal disease states. For discussion purposes, the immaturity of gastrointestinal barrier function will be used to illustrate this circumstance. Epidemiologic studies have shown a striking increase in allergic, infectious, and toxigenic diarrhea during infancy, particularly in premature infants (33). This increased incidence has been ascribed to immature mucosal host defenses against antigen attachment and penetration. A prototypic infectious disease occurring during this interval is necrotizing enterocolitis (NEC) (34), which is directly related to mucosal barrier deficiency.

During the last several years, a major thrust of our laboratory has been to define the developmental deficiencies in mucosal barrier function during the perinatal period. We have concentrated our efforts on the mucus coat and microvillous surface. Udall et al. (35) noted a striking increase in penetration of intestinal antigens in newborn compared to adult animals. Subsequently, in comprehensive experiments by Pang et al. (36,37), striking differences in microvillous membrane composition and structure were demonstrated between newborn and mature animals. Bresson et al. (14) showed that this immaturity could account for enhanced binding of cholera toxin to the microvillous surface and Stern

Table 2 Disruptions of Mucosal Barrier Function as Causes of Pathologic Uptake of Antigen/Fragments

Immature gastrointestinal function
Malnutrition
Inflammation
Gastrointestinal anoxia
Transient/selective IgA deficiency

ANTIGEN SPECIFIC

IMMATURE
GUT SURFACE

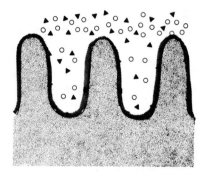

Figure 5 Pathologic antigen interaction with intestinal surface. Intestinal antigens and their antigenic fragments may interact to a greater extent with the immature gut surface because of an absence of protective mucus and an immature composition of the mucosal surface. This enhanced interaction may account for increased antigen uptake in the small intestine of neonates. ○ = Antigen A; ▲ = antigen E.

et al. (15) demonstrated increased antigen attachment at that site, suggesting an association between immaturity and the increased incidence of mechanisms of infectious/allergic disease. In additional studies from this laboratory, Shub et al. (38) have found striking differences in the carbohydrate composition of intestinal mucus from immature and mature rats which could account for the lack of mucus-specific receptor inhibition against bacteria in newborns. Obviously, more studies need to be done to show any specific effect of mucus composition and enhanced bacterial/antigen adherence to microvillous surface in this patient population. Figure 5 depicts the concept of excessive antigen uptake across an immature intestinal surface.

In addition to the immaturity of the intestinal surface of young infants, the mucosal response to antigens is also *abnormal* due to the developmental delay in local immune responsiveness. In the absence of enteric stimuli, principally by bacterial antigens, there is a paucity of IgA-producing plasma cells in the lamina propria. This requires weeks to months of extrauterine existence to establish protective levels in intestinal secretions (39). In addition, the suppressive T-cell function necessary to control a systemic response to enteric antigens is incompletely developed, accounting for systemic responsiveness rather than a state of systemic tolerance. Several studies have demonstrated that the normal response to enteric antigens is a systemic immune response occurring in infancy (40).

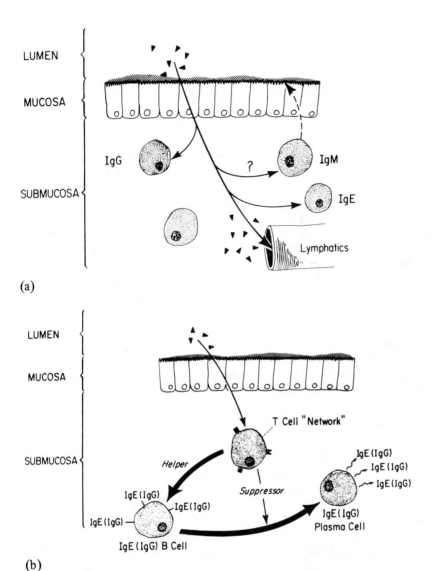

(a)

(b)

Figure 6 Pathologic antigen interactions with the intestinal surface. Under circumstances of pathologic antigen interaction with the intestinal surface (IgA deficiency and/or decreased T suppressor response), an abnormal immune response can occur. In the absence of a local IgA response (IgA deficiency) (a), no IgA antibodies are produced on antigen exposure and excessive antigens can be taken up into the systemic circulation. Alternately, the T modulation of B-cell response (b) can enhance the systemic IgE/IgG response resulting in adverse immune reactions causing allergic disease.

Figure 6 depicts the pathologic local immune response to enteric antigens occurring in infancy.

IV. EFFECTS OF IMMATURE ANTIGEN DIGESTION AND MUCOSAL BARRIER PENETRATION ON THE INITIATION OF IMMUNITY AND TOLERANCE

Identification of factors contributing to the elevated incidence of immune-mediated reactions to dietary antigens and their fragments in infants has been complicated by the array of changes that occur in the function and structure of the gastrointestinal and lymphoid systems throughout this period. Recent work in these areas has advanced from specifying and quantifying potentially relevant factors to defining model systems in which the impact of changes in those factors can be examined in terms of their direct influence on immune responsiveness in developing and mature animals. In particular, useful experimental systems would be based on models that are well-characterized in regard to gastrointestinal and lymphoid maturation, and selected on the basis of evidence that early, physiologic exposures to dietary antigens or fragments lead to enhanced specific immune responsiveness when compared with similar exposures in adults. One such system involves the feeding of ovalbumin, a potent immunogen, to experimental neonatal animals that are genetically defined "high-responders" to this antigen (41). Initial studies of this model have demonstrated that newborn animals show enhanced specific responsiveness ("Priming") if fed 1 mg of ovalbumin per gram of body weight within 2-3 days after birth. Weanlings and adults fed the same dose of antigen develop substantial depression of specific responsiveness (tolerance). These effects are expressed in both cell-mediated immune responses and antibody responses, including IgG and IgE antibody classes (41,42). Models of this kind should prove valuable in characterising the influence of maturational events at the lymphoid and gastrointestinal levels upon tendencies toward increased or decreased immune responsiveness to specific dietary antigens. For example, initial dose–response studies led to proposal of the hypothesis that infant mice, in which luminal digestive processes are poorly developed at birth, may respond to absorbed and injected antigens in a similar manner determined by the systemic concentrations of antigen that are achieved, irrespective of the route of exposure.

This hypothesis, and the results of future testing, are likely to illuminate an as yet poorly understood contribution of the maturation of gastrointestinal digestive processes and the mucosal barrier to differences between infants and adults in the character of absorbed antigens, and in their immunomodulatory effects. Many investigators have shown that immunoreactive antigen—recognizable by specific antibodies—is taken up in greater amounts from neonates than adults when fed under comparable conditions (e.g., 36,41). Little is known, however, about whether the detectable antigenic materials represent molecular forms that are dissimilar or comparable (but absorbed in differing amounts) in neonates and adults. One might expect that relatively inefficient luminal digestion in neonates and greater permeability of the neonatal mucosal barrier, would tend to allow uptake of a greater ratio of relatively intact:fragmented antigen derivatives in neonates. As proposed in the above hypothesis, small or moderate amounts of antigen absorbed from neonatal gut would be expected to enhance specific responsiveness, whereas larger amounts would tend to tolerize, as observed when native antigen is injected parenterally into newborns (41). In contrast, the mature digestive capatitity of adults would be expected to fragment proteins more effectively, encouraging a shift toward increased production of smaller derivatives which, by virtue of their size, could be taken up in significant amounts.

Support for the potential importance of intact antigen:fragment ratios was obtained from a feeding study in which mice were injected parenterally with a small priming dose of native antigen (10 μg) at the time of a tolerizing intragastric feeding of the same antigen (20 mg). Animals given both exposures showed neither tolerance nor priming, which suggested that systematic availability of small amounts of intact antigen overcame the effects of absorbed antigen by providing a positive stimulus of similar magnitude (43). Current studies in our laboratories show that acute prefeeding of a trypsin inhibitor to adult mice before a normally tolerizing feeding of antigen results in substantial (12-fold) increases in the concentration of antigen-specific determinants in the serum, and a reversal in the immunologic effect of antigen feeding from tolerance to priming for specific antibody responses (D. Hanson et al., manuscript in preparation). While these observations have not yet been evaluated regarding the properties of antigen derivatives in the serum, they are consistent with the hypothesis that gastrointestinal processing and uptake of proteins can affect the immunologic outcome of antigen consumption by determining the influence of antigenic derivatives that reach the lymphoid tissues.

Exposure of local and systemic lymphoid cells to absorbed *fragments* of antigen may in turn be of considerable importance for understanding why protein feeding in adults is biased toward induction of tolerance rather than priming. Although a role of digestively produced protein fragments is not yet directly defined in the induction of priming and tolerance by ingested antigens, proteins that are denatured or fragmented in vitro are capable of inducing specific tolerance when injected parenterally (44,45). Some of these fragments cannot be detected by traditional immunoassays that depend upon binding by antibodies specific to the native molecule, and have been shown to produce unresponsiveness through induction of suppressor T cells in vivo. A suppressor T-cell component has been identified in orally induced tolerance to several protein antigens (46–48). Antigen fragments that contain a specific epitope are also capable of depressing the responses of specific helper T cells in vitro (49), consistent with other evidence that absorbed antigen may promote tolerance through more than one mechanism in fed animals (50).

Gastrointestinally processed protein fragments may achieve their effects by interacting differently than native molecules with the lymphoid and accessory cells that participate in immune responses. This is likely in view of studies indicating that B and T lymphocytes bear cell-surface receptors that recognize different features of protein antigens. The immunoglobulin molecules that serve as receptors on B lymphocytes appear to bind conformational "determinants" associated with shapes found on exposed areas of the folded molecule. In contrast, the T-lymphocyte receptor is capable of recognizing "epitopes" on molecular fragments consisting of as few as 15-20 amino acids, when the specific fragments are presented with appropriate histocompatibility markers on the surfaces of antigen-presenting cells (49,51). Whereas shape determinants are likely, in general, to be distorted or destroyed upon exposure to mature gastrointestinal processing that includes gastric acidity and luminal endopeptidase activity, the primary sequence of amino acids comprising an epitope may persist on fragments of various sizes until directly cleaved by endopeptidases or terminal peptidases. Differences in the degree and character of antigen fragmentation in neonatal and adult gut might therefore influence the stimuli available to specific B and T lymphocytes, hence, modifying the pattern of later antibody and cell-mediated immune responses.

The ability of antigen fragments to interact with specific B lymphocytes is related to the retention of determinants that can bind surface immunoglobulin receptors. That retention probably varies widely for different antigens exposed to the same conditions of digestion. Fragments that possess two or more intact determinants can cross-link or "bridge" receptors on individual B cells, a critical event in the activation and clonal proliferation that underlie B-lymphocyte priming (52). Fragments that retain a single determinant may have opposing effects: one is to "blockade" B-lymphocyte receptors by interfering with cross-linking by molecules that are more intact. Antigen fragments can also bind to endogenous plasma proteins after absorption (53); this might create "hybrid" molecules that could cross-link B-cell receptors if more than one fragment were present on the self-protein. Fragments that lack conformational determinants from the native molecules would be unable to interact with specific B lymphocytes, but could retain short, primary sequence epitopes that permit uptake by antigen-presenting cells, and recognition by specific T lymphocytes (51). If absorbed in small amounts, such fragments are capable of specific T-cell priming, but larger quantities may be responsible for depressing helper T-cell responsiveness (49), leading to tolerance.

Additional study will be valuable in defining the components of luminal digestion and properties of the mucosal barrier, that jointly determine the stimulus characteristics of antigens and fragments that are taken up via the gut in infants and adults. Responses to these materials will, in turn, depend on the degree of maturation in lymphoid and accessory cells, and their pattern of distribution in gastrointestinal and other tissues.

V. ROLE OF HUMAN COLOSTRUM IN CLOSURE

As stated earlier, newborns lack many specific and nonspecific intestinal features that are necessary to protect them adequately from the extrauterine environment. Fortunately, "nature" has provided an excellent substitute to protect the vulnerable neonate passively during this critical period. This substitute, human milk, contains many factors that can compensate for processes lacking in the infant and, at the same time, stimulate the maturation of the gut toward independent function.

It is increasingly apparent that human milk contains not only important nutrients and protective factors for the newborn but also factors that can facilitate intestinal maturation. Heird and Hansen (54) have reported that the ingestion of colostrum can facilitate the maturation of mucosal epithelial cells, enhance absorption of digested foods, and perhaps accelerate the development of an intact mucosal barrier. They have also shown that brush-border enzymes (lactase, sucrase, alkaline phosphatase) are enhanced after the ingestion of colostrum (54). Udall et al. (55) have actually demonstrated a decrease in antigen penetration in newborns after colostrum feeding. These investigations have suggested that milk may contain a "mucosal growth factor" which facilitates the early maturation of the gut (closure).

In addition to actively accelerating closure in the newborn, human colostrum/milk provides a passive protection of the gut surface while it is maturing. Specific secretory IgA antibodies exist in milk and these exclude bacteria and luminal antigens. Also present, are additional protective factors that contribute to the protection of the newborn. However, a more prolonged discussion of this topic is beyond the scope of this chapter.

VI. CLINICAL CONDITIONS POSSIBLY ASSOCIATED WITH IMMATURE MUCOSAL BARRIER

Clinical conditions known to be associated with pathologic uptake of antigens are shown in Table 3. The pathophysiologic mechanism(s) of representative conditions discussed in this section will illustrate the association between antigen transport and clinical disease. A comprehensive review of all clinical conditions is beyond the scope of this paper (18).

Table 3 Clinical Conditions Possibly Associated with Immature Mucosal Barrier

---

Newborn and early childhood (immediate clinical response)
   Necrotizing enterocolitis
   Gastrointestinal allergy
   Sudden infant death syndrome
   Dermatitis
   Toxigenic diarrhea
   Malabsorption
Later childhood and adulthood (delayed clinical response)
   Inflammatory bowel disease
   Chronic active hepatitis
   Nephritis
   Autoimmune (immune complex-mediated diseases)

As a result of the pathologic transport of antigens across the small intestine, ingested antigens may traverse the mucosal barrier and predispose to allergic and toxic reactions leading to a number of gastrointestinal diseases. The gastrointestinal diseases possibly associated with antigen absorption are gastrointestinal allergy (56), inflammatory bowel disease (57), celiac disease (58), toxigenic diarrhea (59), chronic hepatitis (60), necrotizing enterocolitis, and autoimmune disease (60). Because the evidence cited to support the hypothesis that intestinal permeability to antigens is involved in the pathogenesis of human disease is largely indirect, one should realize that these comments are somewhat speculative and still remain to be proved by more direct evidence. For purposes of this report, only gastrointestinal allergy will be discussed in detail as a prototype condition.

VII. GASTROINTESTINAL ALLERGY

Probably the most striking association between antigen handling and clinical disease is shown with gastrointestinal allergy. Several clinical symptoms of such allergy have been described and these appear to relate specifically to the ingestion of specific foods (particularly cow's milk). These conditions may be localized to the gastrointestinal tract and present with diarrhea, gastrointestinal bleeding, or protein-losing enteropathy, or they may be represented by systemic manifestations of allergy ranging in severity from exanthema to anaphylaxis. The clinical expression of allergy may relate: (a) to the transport of antigens into the lamina propria alone (local allergic reactions), or (b) into both the lamina propria and the systemic circulation (systemic allergic response). Factors that determine the nature of the allergic response are not entirely understood, but they undoubtedly are related to the degree of sensitivity of the allergic patient and/ or the concentration of allergen ingested. Although the mechanism(s) of gastrointestinal allergy is at present obscure, it would appear that the intestinal transport of allergens is a necessary initial step in the process. In fact, it has been suggested that during the neonatal period when increased antigen permeability exists, susceptible infants may become sensitized to specific ingested protein. With re-exposure at a time when much less macromolecular absorption is occurring, minute quantities of allergen may be absorbed and result in allergic symptoms. These symptoms can then be propagated by further uptake of allergens across a disrupted mucosal surface. In recent experimental studies from this laboratory (61), we reported that intestinal anaphylaxis can lead to increased uptake of nonspecific intestinal allergens, which in turn can evoke an IgG-mediated reaction leading to further propagation of disease. This secondary process occurring with classic IgE-mediated disease may be important in converting a self-limited process into a chronic disease state.

VIII. SUMMARY AND CONCLUSIONS

An important adaptation of the gastrointestinal tract to the extrauterine environment is its development of a mucosal barrier against the penetration of proteins and protein fragments. To combat the potential danger of invasion across the mucosal barrier, the infant must develop within the lumen and on the luminal mucosal surface an elaborate system of defense mechanisms that act to control and maintain the epithelium as an impermeable barrier to the uptake of macromolecular antigens. These defenses include a unique local immunologic system adapted to function in the complicated milieu of the intestine as well as other nonimmunologic processes such as a gastric barrier, intestinal surface secretions, peristaltic movement, etc., all of which help to provide maximum protection for the intestinal surface.

Unfortunately, during the immediate postpartum period, especially for premature and "small-for-date" infants, this elaborate local defense system is incompletely developed. As a result of the delay in the maturation of the mucosal barrier, newborn infants are particularly vulnerable to pathologic penetration by harmful intraluminal substances. The consequences of altered defense are susceptibility to infection and the potential for hypersensitivity reactions and the formation of immune complexes. With these reactions comes the potential for developing life-threatening diseases such as necrotizing enterocolitis, sepsis, and hepatitis. Fortunately, nature has provided a means for passively protecting the "vulnerable" newborn against the dangers of a deficient intestinal defense system: human milk. It is now increasingly apparent that human milk contains not only antibodies and viable leukocytes, but many other substances that can interfere with bacterial colonization and prevent antigen penetration.

REFERENCES

1. Walker, W. A. Gastrointestinal host defense: Importance of gut closure in control of macromolecular transport. *Ciba Found. Symp.* 70, 201-219, 1956.
2. Walker, W. A. Antigen absorption from the small intestine and gastrointestinal disease. *Pediatr. Clin. North Am.* 22, 731-746, 1975.
3. Udall, J. N., and Walker, W. A. The physiologic and pathologic basis for the transport of macromolecules across the intestinal tract. *J. Pediatr. Gastroenterol. Clin. Nutri.* 1, 295-301, 1982.
4. Miller, H. R. P., and Nawa, Y. Immune regulation of intestinal goblet cell differentiation. Specific induction of non-specific protection against helminths? *Nouv. Rev. Fr. Hematol.* 21, 31-45, 1979.
5. Boedeker, E. C. Enterocyte adherence of *Escherichia coli*: Its relation to diarrheal disease. *Gastroenterology* 83, 489-492, 1982.
6. Jones, G. W., and Freter, R. Adhesive properties of *Vibrio cholerae*: Nature of the interaction with isolated rabbit brush border membranes and human erythrocytes. *Infect. Immun.* 14, 240-245, 1976.
7. Forstner, G., Sturgess, J. M., and Forstner, J. Malfunction of intestinal mucus and mucus production. *Adv. Exp. Med. Biol.* 89, 349-358, 1976.
8. Quaroni, A., Kirsch, K., Herscovics, A., and Isselbacher, K. J. Surface-membrane biogenesis in rat intestinal epithelial cells at different stages of maturation. *Biochem. J.* 192, 133-144, 1980.
9. Raul, F., Simon, P., Kedinger, M., and Haffen, K. Intestinal enzymes activities in isolated villus and crypt cells during postnatal development of the rat. *Cell Tiss. Res.* 176, 167-178, 1977.
10. Deboth, N. J., Van Der Kamp, A. W., and Van Dongen, J. M. The influence of changing crypt cell kinetics on functional differentiation in the small intestine of the rat. Nucleotide and protein synthesis. *Differentiation* 4, 175-182, 1975.
11. Lojda, A. Cytochemistry of enterocytes and of other cells in mucosal membrane of the small intestine. In: *Biomembranes* Vol. 4A: *Intestinal Absorption,* Smyth, D. H. (ed.). Plenum Press, London, pp. 43-122, 1974.
12. Etzler, M. E., and Branstrator, M. L. Cell surface components of intestinal epithelial cells and their relationship to cellular differentiation. In: *Development of Mammalian Absorptive Processes.* Excerpta Medica, Amsterdam (Ciba Found Symp. 70), pp. 51-68, 1979.
13. Toofantan, F., Kidder, D. E., and Hill, F. W. The postnatal development of intestinal disaccharidases in the calf. *Res. Vet. Sci.* 16, 382-392, 1975.
14. Bresson, J. L., Pang, K. Y., and Walker, W. A. Microvillus membrane differentiation: Quantitative difference in cholera toxin binding to the intestinal surface of newborn and adult rabbits. *Pediatr. Res.* 18, 984-987, 1984.
15. Stern, M. S., Pang, K. Y., and Walker, W. A. Food proteins and gut mucosal barrier. II. Differential interaction of cow's milk proteins with the mucous coat and the surface membrane of adult and immature rat jejunum. *Pediatr. Res.* 18, 1252-1257, 1984.

16. Tomasi, T. B., Lawson, I. M. Challacombe, S., and McNabb, P. Mucosal immunity: The origin and migration pattern of cells in the secretory system. *J. Allergy Clin. Immunol.* 65, 12–19, 1980.

17. Marsh, M. N. The small intestine: Mechanisms of local immunity and gluten sensitivity. *Clin. Sci.* 61, 497–503, 1981.

18. Walker, W. A. Intestinal transport of macromolecules. In: *Physiology of the Gastrointestinal Tract,* Johnson, L. R., Christensen, J., Grossman, M. I., Jacobson, E. D., and Schultz, S. G. (eds.). Raven Press, New York, pp. 1271–1289. 1981.

19. Allansmith, M. McClellan, B. H. Butterworth, M., and Maloney, J. R. The development of immunoglobulin levels in man. *J. Pediatr.* 72, 276–290, 1968.

20. Selner, J. C., Merrill, D. A., and Claman, H. N. Salivary immunoglobulin and albumin: Development during the newborn period. *J. Pediatr.* 72, 685–689, 1968.

21. Haneberg, B., and Aarskog, D. Human fecal immunoglobulins in healthy infants and children and in some with diseases affecting the intestinal tract or the immune system. *Clin. Exp. Immunol.* 22, 210–222, 1975.

22. Burgio, G. R., Lanzavecchia, A., Plebani, A., Jayakar, S., and Ugazio, A. G. Ontogeny of secretory immunity: Levels of secretory IgA and natural antibodies in saliva. *Pediatr. Res.* 14, 1111–1114, 1980.

23. Cunningham-Rundles, C., Brandeis, W. E., Good, R. A., and Day, N. K. Milk precipitins, circulating immune complexes and IgA deficiency. *Proc. Natl. Acad. Sci. USA* 75, 2287–3389, 1978.

24. Cunningham-Rundles, C., Brandeis, W. E., Good, R. A., and Day, N. K. Bovine antigens and the formation of circulating immune complexes in selective immunoglobulin A deficiency. *J. Clin. Invest.* 64, 272–279, 1979.

25. Owen, R. L., and Jones, A. L. Epithelial cell specialization within human Peyer's patches: An ultrastructural study of intestinal lymphoid follicles. *Gastroenterology* 66, 189–203, 1974.

26. Owen, R. L. Sequential uptake of horseradish peroxidase by lymphoid follicle epithelium of Peyer's patches in the normal unobstructed mouse intestine: An ultrastructural study. *Gastroenterology* 72, 440–451, 1977.

27. Wolf, J. L., Rubin, D. H., Finberg, R., Kauffman, R. S. Sharpe, A. H., Trier, J. S., and Field, B. N. Intestinal M. cells: A pathway for entry of reovirus into the host. *Science* (Wash., D.C.) 212, 471–472, 1981.

28. Walker, W. A., and Isselbacher, K. J. Intestinal antibodies. *N. Engl. J. Med.* 297, 767–773, 1977.

29. Vaz, N. M., Maia, L. C., Hanson, D. G., and Lynch, J. Inhibition of homocytotropic antibody responses in adult inbred mice by previous feeding of the specific antigen. *J. Allergy Clin. Immunol.* 60, 110–115, 1977.

30. Walker, W. A., Wu, M., Isselbacher, K. J., and Bloch, K. J. Intestinal uptake of macromolecules. IV. The effect of pancreatic duct ligation on the breakdown of antigen and antigen-antibody complexes on the intestinal surface. *Gastroenterology* 69, 1223–1229, 1975.

31. Lake, A. M., Bloch, K. J., Sinclair, K. J., and Walker, W. A. Anaphylactic release of intestinal goblet cell mucus. *Immunology* 39, 173–178, 1979.

32. Walker, W. A. Role of the mucosal barrier in toxin/microbial attachment to the gastrointestinal tract. *Ciba Symp.* 112, 34–47, 1985.
33. Virnig, N. L., and Reynolds, J. W. Epidemiological aspects of neonatal necrotizing enterocolitis. *Am. J. Dis. Child.* 128, 186–190, 1974.
34. Lake, A. M., and Walker, W. A. Neonatal necrotizing enterocolitis: A disease of altered host defense. *Clin. Gastroenterol.* 6, 463–480, 1977.
35. Udall, J. N., Pang, K., Fritze, L., Kleinman, R., Trier, J. S., and Walker, W. A. Development of gastrointestinal mucosal barrier. I. The effect of age on intestinal permeability to macromolecules. *Pediatr. Res.* 15, 241–244, 1981.
36. Pang, K. Y., Bresson, J. L., and Walker, W. A. Development of the gastrointestinal mucosal barrier. III. Evidence for structural differences in microvillus membranes from newborn and adult rabbits. *Biochem. Biophys. Acta* 727, 201–208, 1983.
37. Pang, K. Y., Bresson, J. L., and Walker, W. A. Development of the gastrointestinal mucosal barrier. V. Comparative effect of calcium binding on microvillus structure in newborn and adult rats. *Pediatr. Res.* 17, 856–861, 1983.
38. Shub, M. D., Pang, K. Y., Swann, D. A., and Walker, W. A. Age-related changes in chemical composition and physical properties of mucus glycoproteins from rat small intestine. *Biochem. J.* 215, 405–411, 1983.
39. Walker, W. A. Absorption of protein and protein fragments in the developing intestine: Role of immunologic/allergic reactions. *Pediatrics,* 75(suppl), 167–171, 1985.
40. Udall, J. N., and Walker, W. A. Immunologic function of the developing gut. In: *Selected Topics in Developmental Medicine.* Warshaw, J. (ed.). Elsevier Science Publishing Co., New York, pp. 221–238, 1983.
41. Hanson, D. G., Ontogeny of orally induced tolerance to soluble proteins in mice. I. Priming and tolerance in newborns. *J. Immunol.* 127, 1518–1524, 1981.
42. Strobel, S., and Ferguson, A. Immune responses to fed protein antigens in mice. 3. Systemic tolerance or priming is related to age at which antigen is first encountered. *Pediatr. Res.* 18, 588–594, 1984.
43. Hanson, D. G., Vaz, N. M. Rawlings, L., and Lynch, J. M. Inhibition of specific immune responses by feeding protein antigens. II. Effects of prior passive and active immunization. *J. Immunol.* 122, 2261–2266, 1979.
44. Takatsu, K., and Ishizaka, K. Reaginic antibody formation in the mouse. VII. Induction of suppressor T cells for IgE and IgG antibody responses. *J. Immunol.* 116, 1257–1264, 1976.
45. Muckerheide, A., Pesce, A., and Michael, J. G. Immunosuppressive properties of a peptic fragment of BSA. *J. Immunol.* 119, 1340–1345, 1977.
46. Richman, L. K., Chiller, J. M., Brown, W. R. Hanson, D. G., and Vaz, N. M. Enterically induced immunologic tolerance. I. Induction of suppressor T lymphocytes by intragastric administration of soluble proteins. *J. Immunol.* 121, 2429–2434, 1978.

47. Miller, S. D., and Hanson, D. G. Inhibition of specific immune responses by feeding protein antigens. IV. Evidence for tolerance and specific active suppression of cell-mediated immune responses to ovalbumin. *J. Immunol.* 123, 2344–2350, 1979.

48. Silverman, G. A., Peri, B. A., Fitch, F. W., and Rothberg, R. M. Enterically induced regulation of systemic immune responses. II. Suppression of proliferating T cells by an Lyt-1[+], 2[-] T effector cell. *J. Immunol.* 131, 2656–2661, 1983.

49. Lamb, J. R., Skidmore, B. J., Green, N., Chiller, J. M., and Feldmann, M. Induction of tolerance in influenza virus-immune T lymphocyte clones with synthetic peptides of influenza hemagglutinin. *J. Exp. Med.* 157, 1434–1447, 1983.

50. Hanson, D. G., and Miller, S. D. Inhibition of specific immune responses by feeding protein antigens. V. Induction of the tolerant state in the absence of specific suppressor T cells. *J. Immunol.* 128, 2378–2381, 1982.

51. Shimonkevitz, R., Colon, S., Kappler, J. W., Marrack, P., and Grey, H. M. Antigen recognition by H-2-restricted T cells. II. A tryptic ovalbumin peptide that substitutes for processed antigen. *J. Immunol.* 133, 2067–2074, 1984.

52. Pure, E., Isakson, P., Kappler, J., Marrack, P., Krammer, P., and Vitetta, E. S. T cell-derived B cell growth and differentiation factors: Dichotomy between the responsiveness of B cells from adult and neonatal mice. *J. Exp. Med.* 157, 600–612, 1983.

53. Udall, J. N., Pang, K. Y., Scrimshaw, N. S., and Walker, W. A. The effect ous peptide fragments to native proteins: Possible explanation for the overestimation of uptake of intact proteins from the gut. *Immunology* 42, 251–257, 1981.

54. Heird, W. C., and Hansen, I. H. Effect of colostrum on growth of intestinal mucosa. *Pediatr. Res.* 11, 406, 1977.

55. Udall, J. N., Pang, K. Y., Scrimshaw, N. S. and Walker, W. A. The effect of early nutrition on intestinal maturation. *Pediatr. Res.* 13, 409, 1979.

56. Taylor, B., Normal, A. P., and Orgel, H. A. Transient IgA deficiency and pathogenesis of infantile atopy. *Lancet* 2, 111–113, 1973.

57. Ferguson, A. Intraepithelial lymphocytes of the small intestine. *Gut* 18, 921–937, 1977.

58. Shiner, M., and Ballard, J. Antigen-antibody reactions in jejunal mucosa in childhood coeliac disease after gluten challenge. *Lancet* 1, 1202–1205, 1972.

59. Ogra, P. L., and Karzon, D. T. The role of immunoglobulins in the mechanisms of mucosal immunity to viral infection. *Pediatr. Clin. North Am.* 17, 385–389, 1970.

60. Walker, W. A. Antigen absorption from the small intestine and gastrointestinal disease. *Pediatr. Clin. North Am.* 22, 731–746, 1975.

61. Kleinman, R. E., Bloch, K. J., and Walker, W. A. Gut induced anaphylaxis and uptake of a bystander protein: An amplification of anaphylactic sensitivity. *Ped. Res.* 15, 598, 1981.

7

The Regulation of Immunoglobulin Delivery into the Gut

Serem Freier
Shaare Zedek Hospital, Jerusalem, Israel, and International Institute for Infant Nutrition and Gastrointestinal Disease, Children's Hospital of Buffalo, Buffalo, New York

Emanuel Lebanthal
State University of New York at Buffalo and International Institute for Infant Nutrition and Gastrointestinal Disease, Children's Hospital of Buffalo, Buffalo, New York

I. INTRODUCTION

The human gut is in constant contact with bacterial and viral antigens. In addition, it is exposed to a considerable antigenic load of food protein at meal times. In order to deal with these antigens, the body possesses a highly complex apparatus the mechanics of which are only beginning to be unravelled. It is suggested that this process begins with antigen recognition at the special sampling site in the Peyer's patches. Thereafter, a process of maturation and proliferation of plasma cell precursors occurs followed by their entering the effector organ, mainly, the lamina propria of the intestine. It is possible that this homing process is influenced by hormone-induced lymphocyte-binding sites for vascular endothelium. The mature IgA-producing plasma cell in the lamina propria releases this immunoglobulin in its dimeric form joined by the "J" chain. It is believed that this dimer is taken up by the enterocytes by receptor-mediated endocytosis, transported intracellularly, and finally released into the lumen of the intestine. The rate of delivery of IgA, particularly its synchronization with the process of digestion might involve neural as well as hormonal stimuli. It is the purpose of this article to review briefly the known neuro/endocrine–immune interactions regulating the delivery of immunoglobulins to the gut.

II. IMMUNE RECOGNITION

In order to deal with foreign antigens, the body has to recognize them as such and then develop the protection against them. This process begins at the "M" cells overlying the lymphoid tissue of Peyer's patches (1–3). These cells, which possess neither lysosomes nor microvilli, allow antigen to pass undigested to the subjacent lymphoid tissue. Subsequently, the process leading to specific antibody production is initiated. This process is unique for mucosal tissues insofar as the antibody produced belongs predominantly to immunoglobulin class A. As the initial plasma cell precursor in Peyer's patches is an IgM-bearing cell, a number of regulatory mechanisms must come into play in order to bring about the maturation and proliferation of cells producing IgA (4–7). It has been suggested that a specialized T cell switches IgM-bearing cells to cells bearing IgA (6). Such switch T cells appear to be the main factor bringing about the predominance of IgA-bearing cells in Peyer's patches. It is believed that the switch cells are not helper cells but rather cells capable of causing a series of deletions and/or rearrangements of genetic material in order to produce terminal differentiation to IgA-bearing cells (8,9). Some IgA-bearing cells also bear IgE (5). It is believed that the local T-helper and suppressor populations determine which of these immunoglobulins will ultimately be produced (4). As a rule, it is assumed that IgE and IgG production are suppressed in the intestine, while IgA production is encouraged. The concept, therefore, emerges of a number of regulatory cells which at the level of Peyer's patches direct the isotype (immunoglobulin) and idiotype (antibody) specificity of immunoglobulin production.

III. THE IMPORTANCE OF VASOACTIVE INTESTINAL PEPTIDE IN THE "HOMING" OF LYMPHOCYTES

Following the above regulatory mechanism, plasma cell precursors and other lymphocytes leave Peyer's patches and undergo further maturation and proliferation at the level of the mesenteric lymph nodes. Thereafter, B cells "home" preferentially to the intestinal mucosa, while T cells may recirculate to Peyer's patches and mesenteric lymph nodes (10–17). This capacity of lymphocytes and precursor plasma cells to show a predilection for certain tissues is suggested to be conditioned by vasoactive intestinal peptide (VIP). It has been known for some time that the specialized high endothelium of the postcapillary venules of lymph nodes and Peyer's patches is recognized as the site through which lymphocytes leave the blood to enter these tissues (12,17). It is likely, therefore, that some interaction between lymphoid cells and this endothelium has to take place. Ottaway (18) has recently demonstrated that VIP is required. He postulated that the interaction of VIP with receptors on lymphocytic cells alters their surface components in such a manner as to facilitate their interaction with the endothelium of the postcapillary venule. In this context, therefore, the observation that nerves containing VIP have been found in close proximity to small bowel vessels in the gut may be of significance (19). It is possible that the local release of VIP from nerve endings may occur near the postcapillary venules or within other elements of the microvasculature of mesenteric nodes and Peyer's patches encourages the local migration of lymphocytes through the endothelium. Although the above studies were performed in animals, the fact that human T cells possess receptors for VIP (20) suggests that a similar affinity of lymphoid cells for postcapillary venules may be brought about by vasoactive intestinal peptide in humans.

IV. THE ORIGIN OF INTESTINAL ANTIBODIES

While antibodies are produced along the length of the gastrointestinal mucosa they are also found in biliary and pancreatic secretions.

The gastric mucosa has a large population of immunoglobulin-containing cells, and gastric juice in humans contains IgA, IgG, and IgM with IgA predominating at a concentration ranging from 20-500 mg/dl (21). These measurements, however, include salivary secretions. In an acid environment, all immunoglobulins except secretory IgA (s/IgA) are rapidly destroyed. Secretory IgA, however, appears to be acid resistant and may, therefore, participate in the anti-infective mechanisms of the stomach. The transport of polymeric IgA and IgM joined by secretory component (SC) appears to proceed by a mechanism similar or identical to the one which we shall describe when discussing the intestine. Immunoglobulin G is abundant in the gastric mucosa but does not appear to penetrate or traverse the epithelial cells (22). Immunoglobulins E and D have so far not been sought for in gastric juice.

Immunoglobulins G,A,M,E, and D have been found in pancreatic secretions (23-25). It is worthy of note that the IgA in this fluid is of the monomeric 7S type and it is unlikely, therefore, that it plays a part in protecting anything but the pancreas itself (23).

The liver is an important organ for IgA secretion into the gastrointestinal tract. This phenomenon was originally described in rats (26), but has subsequently been found to occur in humans (27). Polymeric IgA in rat serum is bound by hepatocytes. It is suggested that SC is the receptor mediating this uptake by hepatocytes. Secretory IgA is then discharged by the bile ducts into the upper gastrointestinal tract. Its relative importance can be assumed from the observation that the diversion of the bile ducts in rats reduces the IgA content of the upper intestine to one tenth of its normal value (26). In the human, polymeric IgA is also taken up by hepatocytes (28), though the main transport route of IgA in the human appears to be across the epithelium of bile ductules. Here, too, SC appears to be the receptor responsible for the endocytosis of IgA. The human gallbladder is believed to secrete about 400 mg of IgA daily into the upper intestine (27). The greater part of the polymeric IgA taken up by the liver is derived from intestinal lymphoid tissues (29). A small fraction of the sIgA as well as the IgG and IgM found in the bile are believed to be produced within the liver or within the biliary mucosa (29). The sIgA in bile supplies the intestine with specific antibodies. In addition, the liver also clears IgA-antigen complexes from the bloodstream, thus performing an important excretory function (30).

V. RECEPTOR-MEDIATED ENDOCYTOSIS OF IMMUNOGLOBULINS A AND M ACROSS ENTEROCYTES

In the lamina propria, dimeric IgA and pentameric IgM are produced in the plasma cells. J chains are incorporated into these two immunoglobulins within the cells producing them. The addition of J chains to the immunoglobulins endows them with a new configuration allowing them to combine with SC (31). Here, presumably, lies the key to the transport of IgA and IgM. Secretory component itself is produced in enterocytes as shown by its localization in the endoplasmic reticulum. It can, however, also be found in the basolateral membrane of enterocytes (32,33). In this location, SC acts as a receptor for dimeric IgA and pentameric IgM. Subsequently, the sIgA and sIgM are internalized by endocytosis. It is suggested that the endocytic vesicles are transported through the cytoplasm of the enterocytes and discharged at their apical surface (34). Secretory component is present primarily in the columnar cells of the crypts of Lieberkuhn and decreases in concentration in the villous cells (35). This finding might mean that the secretion of immunoglobulins occurs primarily in the crypts. It is in this region too that the main secretion of water and electrolytes takes place. Alternatively, it is possible that the binding of SC to immunoglobulins occurs in the crypt but the secretion is in the level of the villus. Extracellular staining of IgG is usually much more marked than that of IgA. As IgG does not appear to be transported by epithelial cells, it presumably accumulates in the lamina propria and exerts its protective function at that site. On the other hand, IgA and IgM exert their function within the lumen of the gastrointestinal tract. Immunoglobulin E is also found in duodenal fluid (36), but the mechanism of its transport is unknown.

VI. NERVOUS REGULATION OF IMMUNO-GLOBULIN DELIVERY TO THE GUT

It was shown that the injection of pilocarpine, a cholinergic agent, resulted in the release of IgA into the intestine (37). A similar effect was achieved by injecting muscarine and bethanechol. The increase in intestinal IgA secretion induced by pilocarpine was blocked by atropine, suggesting that the effect of pilocarpine is mediated through muscarinic receptors. The same authors (37) found that the basal secretion of IgA in the rat intestine could be reduced by atropine. This might mean that intestinal IgA secretion is subject to permanent nervous stimuli. The mechanism of action of these cholinergic fibers remains to be elucidated. Do they act on IgA release from plasma cells or do they step up the transport of sIgA through the enterocytes? Or is the action merely mechanical, either due to flushing of the crypts by the increased water and electrolyte secretions, or by increased motility, or both?

VII. ENDOCRINE AND PARACRINE EFFECTS ON IMMUNOGLOBULIN SECRETION

It is likely that some endocrine and paracrine neuromodulators of the intestine may produce results similar to cholinergic drugs. So far, only cholecystokinin (CCK) and secretin have been studies in this respect. While analyzing intestinal juice of sick children and healthy adults following intravenous stimulation by CCK, we found a rise in antibodies of the immunoglobulin classes G, A, M, E, and D (38-41). Secretion also enhanced release of IgA and IgM antibodies, but not IgG, IgE, and IgD. From these observations, it could not be determined if all these antibodies arose from the liver, gallbladder, or pancreas, or if there was increased direct translocation of immunoglobulins through the intestinal epithelium. In vivo studies utilizing isolated perfused segment of rat intestine demonstrated that intravenous injection of CCK resulted in the increased release of antibodies of the IgA class from the intestinal epithelium (Freier et al., to be published). This effect began within 2-5 minutes of injecting CCK and persisted for at least 10 minutes. Possible mechanisms include (a) CCK acting as a neuromodulator for greater release of acetylcholine (42) and, this in turn, releasing the immunoglobulin, or (b) CCK acting in a fashion analagous to acetylcholine but using a different receptor. The chemically related peptide gastrin may well have a similar effect. Other neuromodulators with secretory effects will have to be studied for their potential in enhancing IgA release.

VIII. CONCLUSION

The purpose of this chapter was to describe the remarkable integration of the endocrine, neural, and immune systems in the response of the body to foreign antigens in the gastrointestinal tract. In this context, the gastrointestinal tract is no exception; for it is becoming obvious that immune processes elsewhere in the body are clearly influenced by hormones and neuropeptides. Some hormones act as modulators of lymphocyte proliferation (43) and immunoglobulin synthesis (44). On the other hand, lymphokines have been shown to have effects not dissimilar to some hormones (45). It is only by adopting a comprehensive concept of all factors concerned that the synthesis, production, delivery, and synchronization of the availability of the immunoglobulins in the gut can be understood.

REFERENCES

1. Bockman, D. E., and Cooper, M. D. Pinocytosis by epithelium associated with lymphoid follicles in the bursa of Fabricius, appendix, and Peyer's patches: An electron microscopic study. *Am. J. Anat.* 136, 455-478, 1973.

2. Owen, R. L., and Nemanic, P. Antigen processing structures of the mammalian intestinal tract: An SEM study of lymphoepithelial organs. *Scan. Electron. Microsc.* 2, 367-378, 1978.

3. Waksman, B. H., and Ozer, H. Specialized amplification elements in the immune system: The role of nodular lymphoid organs in mucous membranes. *Progr. Allergy* 21, 1-113, 1976.

4. Ngan, J., and Kind, L. S. Suppressor T-cells for IgE and IgG in Peyer's patches of mice made tolerant by the oral administration of oralbumin. *J. Immunol.* 120, 861-867, 1978.

5. Durkin, H. G., Bazin, H., and Waksman, B. H. Origin and fate of IgE-bearing lymphocytes: Peyer's patches as differentiation site of cells simultaneously bearing IgA and IgE. *J. Exp. Med.* 154, 640-645, 1981.

6. Kawaniski, H., Saltzman, L. E., and Strober, W. Mechanisms regulating IgA class specific immunoglobulin production in murine gut associated lymphoid tissues. I. T-cells derived from Peyer's patches that switch sIgM B cells to sIgA B cells in vitro. *J. Exp. Med.* 157, 433-436, 1983.

7. Kawaniski, H., Saltzman, L., and Strober, W. Mechanisms regulating IgA class specific immunoglobulin production in murine gut associated lymphoid tissue. *J. Exp. Med.* 158, 649-656, 1983.

8. Horgo, T., and Lalaoka, T. Organization of immunoglobulin heavy chain genes and allelic deletion mode. *Proc. Natl. Acad. Sci. U SA* 75, 2140-2144, 1978.

9. Hurwitz, T. C., Coleclough, C., and Cebra, J. J. C_H gene rearrangements in IgM-bearing B cells and in the normal splenic DNA component of hybridomas making different isotypes of antibody. *Cell* 22, 349-359, 1980.

10. Guy-Grand, D., Griscelli, C., and Vassali, P. The gut-associated lymphoid system: Nature and properties of the large dividing cells. *Eur. J. Immunol.* 4, 435-443, 1978.

11. Guy-Grand, D., Griscelli, C., and Vassali, P. The mouse gut T-lymphocyte, a novel type of T-cell: Nature, origin, and haffic in mice in normal and graft-versus-host conditions. *J. Exp. Med.* 148, 1661-1667, 1978.

12. Gowans, J. L., and Knight, G. The route of re-circulation of lymphocytes in the rat. *Proc. R. Soc. Ser. B.* 159, 257-282, 1964.

13. Griscelli, C., Vassali, P., and McCluskey, R. T. The distribution of large dividing lymph node cells in synergic recipient rats after intravenous injection. *J. Exp. Med.* 130, 1427-1451, 1969.

14. Guy-Grand, D., Griscelli, C., and Vassali, P. The gut associated lymphoid system: Nature and properties of the large dividing cells. *Eur. J. Immunol.* 4, 435-443, 1974.

15. McWilliams, M., Phillips-Quagliata, J. M., and Lamm, M. E. Characteristics of mesenteric lymph node cells homing to gut-associated lymphoid tissue in synergic mice. *J. Immunol.* 115, 54-58, 1975.

16. Smith, M. E., Martin, A. F., and Ford, W. L. Migration of lymphoblasts in the rat. *Monogr. Allergy* 16, 203-232, 1979.
17. Marchesi, V. T., and Gowens, J. L. The migration of lymphocytes through the endothelium of venules in lymph nodes: An electron microscopic study. *Proc. R. Soc. Lond.* 159, 283-284, 1964.
18. Ottaway, C. A. In vitro alteration of receptors for vasoactive intestinal peptide changes in the in vivo localization of mouse T-cells. *J. Exp. Med.* 160, 1054-1069, 1984.
19. Jessen, K. R., Saffrey, M. J., Noorden, S., Bloom, S. R., Polak, J. M., and Burnstock, G. Immunohistochemical studies of the enteric nervous system in tissue culture and in situ. Localization of vasoactive intestinal peptide, substance P and enkephalin immunoreactive nerves in the guinea pig. *Neurosciences* 5, 1717-1720, 1980.
20. Danek, A., O'Darisio, M. S., O'Donisio, T. M., and George, J. M. Specific binding sites for vasoactive intestinal polypeptide on nonadherent peripheral blood lymphocytes. *J. Immunol.* 131, 1173-1175, 1983.
21. McClelland, D. B. L., Finlayson, N. D. C., Samson, R. R., Nairn, M., and Shearman, D. J. C. Quantitation of immunoglobulins in gastric juice by electroimmunodiffusion. *Gastroenterology* 60, 509-514, 1971.
22. Volnoes, K., Brandtzaeg, P., Elgo, K., Stove, R. Specific and non-specific humoral defense factors in the epithelium of normal and inflamed gastric mucosa. *Gastroenterology* 86, 402-412, 1984.
23. Brosher, G. W., Dyck, W. P., Hall, F. F., and Spiekerman, A. M. Immunoglobulin characterization of human pancreatic fluid. *Am. J. Dig. Dis.* 20, 454-459, 1975.
24. Bramis, J. P., Messes, J., Nachiero, M., and Dreiling, D. A. The diagnostic significance of immunoglobulin A and M ratios in the pancreatic and duodenal fluid of patients with benign and malignant pancreatic diseases. *Am. J. Gastroenterol.* 69, 565-571, 1978.
25. Goodale, R. L., Condie, R. M., Dressel, T. K., Taylor, T. N., and Gajl-Peczalska, K. A study of secretory proteins, cytology, and tumor site in pancreatic cancer. *Ann. Surg.* 184, 340-344, 1979.
26. Lemaitre-Coehlo, I., Jackson, G. D. F., and Vaerman, J. P. Relevance of biliary IgA antibodies in rat intestinal immunity. *Scand. J. Immunol.* 8, 459-464, 1978.
27. Nagura, H., Smith, P. D., Nakane, P. D., and Brown, W. R. IgA in human bile and liver. *J. Immunol.* 126, 587-595, 1981.
28. Hopf, V., Brantzaeg, P., Hutteroth, T. H., and Meyer-zum-Buscheufelde, K. H. In vivo and in vitro binding of IgA to the plasma membrane of hepatocytes. *Scand. J. Immunol.* 8, 453-459, 1978.
29. Moaning, R. J., Walker, P. G., Carter, L., Barrington, P. J., and Jackson, G. D. F. Studies on the origin of biliary immunoglobulins in rats. *Gastroenterology* 87, 173-179, 1984.
30. Peppard, J. V., Orlans, E., Andrew, A., and Payne, W. R. Elimination into bile of circulating antigen by endogenous IgA antibody in rats. *Immunology* 45, 467-472, 1982.

31. Brantzaeg, P. Transport models for secretory IgA and secretory IgM. *Clin. Exp. Immunol.* 44, 221-232, 1981.

32. Brown, W. R., Isobe, Y., and Nakane, P. K. Studies on the translocation of immunoglobulins across intestinal epithelium. Immunoelectronmicroscopic localization of immunoglobulins and secretory component in human intestinal mucosa. *Gastroenterology* 71, 985-995, 1976.

33. Bos, J., Lobbe, F., Gerry, B., and Griscelli, C. Immunoelectron microscopic localization of immunoglobulin A and secretory component in jejunal mucosa from children with celiac disease. *Scand. J. Immunol.* 9, 44d, 1979.

34. Nagura, H., Nakane, P. K., and Brown, W. R. Translocation of dimeric IgA through neoplastic colon cells in vitro. *J. Immunol.* 123, 2359-2363, 1979.

35. Brandtzaeg, P., and Bakbien, K. Immunohistochemical studies on the formation and epithelial transport of immunoglobulins in normal and disclosed human intestinal mucosa. *Scand. J. Gastroenterol.* 11 (Suppl.), 36, 1976.

36. Bebet, D., Moneret-Vautrin, D. A., Nicholas, J. P., and Grillilot, J. P. IgE levels in intestinal juice. *Dig. Dis. Sci.* 25, 323-333, 1980.

37. Dodd Wilson, L., Soltis, R. D., Olsen, R. E., and Erandsen, S. L. Cholinergic stimulation of immunoglobulin A secretion in rat intestine. *Gastroenterology* 83, 881-888, 1982.

38. Lebenthal, E., and Clark, B. Immunoglobulin concentrations in duodenal fluids of infants and children. II. The effect of pancreozymin and secretin. *Am. J. Gastroenterol.* 75, 436-439, 1981.

39. Park, B. H., and Lebenthal, E. Age related changes in the levels of antibodies to cow's milk proteins as measured by enzyme linked immunosorbent assay (ELISA). *Med. Sci.* 9, 866-867, 1981.

40. Shah, P. C., Freier, S., Park, B. H., Lee, P. C., and Lebenthal, E. Detection of antibodies to cow's milk protein in duodenal fluid. *Gastroenterology* 83, 916-921, 1982.

41. Freier, S., Lebenthal, E., Freier, M., Shah, P. C., Park, B. H., and Lee, P. C. IgE and IgE antibodies to cow milk and soy protein in duodenal fluid: Effects of pancreozymin and secretin. *Immunology* 49, 69-75, 1983.

42. Nilsson, S., Leander, S., Vallgren, S., and Hakanson, R. Gastrins and cholecystokinins release acetyl-choline but not substance P from neurons in guinea pig *Tannia coli*. *Eur. J. Pharmacol.* 90, 245-250, 1983.

43. Payan, D. G., Brewster, D. R., and Goetzl, E. J. Specific stimulation of human T-lymphocytes by substance P. *J. Immunol.* 131, 1613-1616, 1983.

44. Johnson, H. M., Smith, E. M., Torres, B. A., and Blalock, J. E. Regulation of the in vitro antibody response by neuro-endocrine hormones. *Proc. Natl. Acad. Sci. U SA* 79, 4171, 1982.

45. Blalock, J. E. The immune system as a sensory organ. *J. Immunol.* 132, 1067-1070, 1984.

8

Processing and Evaluation of the Antigenicity of Protein Hydrolysates

Ralph J. Knights
Mead Johnson Nutritional Division, Evansville, Indiana

I. INTRODUCTION

A hydrolysate of casein has been manufactured and used by Mead Johnson in the production of a hypoallergenic infant formula since the 1940s. The hydrolysate used in Nutramigen and Pregestimil is made and tested in much the same way as was Amigen, a parenteral grade of protein hydrolysate. The concept of a nonantigenic nitrogen source for allergic infants is relatively spimple: predigest a highly nutritional protein to provide the necessary nitrogen as amino acids and peptides which are small enough to have no interaction with the immune system. The presence of peptides in a nonantigenic product usually raises questions. "How big are they?" "How many are there?" "What are their compositions?" "Do they act as new antigens?" Although providing the answers to all of these questions is beyond the scope of this chapter, we present here the general scheme for the manufacture and testing of protein hydrolysate, for infant formulas as well as recent information on the hydrolysate's molecular weight profile and its interaction with casein-specific antibodies.

II. PROTEIN HYDROLYSIS

A. Method

The hydrolysis of proteins follows the generalized sequence shown in Table 1. Proteins are degraded to proteoses, then to peptones, then small peptides, and

Table 1 Hydrolysate Products and Characteristics

	Average MW[a]	AN:TN[b]
Protein	>20,000	<0.01
Proteose	5000–10,000	<0.1
Peptone	1000–6000	0.1–0.5
Peptide amino acid mix	200–500	0.5–0.8
Amino acid mix	75–200	0.8–0.9

[a]Average molecular weights are offered as guidelines for classifications.
[b]The ratio of AN/TN (or free α-nitrogen to total nitrogen) are the expected values for proteins and proteoses, the reported range for commercial peptones (2), the defined lower limit for parenteral grade hydrolysates containing peptides (1), and the maximum possible value for an amino acid mix, allowing for 10–20% side-chain nitrogen.

finally to amino acids. The classification is somewhat arbitrary and is based on features such as solubility rather than molecular weight. The molecular weight ranges shown in the table are estimates and are offered here only as approximate guidelines for the various hydrolysis products.

Protein hydrolysates suitable for injection are mixes of amino acids and short peptides with an alpha-nitrogen to total nitrogen ratio of 0.50 or greater (1). Peptones, by definition, are to be soluble in saturated ammonium sulfate, and it has been estimated that the upper molecular weight limit is 3000–6000 (2,3). The alpha-nitrogen to total nitrogen ratio for a sampling of commercial peptones range is 0.1–0.5 (2). Proteoses are the products of limited hydrolysis, and they are insoluble in 50-100% saturated ammonium sulfate.

Protein hydrolysis can be achieved by treatment with concentrated acids or with proteolytic enzymes. Acid hydrolysis destroys or modifies essential amino acids and thus gives a product of poor nutritional value. Single enzymes or combinations of enzymes can be used to obtain a variety of finished product characteristics. Mead Johnson uses a mix of proteases derived from pancreas. The enzyme combination simulates intestinal processing of food proteins, and the mix of exo- and endopeptidases provides the necessary extensive hydrolysis and a high yield of small peptides and amino acids.

The process for hydrolysis is not unlike typical laboratory methods to hydrolyze a protein. The substrate, casein, is suspended or dissolved at the desired pH and the enzyme is added. After the desired state of hydrolysis is achieved, the enzyme reaction is quenched, the residual proteins are aggregated, and the hydrolysate is clarified by filtration or centrifugation. The last step in processing is a treatment with activated charcoal.

B. Time Course of Hydrolysis

In following the time course of protein digestion, there is no single quantitative assay which will measure the extent of hydrolysis. We have used both the Coomassie (4) and the trinitrobenzenesulfonic acid (TNBS) (5) assays to respectively provide information on the residual amount of protein and the extent of peptide bond cleavage. Coomassie dye reacts intensely with proteins and large peptides, and it gives no color in the presence of peptides less than about 500 molecular weight (4, Manes and Knights, unpublished observations). It is ideal for following the initial hydrolysis of proteins to yield small peptides. The TNBS assay measures the increase in free amino groups generated by peptide bond hydrolysis.

Figure 1 shows these measurements for a typical casein hydrolysate. Coomassie-reactive material diminishes very rapidly. After about 20% of the total allowed time for hydrolysis, the Coomassie value has been reduced to less than

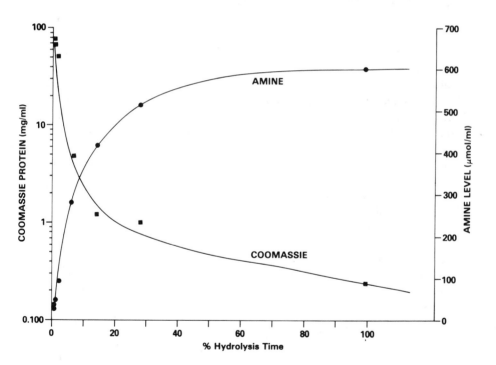

Figure 1 Time course of casein hydrolysis using the Coomassie dye reaction (□) and the TNBS assay (x) to follow the loss of protein and the increase in amine level, respectively. Coomassie protein units are mg of protein per ml with bovine serum albumin used as the standard; TNBS units are μmol of amine per ml, with leucine used as a standard. Units of time are proprietary.

1% of the initial value; further changes are very slow. In contrast, the TNBS value increases steadily over almost the entire time course of digestion. In reference to the Coomassie value above, and at 20% of the allowed hydrolysis time, the TNBS value has reached about 80% of its final value.

The concentration of amino groups produced by hydrolysis and the initial concentration of protein can be used to calculate an average peptide molecular weight. Extensively hydrolyzed casein used in Nutramigen typically has a calculated average molecular weight of around 200.

Measurements like these are helpful to the processor in assuring that production is reproducible. They are helpful in assessing improvements to processing, and they add to an understanding of the meaning of other measurements, such as the free amino acid levels or the alpha-nitrogen to total nitrogen ratio obtained from formol titrations.

III. ANTIGENICITY MEASUREMENT

A. Methods

Low antigenicity, however, is the key issue in quality control and in clinical application of these hydrolysates. There are a number of techniques used to evaluate the antigenic character of food proteins and hydrolysates. The Shultz Dale technique has been used to test for casein and casein proteoses (6); passive cutaneous anaphylaxis (PCA) and PCA inhibition have been used to qualify nonantigenic hydrolysates of casein and whey proteins (7,8). These assays are, at best, semiquantitative, and they are several orders of magnitude less sensitive than those using isolated antibodies. Radioallergosorbent test (RAST) inhibition and radioimmunoassay (RIA) inhibition have been employed for measuring the binding of peptides to antibodies elicited to intact peanut protein and bovine serum albumin (BSA) (9,10).

For many years, Mead Johnson has used the anaphylaxis test described in the *U.S. Pharmacopeia* for "Hydrolysates to Be Used for Injection" (1). For this assay, guinea pigs are immunized with a partial digest of the protein and then challenged with the finished product. The sensitized animals are capable of detecting both intact casein and the peptides present in the partial digest used for the immunization.

B. Immunosorbent Inhibition

Recently, we have utilized an immunosorbent assay for the detection of hydrolysate components that retain the capacity to bind to casein-specific rabbit or human IgG. Inhibition curves for hydrolysates are compared to a standard casein inhibition curve in order to calculate the caseinlike determinants remaining in the hydrolysate. Figure 2 shows that inhibition lines for a partial and a finished

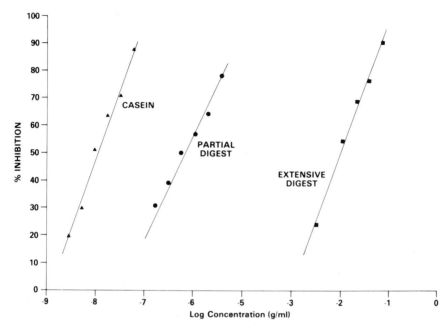

Figure 2 ELISA inhibition curves. Inhibition of the binding of rabbit anti-casein IgG to casein-coated microtiter plates in the presence of casein (△), a partial hydrolysate of casein (x), and an extensive hydrolysate of casein (□). Inhibition by the extensive hydrolysate required 10^6 times higher concentration than inhibition by casein.

hydrolysate lie parallel to the inhibition line for casein, but at higher concentrations. The inhibition line for the hydrolysate used in Nutramigen is positioned on the concentration scale roughly six orders of magnitude higher than that for casein. This is interpreted as a measure of about 1 µg of "casein equivalent" determinants per gram of casein hydrolysate. There is some additional evidence (not shown here) which suggests that these hydrolysate determinants are not due to residual protein, but rather due to peptides, less than 1200 MW, which retain some capacity to bind weakly to the casein-specific antibodies.

C. Time Course of Antigenicity Loss

The time course of hydrolysis has also been followed using the immunosorbent inhibition assay. Figure 3 shows both the residual determinants and the amine content at various times of casein digestion with pancreas-derived enzymes. There is an initial rapid loss in determinants with a change by a factor 10^{-4} to

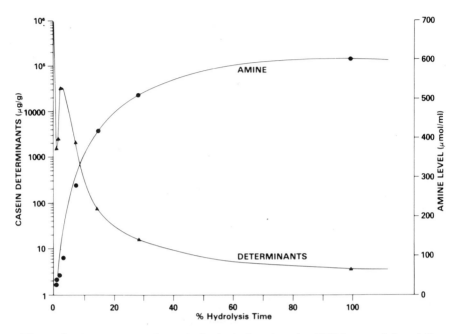

Figure 3 Time course of casein hydrolysis using the TNBS assay (x) and the inhibition of antibody binding (△). ELISA units are calculated as µg of casein equivalents per gram of dry weight.

10^{-5} within the first 20% of the allowed digestion time. The slow loss thereafter is quantifiable, reproducible, and significant in obtaining finished hydrolysates with the lowest possible antigenic character.

We have found that treating the hydrolysate with activated carbon further reduces the level of residual determinants in extensive hydrolysates. Before carbon treatment, hydrolysates have 2–4 µg of determinant equivalents per gram of solids, and after carbon treatment the value is 1–2 µg/g.

All commercial enzymatic hydrolysates are not the same; they vary in the extent of hydrolysis, the post hydrolysis treatment, and the level of determinants measured by the immunosorbent assay. A small sampling of hydrolysates, sold principally for use as microbial growth media, were compared to the Mead Johnson hydrolysate (see Table 2). The lowest value for residual caseinlike determinants was measured for the carbon-treated Mead Johnson product with other hydrolysates containing 10- to 1000-fold more residual determinants.

Table 2 Casein Determinants Measured in Casein Hydrolysates

Source	Description	Casein equivalent[a] μg/g
MJ	Casein hydrolysate	
	No treatment	2.4
	Carbon treated	1.3
A	Casein enzymatic digest	21
B	Pancreatic digest of casein	47
C	Pancreatic casein hydrolysate	230
C	Pancreatic casein hydrolysate	3200

[a]Measured by ELISA inhibition and using casein as a standard for quantitation.

IV. MOLECULAR WEIGHT PROFILES

A. Method

Knowledge of the molecular weight of peptides in a hydrolysate should provide some insight into the potential antigenic or immunogenic nature of the hydrolysate. Intact proteins of molecular weight 20,000–60,000 appear to be the most common antigens. Peptones, which range up to a few thousand in molecular weight, have been shown to produce peptone shock or anaphylaxis in sensitized animals (11). Synthetic peptides greater than about 1600 MW were shown to be immunogenic on injection into a responder strain of mice (12), but peptides of 1000 MW or less must be covalently coupled to carrier proteins in order to elicit antigen-specific antibodies (13). The linear peptide determinants recognized by antibodies, T cells and B cells, are contained in peptides between 12 and 20 amino acids long; the lower limit of determinant size is not known (14). Based on molecular weight alone, nonantigenic hydrolysates should probably contain no peptides that are greater than 1200 MW, and should have a distribution favoring free amino acids and small peptides.

For molecular weight profiles of hydrolysates, we have adapted a high-performance liquid chromatographic (HPLC) method described by Richter et al. (15) because of the good separation of peptides and a linear correlation of retention time with log MW. Two columns of TSK-125 were used (Bio Rad, 300 × 7.5 mm each). The solvent was 6 M guanidine hydrochloride (GuHCl) and, at a flow rate of 1 ml/min, the separations were complete in 30 minutes. Dried samples of standards and hydrolysates were reconstituted at 10 mg/ml of 6 M GuHCl. The proteins and peptides used as standards were: bovine serum albumin (67,000), ovalbumin (44,000), chymotrypsinogen (25,000), ribonuclease A

(13,700), insulin (6000), insulin A chain (2530), sleep-inducing peptide (849), N-succinyl-Ala-Ala-Ala-p-nitroanilide (451), tryptophan (204), phenylalanine (165), and glycine (75).

The column effluent was monitored for refractive index changes and for UV-light absorption at 280 nm. Signals from the monitors were processed by gel permeation chromatography software from Nelson Analytical (Palo Alto, CA). Ninhydrin, Lowry, and Coomassie assays provided no additional information on the peptide distribution.

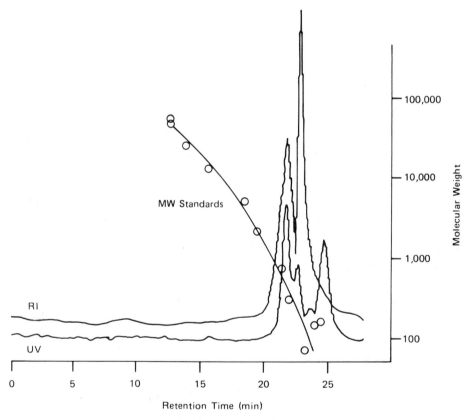

Figure 4 Gel permeation chromatography of an extensive casein hydrolysate on TSK-125 with continuous monitoring of refractive index (RI) and 280 nm (UV) absorption changes. Overlay shows the retention times for standards and the standard curve for retention time vs. MW.

Table 3 Area Percentages from Gel Permeation Chromatography[a]

Molecular weight	Antigenic hydrolysate[b]	Nonantigenic hydrolysate[c]
<500	61.4	67.0
500–1000	28.0	32.5
1000–1500	6.4	0.5
1500–2000	2.4	0
2000–2500	1.0	0
2500–3500	0.5	0
3500–5000	0.3	0
>5000	0	0

[a]Chromatography on TSK-125 using 6 M GuHCl; area percentages using GPC software from Nelson Analytical.
[b]Incomplete hydrolysate and no post hydrolysis treatment. Positive anaphylaxis in 5/5 animals sensitized to a partial digest of casein; measured 90 µg of casein determinant equivalents per gram by ELISA inhibition.
[c]Finished hydrolysate ingredient. Anaphylaxis in 0/5 animals sensitized to a partial digest of casein; measured 1–2 µg casein determinant equivalents per gram by ELISA inhibition.

B. Profiles for Hydrolysates

The molecular weight profile for casein hydrolysate is shown in Figure 4 along with the retention times for the proteins and peptide standards. The chromatograph shows no material greater than 1200 MW. If one allows for a peak width of about 2 minutes, then one might argue that the profile shows there is no material greater than about 1000 MW. Approximately two-thirds of the hydrolysate has a molecular weight less than 500 with the other one-third being peptides with molecular weight between 500 and 1200.

A hydrolysate, which provoked anaphylaxis in sensitized animals and which had a determinant level of about 90 µg of casein equivalents per gram, gave a molecular weight profile significantly different from nonantigenic hydrolysates. Table 3 shows the integrated area percentages between selected molecular weights (retention times) for the two hydrolysates. It is apparent that even a small amount of peptide with molecular weight between 1300 and 5000 will prime the guinea pigs and provoke symptoms of anaphylaxis in animals sensitized by the U.S. Pharmacopeia test (1).

The results reported here were obtained by chromatographing and analyzing the casein hydrolysate raw material used in Nutramigen, Pregestimil, and Critiicare HN. Comparable analyses of the formula products, or extracts of these products, require consideration of the various ingredients which would interfere with the assays and with the molecular weight profiles described here. For instance, vitamin B_{12} (MW 1355) is water soluble and would be extracted from the formula along with the hydrolysate; the vitamin contains a number of amide groups and has a strong UV absorption coefficient. Some of the carbohydrates that could be extracted might retrograde or reassociate to large complexes under some of the assay conditions; this would give the appearance of large molecular weight materials and could possibly be misinterpreted as the appearance of precipitating proteins. It is not unlikely that the fat source and the emulsifiers could form microemulsions and also give the apperance of water-soluble, high molecular weight components. Calcium or magnesium salts could be extracted in slightly acid media and be subsequently precipitated in neutral media or on removing ligands during chromatography. Thus, chemical analysis of the hydrolysate extracted from a complete formula, such as Nutramigen, would be fairly difficult to interpret.

V. CONCLUSIONS

The protein hydrolysate used in Nutramigen and Pregestimil is manufactured under controlled conditions which provide a nitrogen source with the following features: (a) excellent nutritive value and nitrogen utilization (16,17), (b) a calculated average molecular weight of 200, (c) no peptides greater than 1200 MW, (d) no anaphylaxis symptoms in the sensitive U.S. Pharmacopeia test, and (e) trace levels of caseinlike determinants as measured by a very sensitive immunosorbent inhibition assay. It should be noted that these analyses were performed using the hydrolysate ingredient. This assures that trace amounts of low molecular weight peptides can be detected without interference due to the presence of large quantities of carbohydrates, some relatively large molecular weight vitamins, and the insoluble fat, minerals, and emulsifiers present in finished product.

ACKNOWLEDGMENTS

Mead Johnson is grateful to Dr. Irene Cheung of I. C. Biomedical Consultants (Cleveland, OH) for the development of a very sensitive immunosorbent inhibition assay used to measure caseinlike peptides in hydrolysates.

Mr. J. D. Manes and Ms. R. B. Nellis of Mead Johnson performed the chemical analyses and provided the gel permeation chromatography data.

REFERENCES

1. Protein Hydrolysate Injection. In: *United States Pharmacopeia XX.* 687–688, 1980.

2. U. S. Dept. of Commerce, Publication PB82-155466. *Evaluation of the Health Aspects of Peptones as Food Ingredients.* Prepared by the Federation of American Societies of Experimental Biology, Bethesda, MD, 1981.

3. Nixon, J. E., and Mawer, G. E. The digestion and absorption of protein in man. The form in which digested protein is absorbed. *Br. J. Nutr.* 24, 241–258, 1970.

4. Bradford, M. M. A rapid and sensitive method for the quantitation of microgram quantities of protein utilizing the principle of protein-dye binding. *Anal. Biochem.* 72, 248–254, 1976.

5. Synder, S. L., and Sobocinski, P. Z. An improved 2,4,6-trinitrobenzene-sulfonic acid method for the determination of amines. *Anal. Biochem.* 64, 284–288, 1975.

6. Stull, A., and Hampton, S. F. A study of the antigenicity of proteoses. *J. Immunol.* 41, 143–160, 1941.

7. Takase, M., Fukuwatari, Y., Kawasi, K., Kiyosawa, I., Ogasa, K., Suzuki, S., and Kuroume, T. Antigenicity of casein enzymatic hydrolysate. *J. Dairy Sci.* 62, 1570–1576, 1979.

8. Pahud, J. J., and Schwarz, K. Research and development of infant formulae with reduced allergenic properties. *Ann. Allergy* 53, 609–614, 1984.

9. Nordlee, J. A., Taylor, S. L., Jones, R. T., and Yunginger, M. D. Allergenicity of various peanut products as determined by RAST inhibition. *J. Allergy Clin. Immunol.* 68, 376-382, 1981.

10. Wright, R. N., and Rothberg, R. M. The reaction of pepsin and pepsin trypsin digestion products of bovine serum albumin with antisera from rabbits ingesting this protein. *J. Immunol.* 107, 1410-1418, 1971.

11. Dailey, R. Monograph on Peptone. U. S. Department of Commerce, National Technical Information Service PB-284 882, Washington, D.C., 1978.

12. Singh, B., Lee, K. C., Fraga, E., Wilkinson, A., Wong, M., and Barton, M. A. Minimum peptide sequences necessary for priming and triggering of humoral and cell-mediated immune responses in mice. Use of synthetic peptide antigens of defined structure. *J. Immunol.* 124, 1336-1343, 1980.

13. Butler, V. P., and Bieser, S. M. Antibodies to small molecules. In: *Advances in Immunology 17*, Dixon, F. J., and Hunkel, H. G. (eds.). Academic Press, New York, 1973, p. 256.

14. Bixler, G. S., and Atassi, M. Z. T cell recognition of proteins: Conclusions from the localization of full T cell recognition profiles of two native proteins. *BioTechnology* 47-54, January 1985.

15. Richter, W. O., Jacob, B., and Schwandt, P. Molecular weight determination of peptides by high performance gel permeation chromatography. *Anal. Biochem.* 133, 288-291, 1983.

16. Smith, J. L., Artega, C., and Heymsfield, S. B. Increased ureagenesis and impaired nitrogen use during infusion of a synthetic amino acid formula. *N. Engl. J. Med.* 306, 1013-1018, 1982.

17. Albina, J. E., Jacobs, D. O., Melnik, G., Settle, R. G., Stein, T. P., Guy, D., and Rombeau, J. L. Nitrogen utilization from elemental diets. *J. Parent. Enterol. Nutr.* 9, 189-195, 1985.

CLINICAL USE

9

Preclinical and Clinical Evaluations with Casein Hydrolysate Products

Angel Cordano and David A. Cook
Mead Johnson Nutritional Division, Evansville, Indiana

I. INTRODUCTION

In this era of cost containment, the existence of casein hydrolysate (CH) formulas for enteral nutrition is undoubtedly helpful in reducing the excessive use of total parenteral nutrition (TPN). It is widely accepted that enteral feedings should be utilized when the gastrointestinal tract is functional.

Although few physicians think of special infant formulas as essential products in the control or management of certain illnesses, the information presented in this chapter documents the importance of these products in clinical practice.

Between 1912 and 1916 there were several reports describing utilization of amino acids prepared by digestion of casein. Prior to 1940 the only substances available in parenteral feedings were glucose, electrolytes, and vitamins. Amigen, a parenteral grade of protein hydrolysate made by digestion of casein through pancreatic enzymes, was the first hydrolysate used parenterally, and over 400 papers were published on its use.

In the late 1930s and early 1940s, this nonantigenic protein hydrolysate was also used as the nitrogen source in formulas for oral feedings. In 1942 Nutramigen was introduced for management of infants with cow's milk allergy. In the 1950s it was shown that by treating CH with charcoal under carefully defined conditions, most of the aromatic amino acids (phenylalanine, tyrosine, and tryptophan could be removed. The last two were replaced, and methionine was added to compensate for its partial loss in processing. By this process, Lofenalac, for dietary management of phenylketonuria, was made available in 1958 and an offspring product called Low PHE/TYR Diet Powder (Product 3200-AB) low in phenylalanine and tyrosine was introduced for dietetic management of tyrosinosis.

In the late 1960s a formula was developed and clinically tested in subjects intolerant of intact proteins or with malabsorption of lactose, sucrose, or conventional dietary fats. This product, commercially marketed in 1971 as Pregestimil, contained amino acids as CH, dextrose as the major carbohydrate, and medium chain triglycerides (MCT) as the primary fat. A reformulated version of Pregestimil with lower osmolality was introduced in 1979.

Because intestinal mucosa insult may result in monosaccharide intolerance, in 1978 a mono- and disaccharide-free CH product (Product 3232-A) was made available to the therapeutic arsenal of special formulas. In the adult area, CH products have not been utilized to full potential; the first one, Flexical, was introduced in 1973. In 1981 Criticare HN, the first and to date only ready-to-use enteral diet based on HC, was made available for general use.

An important feature of the CH formulas developed over 40 years ago was to have a nonantigenic nitrogen source for infants suffering from allergy due to intact protein. Years later (1978) Eastham and co-workers (3) noted that casein hydrolysate formulas appear to afford some of the benefits of breast milk with regard to subsequent antibody production to ingested protein. This fact has seemingly been confirmed in clinical and immunological studies by Hamburger (4), involving large numbers of infants from atopy-prone families.

II. PRECLINICAL TESTING

A. Protein Quality

Consistency of the nutritional quality of the protein used in formulas containing protein hydrolysate is verified on multiple batches of CH at regular intervals using the official protein efficiency ratio (PER) test of the Association of Official Analytical Chemists. This assures the bioavailability of amino acids in the ingredients and in processed formulas and also that little or no loss of protein quality occurs during processing due to the Maillard reaction between reducing sugars and reactive amino groups in the protein. Typical results of PER values expressed as a percentage of casein are 100–110 for casein hydrolysate, and 115–125 for the hydrolysate supplemented with selected amino acids. These results represent the range of typical response of many unpublished studies conducted over the past several decades.

B. Trace Mineral Bioavailability

Animal models are useful for assessing the bioavailability of various nutrients, including major and trace minerals. For example, recent studies at Mead Johnson (34) demonstrated the high bioavailability of the naturally occurring selenium in infant formulas based on either casein hydrolysate or whey and milk. The level of naturally occurring selenium in Nutramigen is near the lower end of the range of that found in human milk, and the biological availability is very good as measured by the activity of blood and of liver glutathione peroxidase in weaning rats fed diets containing the infant formula as the sole source of selenium but adequate in every other nutrient.

C. Reproduction and Lactation

Since a few patients may be required to subsist on diets or formulas containing casein hydrolysate as the sole source of nutrients for relatively long periods of time and during the important growth phase of infancy, the safety and adequacy of casein hydrolysate have been evaluated by feeding diets containing casein hydrolysate as the sole source of protein to rats from weaning of the F_0 generation through the rapid growth phase of the F_1 generation. Results of these unpublished studies demonstrate that the growth, caloric efficiency, body composition, organ weight, litter size, birth weight, survival, and other parameters of health status of rats on a diet with protein hydrolysate as the sole source of protein were equal to that of rats fed diets with casein.

D. Antigenicity

The USP guinea pig test for antigenicity has been used for many years to assure the nonantigenic nature of the casein hydrolysate intended for intravenous use. The same test has been applied to casein hydrolysate made for use in Nutramigen, Pregestimil, and other formulas containing casein hydrolysate as the nitrogen source. The highly sensitive guinea pig test may in time be superseded by a more rapid, less expensive, and equally sensitive in vitro enzyme-linked immunosorbent assay (ELISA).

III. CLINICAL STUDIES AND USAGES

A. In Pediatrics

1. Protein Quality and Malnutrition

Although Nutramigen has a history of over 40 years of successful clinical use in widely diverse conditions, each time Mead Johnson develops a new product containing CH, or modifies current formulas, multiple studies are conducted involving clinical situations for which the product is intended (5).

Hartmann and colleagues (1,2) published their experience in metabolic balance studies and uses in different clinical situations. Shohl (6) in 1943 published the first metabolic balance study with a formula consisting of CH, Dextri-Maltose, starch, olive oil, brewer's yeast, and salts. Based on his evaluation in 20 infants he stated that "acute gastro-intestinal disturbances does not hinder retention of nitrogen when administered in proper form and amount. The fact that these infants had good nitrogen balances when CH was given, but did not when saline-glucose solution or milk was given, is sufficient proof that CH administration is desirable." It is interesting to observe that 40 years later pediatricians are again looking into CH feeding during diarrhea episodes.

Two more recent reports on Nutramigen include one by Eastham (3) showing that infants fed CH formula for the first 3 months of life had lower antibody (hemagglutinins) to subsequent milk-based or soy-based protein than those given these formulas from birth. The second is by Powell (7) on uses of the product in infants with cow's milk or soy-induced enterocolitis and in infants with chronic diarrhea not due to cow or soy sensitivity.

Protein quality, effectiveness, and tolerance in the management of severe cases of protein-calorie malnutrition were reported in 1973 by Graham et al. (8). This study included 9 infants with marasmus and 1 with kwashiorkor who received the product as their only source of diet for a period of 10–105 days. The results proved the establishment of tolerance and weight gain, while showing improvement of serum albumin. The authors added that the increase in albumin levels was more prompt than was usually experienced in their unit with other diets given in similar fashion.

Because of some reports of intolerance, probably due to the high osmolality of the initial formulation of Pregestimil (>600 mOsm/kg of water), the product was modified by replacing dextrose with corn syrup solids, slightly reducing the content of hydrolysate (from 13 to 11% of calories as protein, adding cystine, tyrosine, and tryptophan to improve the amino acid profile) and replacing a portion of the MCT with corn oil (from 88 to 40%). An osmolality of 338 mOsm/kg water was thereby achieved. A study by Graham et al. (9) on this reformulated product (clinically tested as 3240-D) demonstrated the nutritional value of its protein as well as its effectiveness in the recovery of infants with severe protein-calorie malnutrition.

As in other studies by Graham et al., the product was fed at a level of protein similar to the content in breast milk to infants who already were recovered from acute stage malnutrition and who were steadily gaining not less than 30 g of weight per day. In order to achieve the protein levels of breast milk, the product

Table 1 Digestibility and Utilization

| Case/age (mo.) | Diet | Nitrogen balance | | | Fat ABS (%) |
		Intake (mg/day)	ABS (% intake)	RET (% intake)	
497/14	Casein-1	2569	91.0	28.5	93.0
	3240-D	2627	87.0	34.5	87.3
	Casein-2	2713	86.5	34.5	92.9
541/12	Casein-1	2011	82.0	24.0	89.3
	3240-D	2109	85.5	40.0	81.8
	Casein-2	2208	84.0	32.0	82.5
545/6	Casein-1	1667	81.5	31.0	89.8
	3240-D	1786	90.5	42.5	95.1
	Casein-2	1865	94.0	42.0	94.4

Source: From Ref. 9.

was diluted with soy-cottonseed oils and cane sugar to yield 6.4% protein calories and was compared with preceding and following periods of isonitrogenous, isocaloric casein formulas. Feeding the formula at a reduced protein level provides a more rigorous assessment of protein quality than if fed at its normal protein concentration of 11% calories as protein.

As seen in Table 1, apparent absorption and retention of nitrogen from the diluted test product (3240-D) were not different from those of the preceding and following casein periods. Retentions were higher than those of the preceding period in all three children, but higher than in the follow-up period in only one. The values of absorption above 85% and retentions close to 40% for product 3240-D (Pregestimil) are also comparable to those reported by the same unit with routine infant formulas. Fat absorption was close to 90% in the control and in the test product.

As part of the protein quality evaluation, plasma amino acids at fasting and at 3 and 4 hr postprandial were obtained during the metabolic balance study with diluted product at 6.4% protein as calories and also after 30 days usage of full-strength test formula given for the management of protein-calorie malnutrition. In both circumstances the values were characteristic of those seen with milk protein at similar ratios.

Stegink and Schmitt (10) in 1971 published comparative amino acid values from a study of infants fed routine infant formula or Nutramigen, and also found that values were within normal limits for both groups.

In an unpublished study in 6 infants by Graham (11) a ready-to-use liquid version of Pregestimil was evaluated both by diluting product to provide similar protein as percent of calories as breast milk and also evaluated at full strength. At the 6.4% protein calories, absorption and retention of N_2 in the casein control were 86.5% and 39.5%, respectively, while on the test product, absorption and retention were similar with values of 82 and 39%, respectively. The fat absorption was 86% for the control formula and 95% for the test product.

When the ready-to-use test product was given at full strength the N_2 absorption was 85% with retention of 38% and fat absorption of 95%. Amino acids were within the range of those found for casein at the same levels.

2. Casein Hydrolysate in Prematures

Some clinicians have fed formulas with casein hydrolysate to premature infants, usually with gastrointestinal problems or with some type of short gut syndrome.

An unpublished metabolic balance study (nitrogen, Ca, P, and fat) with a ready-to-use formula similar to Pregestimil, by O'Donnell (12), involved 5 premature infants (weight 1050–1650 g). Nitrogen absorption was 74.2% with a retention of 53.4%, while Ca and P absorptions were 75 and 87.6%, respectively, with a total retention of Ca of 73 mg/kg per day and 44 mg/kg per day of P. Fat balance showed 82% absorption and weight gains were adequate (between 19.5 and 23 g/day).

Moran et al. (13) in 1979 reported 19 prematures who were fed either Pregestimil or a routine milk-based formula. Fat absorption with the CH formulas was 93.4% versus 85.1% with routine formula. Likewise, weight gain on CH formulas was 13.1 g/day versus 10.2 g/day with routine formula.

In a large study conducted in the late 1970s involving multiple neonatal intensive care units, a formulation very similar to Pregestimil was utilized as the initial oral feeding in stressed low birth weight (LBW) infants and compared with various other formulas routinely used in each study unit. No significant advantage in benefit/risk evaluation was identified with use of the CH product. It was concluded that actual CH formulas should not be used as routine formulas for the initial feedings of stressed prematures (Chapter 16).

3. Intractable-Protracted Diarrhea

Another formula with CH that has been utilized in the management of this condition is Mono- and Disaccharide-Free Diet Powder (known also as 3232-A from Mead Johnson). This formula has 88% of its fat as MCT, and it has tapioca starch as a stabilizer without any other carbohydrate. Bobo and Groothuis (15)

Table 2 Intractable Diarrhea: Enteral vs. TPN R_x

	#	Weeks to D-XYL $>$ 15	Days enteral predischarge	Days to discharge
Severe	TPN (4)	7 (2-13)	23 (12-31)	73 (47-86)
	ENT (4)	2 (2-5)	21 (16-24)	21 (16-36)
Moderate	ENT (2)	1 (1-1)	15 (15-15)	15 (15-15)
	Bolus (3)	1 (1-1)	17 (4-24)	17 (4-24)

Adapted from Ref. 16.

reported their experience in 10 infants, concluding that it is a valuable adjunct in the treatment of such conditions, and helps eliminate the potential complications of central hyperalimentation, while oral feedings stimulate gastrointestinal trophic hormones.

A 1985 report by Orenstein (16) described results in 13 infants with intractable diarrhea who were classified as severe (with D-xylose$<$10) and moderate (with D-xylose$>$10). The severe cases were randomized to continuous nasogastric Pregestimil (ENT) or to TPN, while the moderate cases were given ENT or oral bolus (ORL). Both enteral groups were allowed intravenous stool volume replacement with 10% dextrose solution.

Table 2 adapted from Orenstein shows that all TPN patients failed to normalize D-xylose absorption after a mean of 39 (35-51) days of TPN, and because of that, were switched to enteral feedings. The preceding TPN did not shorten their enteral period. One patient of the severe group who was fed enterally for a week continued to lose weight and, as per protocol, was switched to TPN; however, four days later central line sepsis led to a successful return to the enteral group. Between the two enteral feedings in the moderate group there was no difference. The author concluded that enteral therapy of intractable diarrhea can produce comparable correction of malnutrition to TPN, with better correction of malabsorption, shorter hospitalization, and fewer complications.

Pregestimil has been widely utilized for the dietary management of this severe condition (administered by nasogastric drip or by bolus feedings) either as the initial therapeutic measure, or following TPN or along with TPN in the most severe cases (Chapters 13-15).

Other uses of CH products in pediatrics for management of colic, in nutritionally depleted patients suffering from cystic fibrosis, in protein sensitivity, in diarrhea and malnutrition, in children of high-risk allergic families, etc. are covered in other chapters of this book.

B. CH in Adults

Pediatricians were using different CH products for over 25 years before early trials with elemental diets (ED) were undertaken. These formulas allowed new opportunities to feed patients with poor digestive and absorptive capacities. Successful nutritional management with Flexical, an early ED utilizing CH as the protein source, occurred in patients with abdominal radiation (17), short gut (18), gastrointestinal fistula (19), during chemotherapy for cancer (20), as a pre-op bowel prep (21), with pancreatitis (22), with inflammatory bowel disease (23), in children with cystic fibrosis (24), and as postsurgical nutritional support (25). Most of these reports were not randomized trials nor did many compare the use of CH diets to other modes of nutritional support. Several authors have reviewed the literature on elemental diets, and the most complete of these, by Koretz and Meyer (26), provides excellent insights into the use of the protein hydrolysate diets.

Until recently, all EDs, whether based on CH or crystalline amino acids (CAA), were available only as powders to be mixed with water. Criticare HN, introduced in 1981, was the first nutritionally complete, ready-to-use ED. Through the use of appropriate manufacturing techniques, it became possible to terminally sterilize products containing glucose polymers (mono, di, tri, tetra and polymer of glucose), amino acids, and small peptides without inducing a significant Maillard reaction and a subsequent decrease in protein quality. This new development required extensive testing for protein quality as well as safety and acceptance. In these clinical trials, Criticare HN with CH was compared to Vivonex HN, a commercially available diet using only CAA as its protein source. Several examples follow.

In a randomized cross-over design study, the effect of Criticare HN on the intake, absorption, output, and retention of nitrogen and energy was compared to Vivonex HN in malnourished (85% of ideal body weight) Crohn's disease patients (27). The diets were almost identical except for their sources of protein, CH or CAA, respectively. Energy absorption for both diets was excellent (96% and 97% for the CH formula and CAA, respectively) and better than the energy absorption from a solid food diet containing 100 g fat. Nitrogen retention, however, was much better on the casein hydrolysate diet (4.4 g/day) than on the CAA diet (0.5 g/day), even though nitrogen absorption was slightly lower (86%) on the CH diet than the CAA diet (92%).

In a second study, 8 patients with radiation enteritis were studied in a similar manner. All subjects had steatorrhea and were 85% of standard for weight. The apparent digestibility of energy and nitrogen of the CH diet was 93% that of the CAA diet. Nitrogen retention, on the other hand, was three times greater on the CH diet (28).

Albina et al. (29), using chair-adapted malnourished primates made identical observations. Nitrogen balance was significantly better in the CH-fed animals than in the CAA-fed animals. Although there was no difference in digestibility and the protein turnover rates were not significantly different between the two groups of animals, the parameters of protein-calorie malnutrition, albumin, transferrin, and total iron-binding capacity were significantly better in the CH-fed animals than in the CAA-fed animals.

Other investigators have studied malnourished head and neck cancer patients with no evidence of malabsorption (30) and malnourished patients with chronic pancreatic insufficiency (31). Both found that diets based on CH resulted in a significantly better improvement of nutritional status, measured by increases in body weight and serum albumin.

Several authors (32,33) have proposed that di- or tripeptides may be more efficiently utilized than crystalline amino acids. The CH used in these studies are approximately 30% di- or tripeptides. There appeared no obvious advantage in absorption in malabsorbers when a commercially prepared diet with CH was compared to commercial CAA diets (27,28,30). In the studies where there was no evidence of malabsorption (29,30), the better nitrogen retention with hydrolysate could not be attributed to a possible better absorption of di- and tripeptides. To date, it is unclear why diets containing CH support significantly better nitrogen retention and general improvement of nutritional status than diets containing CAA. The data published, however, suggest that there is a distinct advantage of using CH over a diet containing CAA in renourishing the malnourished adult patient, regardless of his or her digestive and absorptive capacity.

IV. SUMMARY

The basic concept that led over 40 years ago to development of CH products was to have a nonantigenic source of nitrogen for infants suffering from allergy to intact protein.

Over the years, several CH products have contributed to improve the treatment of severely allergic infants as well as of children with inborn errors of metabolism. Today, the uses of CH are numerous and include management of intractable diarrhea; nutritional support in cystic fibrosis; feeding colicky infants when dietary management is indicated; managing malabsorption which accompanies gastrointestinal disturbances including short gut and other similar situations. We believe that there is sufficient evidence in cases where severe diarrhea lasts over a week without adequate response. Its use may prevent further deterioration and may decrease the need for TPN. In addition, patients with severe protein-calorie malnutrition and chronic acute superimposed diarrhea who show milk intolerance when orally fed may benefit from a CH formula.

With recent information showing that CH formulas appear to afford some of the benefits of breast milk with regard to subsequent antibody production to ingested protein (4), we are at a point when the use of CH products has to be considered when treating IgE-mediated disorders in atopy-prone families.

Casein hydrolysate products have undoubtedly acquired importance worldwide as part of the nutritional rehabilitation of sick infants and children.

Recent developments in nutritional research may expand the uses of protein hydrolysate to new areas of exciting proportions.

REFERENCES

1. Hartmann, A. F., Meeker, C. S., Perley, A. M., and McGinnis, H. G. Utilization of an enzymatic digest of casein. *J. Pediatr.* 20, 308-324, 1942.

2. Hartmann, A. F., Lawler, H. J., and Meeker, C. S. Studies of amino-acid administration. II. Clinical uses of an enzymatic digest of casein. *J. Pediatr.* 24, 2371-386, 1944.

3. Eastham, J. E., Lichauco, T., Grady, M. I., and Walker, A. Antigenicity of infant formulas: Role of immature intestine on protein permeability. *J. Pediatr.* 93, 561-564, 1978.

4. Hamburger, R. N. Diagnosis of food allergies and intolerances in the study of prophylaxis and control groups in infants. *Ann. Allergy* 53, 673-677, 1984.

5. Cordano, A. Pre-clinical and clinical evaluation of new infant formulas. *Nutr. Res.* 4, 1984.

6. Shohl, A. Nitrogen storage following I.V. and oral administration of casein hydrolysate to infants with acute gastrointestinal disturbance. *J. Clin. Invest.* 22, 257-263, 1943.

7. Powell, G. K. Milk and soy induced enterocolitis of infancy. *J. Pediatr.* 93, 553-560, 1978.

8. Graham, G. G., Baertl, J. M., Cordano, A., and Morales, E. Lactose-free, medium-chain triglyceride formulas in severe malnutrition. *Am. J. Dis. Child.* 126, 1973.

9. Graham, G. G., Klein, G. L., and Cordano, A. Nutritive value of elemental formula with reduced osmolality. *Am. J. Dis. Child.* 133, 1979.

10. Steginik, L. D., and Schmitt, J. Post-prandial serum amino acid levels in young infants fed casein hydrolysate-based formulas. *Nutr. Rep. Int.* 32, 93-99, 1971.

11. Graham, G. G. Unpublished data on file at Mead Johnson, 1980.
12. O'Donnell, A. Unpublished data on file at Mead Johnson, 1980.
13. Moran, J. R., Terry, A. B., Dunn, G. D., and Greene, H. L. A hydrolyzed formula for feeding infants less than 1250 g.: A controlled clinical trial. *Abstr. Am. Fed. Clin. Res.* 1979.
14. Darling, G., Lepage, Tremblay, P., Collet, S., Kien, L. C., and Roy, C. C. Protein quality and quantity in pre-term infants on the same energy intake. (Submitted for publication.)
15. Bobo, R. C., and Groothuis, 3232A formula for the management of intractable diarrhea of infancy. *Am. Coll. Nutr.* Abstract #13, 1980.
16. Orenstein, S. R. Intractable diarrhea of infancy (IDI): Prospective, randomized study of enteral vs. parenteral therapy. *Abstract 710, S.P.R.,* 1985 - Presented.
17. Bounous, G., Le Bel, E., Shuster, J., Gold, P., Tahan, W. T., and Bastin, E. Dietary protection during radiation therapy. *Strahlentherapie* 149, 476-483, 1974.
18. Voitk, A. J., Echave, V., Brown, R. A., and Gurd, F. N.: Use of elemental diet during the adaptive state of short gut syndrome. *Gastroenterology* 65(3), 419-426, 1978.
19. Voitk, A. J., Echave, V., Brown, R. A., McArdle, A. H., and Gurd, F. N. Elemental diet in the treatment of fistulas of the alimentary tract. *Surg. Gynec.* 137(1), 68-72, 1973.
20. Cousineau, L., Bounous, G., Rochon, M., Shuster, J., Gold, P., and Tahan, W. The use of an elemental diet during treatment with anticancer agents (abstr.). *Clin. Res.* 21(5), 1067, 1973.
21. Cooney, D. R., Wassner, J. D., Grosfeld, J. L., and Jesseph, J. E. Are elemental diets useful in bowel preparation. *Arch. Surg.* 109(2), 206-210, 1974.
22. Voitk, A., Brown, R. A., Echave, V., McArdle, A. H., Gurd, F. N., and Thompson, A. G. Use of an elemental diet in the treatment of complicated pancreatitis. *Am. J. Surg.* 125(2), 223-227, 1973.
23. Voitk, A. J., Echave, Feller, J. H., Brown, R. A., and Gurd, F. N. Experience with elemental diet in the treatment of inflammatory bowel disease. Is this primary therapy? *Arch. Surg.* 107(2), 329-333, 1973.
24. Courtney, M. E., Greene, H. L., Donald, W. D., Dunn, G. D., and Hutchinson, A. Nocturnal tubefeeding in cystic fibrosis. *Pediatr. Res.* 17, 186A, 1983.
25. Revard, J. Y., and Lapointe, R. Clinical experience in using elemental diet in the management of various surgical nutritional problems. *Canad. J. Surg.* 18, 90-96, 1975.
26. Koretz, R. L., and Meyer, J. H. Elemental diets—facts and fantasies. *Gastroenterology* 78, 393-410, 1980.
27. Smith, J. L., Arteaga, C., and Heymsfield, S. B. Increased ureagenesis and impaired nitrogen use during infusion of a synthetic amino acid formula. *N. Engl. J. Med.* 306, 1013-1016, 1982.

28. Beer, W. H., Fan, A., and Halsted, C. H. Clinical and nutritional implications of radiation enteritis. *Am. J. Clin. Nutr.* 41, 85-91, 1985.

29. Albina, J. E., Jacobs, D. O., Melnuk, G., Settle, R. G., Stein, T. P., Guy, D., and Rombeau, J. L. Nitrogen utilization from elemental diets. *J. Parent. Ent. Nutr.* 9, 189-195, 1985.

30. Meguid, M. M., Landel, A. M., Terz, J. J., and Akrabawi, S. S. Effects of elemental diet on albumin and urea synthesis: Comparison with partially hydrolyzed protein diet. *J. Surg. Res.* 37, 16-24, 1984.

31. Nasrallah, S. M., and Martin, D. M. Comparative effects of Criticare HN and Vivonex HN in the treatment of malnutrition due to pancreatic insufficiency. *Am. J. Clin. Nutr.* 39, 251:254, 1984.

32. Adibi, S. A. Intestinal transport of dipeptides in man. Relative importance of hydrolysis and intact absorption. *J. Clin. Invest.* 50, 2266-2275, 1971.

33. Silk, D. B. A., Fairclough, P. D., Clark, M. L., Hegarty, J. E., Marrs, T. C., Addison, J. M., Burston, D., Clegg, K. M., and Mathews, D. M. Use of a peptide rather than a free amino acid nitrogen source in chemically defined "elemental" diets. *J. Parent. Ent. Nutr.* 4, 548-553, 1980.

34. Litov, R. E. Evaluating the bioavailability of selenium from nutritional formulas for external use. In: *Proceedings of the 3rd International Symposium on Selenium in Biology and Medicine*, Combs, G. F. Jr., Spallholz, J. E., Levander, O. A., Oldfield, J. E. (eds.). AVI Publishing, Westport, Connecticut, in press.

10

Use of Casein Hydrolysate Formulas in the Diagnosis and Management of Gastrointestinal Food Sensitivity in Infancy

Geraldine K. Powell
University of Texas Medical Branch at Galveston, Galveston, Texas

I. INTRODUCTION

Food sensitivity seems to be a fairly common problem with an estimated incidence of 1-3% in infancy (1). Diagnosis and management of this problem are complicated by the following three problems:

1. It is pleomorphic in presentation, responsible for a variety of syndromes as well as considered potentially involved in a variety of symptoms.
2. There is no laboratory test available that is diagnostic of food sensitivity as such, independent of the symptom or syndrome; diagnosis depends on eliminating other causes of the syndrome or symptom and demonstrating that the problem disappears with removal of the offending antigen, and reoccurs with reintroduction.
3. Diagnosis and management depend on identifying the offending antigen(s).

These problems will be discussed one by one starting with pleomorphism. A host of symptoms have been ascribed to food sensitivity in infancy and childhood, including so called "atopic" symptoms (rhinitis, asthma, urticaria, eczema, and anaphylaxis), gastrointestinal symptoms, and a variety of other conditions including migraine, seizures, and hyperactivity. In fact, one sometimes wonders whether the diagnosis of "food allergy" hasn't replaced "demonic possession" as an explanation for any behavior or symptom that might cause concern to a child's parents, school, or physician! Since this chapter focuses on the use of casein hydrolysate formulas in food sensitivity, a strategy utilized most often in younger infants and children (less than 2 years of age), and is being written from the experiential vantage point of a gastroenterologist, the gastrointestinal symptoms associated with food sensitivity in infants will be described in more detail. However, the principles used in diagnosis and management of the gastrointestinal problems can also be applied to the diagnosis of other symptoms.

III. GASTROINTESTINAL FOOD SENSITIVITY (GFS)

In addition to less specific gastrointestinal symptoms, such as vomiting, diarrhea, and colic, there are four gastrointestinal syndromes that occur in infants or children, and have been characterized carefully enough, including diagnostic challenges, to be considered as hypersensitivity responses. These will be described in more detail, since they serve as a model for characterizing other symptoms and symptom complexes (Table 1).

A. Protein-Losing Enteropathy

Protein-losing enteropathy (PLE) has been described most clearly by Waldmann et al. (2) in patients who presented with edema which was secondary to a low serum albumin. Gastrointestinal symptoms were minimal. Fecal loss of serum protein, as estimated from the excretion of intravenously injected radiolabelled albumin, was increased, became normal when cow's milk was withdrawn from the diet, and increased again within 3–4 days after reintroduction of cow's milk.

B. Iron Deficiency Anemia Associated with Gastrointestinal Blood Loss

Wilson et al. (3) described a severe iron (Fe) deficiency anemia (hemoglobin < 7.0 g/dl) with occasional guaic-positive stools that occurs in infants between 6 to 25 months of age. Intravenously injected radiolabelled red blood cells were recovered in stools in amounts greater than normal. This abnormal loss of red blood cells decreased when cow's milk was withdrawn from the diet and reappeared when it was reintroduced. Many of these infants also demonstrated slight decreases in serum protein levels, and in a group of infants with similar findings, fecal excretion of intravenously injected radiolabelled plasma proteins was also increased (4).

C. Colitis-Enterocolitis

Food protein-induced enterocolitis (FPIE) was first reported as "allergic intestinal bleeding" by Rubin (5) in 1942. Gryboski (6) characterized eight infants

Table 1 Comparative Features of the Four Syndromes of Gastrointestinal Food Sensitivity

	PLE	Iron deficiency anemia	FPIE	Malabsorption
Age	2 mos.–14 yr.	6–25 mos.	3 days–9 mos.	1 wk–2 yr.
Symptoms: Vomit, diarrhea	"mild"	0	+++	++++
Anemia (Hgb < 10.0 g/dl)	+++	++++	+	++
Fecal blood-obvious	0	0	++	+
Fecal blood-occult	+++	+++	+++	NM
Fecal ^{51}Cr RBC	ND	++++	ND	ND
↓Serum albumin[a]	++++	+++	++[b]	++[b]
↑Fecal protein	++++	+++	++	++
PMN leukocytosis	0	NM	+++	ND
Fecal leukocytes	NM	ND	++++	ND
Blood eosinophilia	+++	NM	+	++
Fecal eos., eos. debris	+++	ND	++++	ND
Villous atrophy	0[c]	ND	ND	++++
CHO malabsorption	ND	ND	++++	++++

[a]Decreased serum albumin–total protein <6.0 g/dl.
[b]Some patients in these groups were also malnourished.
[c]Normal villous architecture; 3/5 eosinophilic infiltrate.
0 = rare <5% of patients; + = uncommon <15% of patients; ++ = occasional <30% of patients; +++ = frequent 30–80% of patients; ++++ = almost always >80% of patients; ND = not done; NM = not mentioned; CHO = carbohydrate.

with colitis, describing findings on proctoscopy that ranged in severity from friability to ulcerations. Rectal biopsies showed acute and chronic inflammation and crypt abscesses. More recently, other descriptions of this syndrome have suggested that the clinical presentation is more of an "enterocolitis," with evidence not only of colitis, but also damage to the small bowel mucosa, as manifested clinically by carbohydrate malabsorption (7). The majority of these infants are seen between 2 weeks and 3 months of age, and have a history of vomiting followed by increasing diarrhea. Analysis of stool specimens discloses carbohydrates (Clinitest positive) and blood, either obvious or occult; analysis of smears of stool mucus treated with Hansel's stain (8) reveals leukocytes, eosinophils, and eosinophilic debris. Infants in this clinical presentation group (including prematures with necrotizing enterocolitis due to milk or soy protein sensitivity) (9) respond to a single oral challenge by developing objective symptoms (vomiting or diarrhea), and laboratory studies yield four objective findings: blood, leukocytes, and eosinophils, or eosinophilic debris, which were not present in baseline stools, appear in the stools following a positive challenge, and polymorphonuclear leukocytosis in blood occurs 6-8 hours after challenge (7).

D. Malabsorption Syndrome Associated with Villous Atrophy

Patients with this entity come to medical attention because of chronic diarrhea associated with poor weight gain. Malabsorption is demonstrated, and small intestinal biopsy demonstrates villous atrophy, ranging in severity from "partial" or "patchy" to total, similar to that seen in gluten-induced enteropathy (10). Diagnostic challenge in these patients requires either a repeat intestinal biopsy after a chronic exposure to the formula in question (11) or laboratory demonstration of the reappearance of the malabsorption syndrome, either by fat balance studies or D-xylose absorption tests (12).

III. DIAGNOSTIC CONSIDERATIONS

The pleomorphism of food sensitivity provides a problem in defining an adequate challenge response. For example, in the better defined syndromes, such as enterocolitis (FPIE), one can follow the response to therapy using not only the two symptoms, vomiting and diarrhea with melena, but four more specific criteria, capable of being evaluated double blind (see Table 2). For the PLE syndrome, one can follow stool excretion of radiolabelled albumin, for the Fe deficiency syndrome, stool excretion of radiolabelled red blood cells, for the villous atrophy group, changes in intestinal morphology, or indirectly, changes in fat or D-xylose absorption. A different set of criteria is necessary for each syndrome. But, the problem really becomes difficult when evaluating responses to therapy of symptoms like abdominal pain, colic, or hyperactivity, and study designs become complex.

The second problem in diagnosis and management of this condition relates to the fact that there is no laboratory test that is specific to the diagnosis of food sensitivity. This is most striking in regard to the gastrointestinal food sensitivity problems, where no single laboratory test independent of the presenting symptoms can predict whether the patient's symptoms or syndrome are due to food sensitivity. Reviews have suggested that obtaining a family history of atopy or allergy is helpful. However, since some studies have estimated the incidence of positive family history for allergy to be 43% in atopic individuals, and 28% in normals (13), this particular clue must be considered more in the realm of a "helpful hint" than a compelling diagnostic argument.

A similar argument can be made for the presence of "other allergic symptoms," which, although common in some patients with gastrointestinal food sensitivity, have often not yet occurred in infants with this problem, and in addition, are not uncommon in the population as a whole, and in patients with other gastrointestinal diseases, such as gluten-induced enteropathy and Crohn's disease. In regard to the diagnostic usefulness of serum IgE levels, these are either described as normal in some of the gastrointestinal syndromes, have not been studied in others, and are frequently elevated in patients with inhalant sensitivity rhinitis, and thus are not much help in deciding whether a gastrointestinal syndrome or symptom in a patient is due to GFS. A similar pattern exists for blood eosinophilia; although common in the PLE group, as well as in patients with nongastrointestinal atopy and those with parasites, it is less common in FPIE or in the malabsorption syndrome, and not mentioned in the iron deficiency anemia syndrome.

Thus diagnosis rests on evaluating the constellation of symptoms, eliminating other causes of the problem, and noting the response to withdrawal of the offending antigen and, if improvement occurs, noting the response to reintroduction of the antigen into the diet. This however brings us to the third problem complicating the diagnosis and management of GFS. How does one identify the antigen(s) responsible for the problem?

The difficulty in isolating the offending antigens lies not only in the complexity of the diet most infants receive, but also in the ubiquitous distribution of non-food antigens—preservatives, dyes, and medications. In addition, food protein sensitivity frequently involves more than one food protein, with varying clinical responses even within the same patient. Although dietary history is essential, and sometimes helpful, it is also notoriously unreliable. For example, in a study on serum food antibody levels, we included only infants whose diet has been restricted to formula (14). According to the history obtained from their parents, these infants, all less than 6 months of age, had *never received even a taste of any other food* and had received no medications. Despite this adamant history, 35% had serum antibodies of the IgM and IgA class (nonmaternal) directed against egg white, a relatively rare component of most baby foods, suggesting exposure to a wide range of dietary antigens, all capable of producing sensitivity. Probably this reflects not only parental bias, but also the large number of caretakers and feeders of many young infants.

Skin tests have frequently been used to pinpoint the offending antigens in patients with GFS, but in general, when studied in combination with diagnostic food challenges, correlate poorly with challenge response. In a study by Goldman's group, correlating diagnostic oral milk protein challenges with skin tests to the same antigens, 59% of infants with positive milk challenge and 68% of infants with negative milk challenge had positive skin tests to one or more milk proteins (15). Tests based on IgE antibodies directed against food antigens (radioallergosorbent test [RAST], histamine release) and used to diagnose immediate hypersensitivity reactions have not been tested carefully in the gastrointestinal syndromes. Since most of these would probably fall within the "nonreaginic" group (16) the poor correlation of RAST with diagnostic food challenges (17) is probably not surprising.

Elevated serum antibodies of the IgG and IgA class directed against foods to which the infants are sensitive have been found in some groups of infants with GFS, but the overlap with normals is significant enough to limit the diagnostic usefulness of these determinations for any one infant (14). Blood lymphocytes from patients with the FPIE syndrome show blast transformation (as measured by radioactive thymidine incorporation) when cultured in vitro with the antigens to which the infant reacts positively on oral challenge (18). Although this is a sensitive and specific test for the offending antigen in this particular syndrome, it is not widely available, nor is a test involving production of lymphokine by lymphocytes that have been cultured with food antigens (19).

IV. ELIMINATION DIETS

Since there is no simple laboratory test to pinpoint the antigens involved, two major clinical strategies have been devised. The first is the use of "elimination diets." This particular strategy has been proposed in many forms, but basically the diet is usually limited to perhaps 12 "hypoallergenic" foods that are the mainstay, allowing small amounts of others, and totally eliminating another group. If the symptoms continue, the "in" foods are changed. For success, this would appear to require a complex computer program, as well as a robot to follow the child around estimating and analyzing everything that goes into his or her mouth. Although this may be the only feasible approach for an older child, there is another choice presently available for younger patients. This alternative is to remove all possible antigens from the diet, and show that the problem disappears, then add back food antigens one by one. This is most readily implemented in well-described syndromes where there is a constellation of symptoms and objective laboratory findings to follow and a known time course for response. It is obviously more difficult to implement in cases with a single symptom such as colic, vomiting, or diarrhea.

The question remains, however, how to remove all antigens short of starvation or a course of parenteral alimentation. Although we cannot totally remove all antigens, formulas containing only trace amounts of antigen can be used effectively in most cases. These include breast milk, elemental formulas such as Vivonex, and infant formulas based on hydrolysates of cow milk casein. For the initial "antigen withdrawal trial," breast milk is rarely an option, since it is difficult to obtain on short notice. Elemental formulas such as Vivonex with their minimal fat and resultant high carbohydrate content (16%, approximately twice as high as most infant formulas) often result in diarrhea secondary to carbohydrate malabsorption, especially in situations where intestinal damage has already occurred. They are also not tailored to meet infant nutritional needs, and the long-term effects of a high-carbohydrate, negligible-fat diet on infant growth and nutrition are not known. Addition of the "flavor packs" to make these more palatable adds yet other potential antigens. Therefore, at the present time, probably the best choice for an "antigen withdrawal test" in infants is one of the casein hydrolysate formulas, either Nutramigen or Pregestimil. Long experience with these formulas (15 years, at least 30 patients per year) on our service suggests that infants thrive on Nutramigen, growing at normal rates on 120 kcal/kg body weight, and no nutritional deficiencies have yet been noted. For infants who have no other medical problems complicating their GFS problem, Nutramigen is my preference. The medium-chain triglycerides provided by Pregestimil are not necessary, and any carbohydrate malabsorption still present from residual intestinal mucosal damage can be followed more easily on the sucrose-containing formulas (using the routine Clinitest after boiling with HCl) than on a formula containing glucose polymers, where Clinitest markedly underestimates the severity of carbohydrate malabsorption. Finally, loose stools containing blood (guaiac positive) and eosinophils have occurred in some of the patients we have followed with FPIE while they were receiving Pregestimil, only to resolve when the formula was changed to Nutramigen. This suggests there may be an antigen in Pregestimil not present in Nutramigen (corn syrup solids?). For more complicated patients, such as those with GFS in addition to chronic cholestatic liver disease or short bowel syndrome (not an uncommon combination), where the medium-chain triglycerides are more important for optimal nutritional management and the corn syrup solids less osmolar, Pregestimil might be a better choice.

It is essential however, whichever the choice, that formula only be used, with *no additional foods, beverages, or medications.* Medications such as Bentyl, antibiotics, antihistamines, pseudoephedrine, etc, not only contain their pharmacologically active ingredient—potentially antigenic—but, in children's preparations, additional antigens in the form of dyes, flavors, preservatives, and suspending agents, that complicate interpretation of the antigen withdrawl test results. Each year, we evaluate at least 10 infants with chronic diarrhea that "continued on Nutramigen with nothing added" only to find out, when the diarrhea disappears with a hospital-enforced Nutramigen-only regime and the parents are again questioned, that many additional foods, home remedies, or medications were being given in addition to the formula.

Many physicians dealing with suspected GFS in an infant on cow's milk-based formulas would not "withdraw all antigens" but rather, "change antigens" by a switch to soy-based formula. This may be practical in a very young infant whom one can be certain has not been exposed previously to soy, either in a formula or in foods (such as rice cereal). However, it can confuse the picture, delaying diagnosis if there has been a previous exposure, or if, as in 20% of cases, the infant becomes intolerant to soy (if this occurs, it usually does so within 4–10 days of beginning soy for the first time). Therefore, the simplest expedient is probably to try a low-antigen formula, an antigen withdrawal test, and if the infant responds to this, make the decision about a more permanent formula after the diagnosis is made.

Our most common use of the antigen withdrawal test, using Nutramigen, is in young infants with enterocolitis (FPIE). This will be detailed as an example.

These patients usually present with vomiting and diarrhea, frequently severe enough to be associated with dehydration. Stools are guaiac positive and contain leukocytes and eosinophilic debris; they are also frequently watery and Clinitest positive. Polymorphonuclear leukocytosis, suggesting a diagnosis of sepsis or bacterial gastroenteritis is often present. Stool examinations for parasites, bacterial pathogens, and rotovirus are negative. Vomiting, diarrhea, and melena disappear within 48 hours of food and formula withdrawal, and do not recur when the infant is placed on oral electrolyte solution or Nutramigen. These patients are discharged with a diagnosis of "suspected FPIE" with instructions to remain on Nutramigen for one month, and, if during that month they have been asymptomatic, with normal weight gain and stool consistency, they are readmitted for diagnostic challenge. As part of an effort to elucidate the mechanism of this condition, we studied a number of these infants at the time of readmission. Since we challenged only with milk, soy, and ovalbumin, we could not eliminate the possibility that infants with negative challenges to all three of these foods were not sensitive to other foods. We judged the challenges by five criteria which could be assessed double blind (Table 2) and rated a challenge as "positive" if three or more criteria were present, "negative" if none or one. Nine each of the milk and soy challenges were positive, and 13 were negative. Of note, 4 of the 20 challenges with ovalbumin (the "negative control" antigen) were positive, despite a negative history of *any* solid food ingestion!

Table 2 Criteria for Positive Reaction to Acute Challenge

Evaluated for 24 hours following oral ingestion of formula or food.

(a) Symptoms: vomiting or diarrhea

(b) Increase in peripheral blood polymorphonuclear leukocyte count of $>4000/mm^3$ (between that in a blood sample drawn immediately before oral challenge and that in a sample drawn 6–8 hr after challenge)

(c) Blood (Hemoccult) in the stool—not present in baseline stool

(d) Leukocytes in Hansel-stained smears of stool mucus not present in baseline stool

(e) Charcot-Leyden crystals or eosinophilic debris in stool mucus not present in baseline stool

As can be seen from this experience, it is well worth confirming the diagnosis in cases of "suspected GFS" to milk and soy, since a significant percentage of these patients have negative responses to challenge, despite an apparent positive response to the antigen withdrawal test. Of course, one cannot eliminate the possibility that these patients were sensitive to a food not tested, or that they "outgrew" the problem in the intervening months; in any event, since most younger infants derive the majority of their caloric and nutritional requirements from the formula portion of their diet, a negative response to one of these standard formulas simplifies further dietary management. Conversely, a positive response tends to have the effect of certifying the diagnosis, in the minds of the physicians as well as the family, which is an equally important outcome in a situation which will require long-term dietary compliance for proper management.

V. THERAPEUTIC APPROACH

Based on our experience with patients with FPIE, we recommend the following approach for suspected GFS:

1. Place the infant on Nutramigen only.
2. Show normalization of stool frequency, consistency, absence of blood, cells, and eosinophils, and normal weight gain with normal caloric intake for at least 1 month. (If height and weight have fallen below the 5th percentile, we usually do not consider a diagnostic challenge until the infant is back up to the percentile growth level achieved prior to the illness.)
3. Diagnostic oral milk and soy challenges (most infants have been exposed to both milk and soy proteins).
4. If both challenges are negative, we place the infant on a cow's milk-based formula and ask the parents to add no other foods until we evaluate chronic tolerance at a clinic visit one to two months later. (See Table 3 for criteria

Table 3   Criteria for Chronic Formula Tolerance

Evaluated after receiving only the challenge formula for one–two months
1. Absence of gastrointestinal symptoms (vomiting or diarrhea)
2. Weight gain appropriate for caloric intake
3. Normal stool frequency and consistency (by history)
4. Normal results from stool examination on follow-up clinic visit (consistency, absence of blood, leukocytes, and eosinophilic debris)
5. No change in serum albumin
6. Normal white blood count and differential
7. Normal D-xylose absorption test

---

for chronic tolerance.) To date, all infants with the FPIE syndrome less than 9 months of age at the time of challenge have tolerated the formula chronically, if they had a negative acute challenge. A negative acute challenge is less predictive of chronic tolerance in older infants with this syndrome, and it may be very different for other syndromes and symptoms. If the formula is tolerated chronically, we suggest the addition of solid foods, one new one each week (after 6 months of age).

5. If milk challenge is negative, but soy positive, we use the same strategy as above, but suggest that introduction of solid food be delayed until the infant reaches 1 year of age.

6. If both challenges are positive, we suggest a low-antigen formula regime be maintained until 1 year of age with introduction of solid foods delayed until then. Although Nutramigen is most often utilized for the initial antigen withdrawal trial, if the low-antigen regimen is to be extended over a greater length of time, the possibility of the mother's beginning to breast feed again should be discussed with the parents. The financial, nutritional, and immunological advantages of breast milk over Nutramigen are obvious. However, reinduction of breast feeding in the infant's mother is not always feasible in the context of the family's lifestyle, baby's age, etc.

A potential contraindication to breast feeding of infants with GFS are the recent reports of what appear to be GFS in breast-fed babies. The best documented report of this problem, the combined experience of two large medical centers over a 5-year period, describes six infants with mild chronic diarrhea associated with melena. Colitis, documented by proctoscopy and fecal leukocytes, disappeared when breast milk was withdrawn and reappeared when it was reintroduced. In none of the cases was the diarrhea severe enough to result in dehydration or failure to gain weight (20). A mechanism for the GFS in breast-fed infants is suggested by the finding of small amounts of dietary protein, antigenically intact, in some breast milk samples. Despite this, it is quite rare for this problem to be of sufficient magnitude to result in *any* symptoms, and in the rare cases that it does, the symptoms are most often milder than those described above. On the other hand, the amount of unhydrolyzed, intact casein in Nutramigen varies from batch to batch. Despite this, more than 95% of our patients with GFS receiving Nutramigen tolerate the small varying amount of antigen quite well clinically.

Although the antigen withdrawal and rechallenge method has been detailed for only one syndrome of GFS, namely, FPIE, a similar approach can be used for the other syndromes, choosing from the constellation of findings one or two of the simplest but most objective measures to follow. For less specific symptoms, such as colic, vomiting, or nonspecific diarrhea, it may be wise to look for additional associated signs, since it is much more difficult to evaluate a challenge result that depends on a single subjective symptom. For example, a number of infants we see with vomiting as a symptom of GFS also have eosinophils in their stools. Also, in Lothe's study (21) of 60 infants with colic symptoms which responded to withdrawal of antigen (Nutramigen), although no other gastrointestinal symptoms were described at presentation, 10 of the 11 infants who underwent an official diagnostic challenge by the authors developed vomiting and diarrhea in addition to "colic" following challenge. In the case where only a single nonspecific symptom ("fussiness-colic") with no associated findings is available, it may be necessary to follow Goldman's original dictum of three separate challenges with the same symptom response and time course following each challenge (22).

Finally, there are perhaps three disadvantages to long-term use of Nutramigen. The first and most obvious is its cost—at least 2 1/2 times the cost of milk or soy. Added to this is the difficulty in obtaining it widely. It is not usually a "stock item" at most pharmacies or groceries. Finally, there is the concern about the potential effect on neurological development of the high levels of some plasma amino acids described in infants on predominately casein-containing formulas (23), as the amino acids in Nutramigen are totally casein derived. This may be of importance only in very young infants; more research will be necessary before this can be answered definitively.

ACKNOWLEDGMENTS

Studies described here were carried out at the Clinical Research Center, University of Texas Medical Branch supported by a grant (RR-73) from the General Clinical Research Center Program of the Division of Research and Resources, National Institutes of Health. These studies also were supported by the National Institutes of Health, National Institute of Child Health and Human Development, NOI HD 92834.

REFERENCES

1. Bachman, K. D., and Dees, S. C. Milk allergy I. Observations on incidence and symptoms in "well" babies. *Pediatrics* 20, 393–399, 1957.

2. Waldmann, T. A., Wochner, R. D., Laster, L., and Gordon, R. S., Jr. Allergic gastroenteropathy a cause of excessive gastrointestinal protein loss. *N. Engl. J. Med.* 276, 761–769, 1967.

3. Wilson, J. F., Lahey, M. D., and Heiner, D. C. Studies on iron metabolism. V. Further observations on cow's milk-induced gastrointestinal bleeding in infants with iron-deficiency anemia. *J. Pediatr.* 84, 335–344, 1974.

4. Woodruff, C. W., and Clark, J. L. The role of fresh cow's milk in iron deficiency I. Albumin turnover in infants with iron deficiency anemia. *Am. J. Dis. Child.* 24, 18–23, 1972.

5. Rubin, M. I. Allergic intestinal bleeding in the newborn: A clinical syndrome. *Am. J. Med. Sci.* 200, 385–390, 1940.

6. Gryboski, J. D. Gastrointestinal milk allergy in infants. *Pediatrics* 40, 354–362, 1967.

7. Powell, G. K. Milk-and-soy induced enterocolitis of infancy: Clinical features and standardization of challenge. *J. Pediatr.* 93, 553–560, 1978.

8. Hansel, F. K. Cytologic diagnosis in respiratory allergy and infection. *Ann. Allergy* 24, 564–659, 1966.

9. Powell, G. K. Enterocolitis in low-birth-weight infants associated with milk and soy protein intolerance. *J. Pediatr.* 88, 840–844, 1976.

10. Kuitunen, P., Visakorpi, J. K., Savilahti, E., and Pelkonen, P. Malabsorption syndrome with cow's milk intolerance: Clinical findings and course in 54 cases. *Arch. Dis. Child.* 50, 351–356, 1975.

11. Iynkaran, N., Robinson, M. J., Prathap, K., Sumithran, E., and Yadav, M. Cow's milk protein-sensitive enteropathy. Combined clinical and histological criteria for diagnosis. *Arch. Dis. Child.* 53, 20–26, 1978.

12. Morin, C. L., Buts, J. P., Weber, A., Roy, C. C., and Brochu, P. One-hour blood-xylose test in diagnosis of cow's milk protein intolerance. *Lancet* i, 1102–1104, 1979.

13. Bendal, S., Chan-Yeung, M., Ashley, M. J., Enarson, D., and Lam, S. C. Does a family history of allergy predict immediate skin reactivity? *Can. Med. Assoc. J.* 132, 34–37, 1985.

14. McDonald, P. J., Goldblum, R. M., Van Sickle, G. J., and Powell, G. K. Food protein-induced enterocolitis: Altered antibody response to ingested antigen. *Pediatr. Res.* 18, 751–755, 1984.

15. Goldman, A. S., Sellers, W. A., Ralpern, S. R., Anderson, D. W., Furlow, T. E., Johnson, C. H., and collaborators. Skin testing of allergic and normal children with purified milk proteins. *Pediatrics* 32, 572–579, 1963.

16. Bock, S. A., and May, C. D. True manifestations of sensitivity reactions to foods and the associated immunologic findings. In *The Mucosal System in Health and Disease. Report of the Eighty-First Ross Conference on Pediatric Research.* Ogra, P. L., and Bienenstock, J. (eds.). Ross Laboratories, Columbus, Ohio, 1981, pp. 114–118.

17. Kletter, B., Gerg, I., Freier, S., Noah, Z., and Davies, M. A. Immunoglobulin E antibodies to milk proteins. *Clin. Allergy* 1, 249–255, 1971.
18. Van Sickle, G. J., Powell, G. K., McDonald, P. J., and Goldblum, R. M. Milk and soy protein-induced enterocolitis: Evidence for lymphocyte sensitization to specific food proteins. *Gastroenterology*, in press, 1985.
19. Ashkenazi, A., Levin, S., Idar, D., Ayala, O., Rosenberg, I., and Handzel, Z. T. In vitro cell-mediated immunologic assay for cow's milk allergy. *Pediatrics* 66, 399–402, 1980.
20. Lake, A. M., Whitington, P. F., and Hamilton, S. R. Dietary protein-induced colitis in breast-fed infants. *J. Pediatr.* 101, 906–910, 1982.
21. Lothe, L., Lindberg, T., and Jakobsson, I. Cow's milk formula as a cause of infantile colic: A double-blind study. *Pediatrics* 70, 7–10, 1982.
22. Goldman, A. S., Anderson, D. W., Sellers, W. A., Saperstein, S., Kniker, W. T., Halpern, S. R., and collaborators. Oral challenge with milk and isolated milk proteins in allergic children. *Pediatrics* 32, 425–443, 1963.
23. Raiha, N. C. R., Heinonen, K., Rassin, D. K., and Gaull, G. E. Milk protein quantity and quality in low-birth-weight infants: 1. Metabolic responses and effects on growth. *Pediatrics* 57, 659–674, 1976.

11

Carbohydrate Malabsorption

Jay A. Perman
Johns Hopkins University School of Medicine and Johns Hopkins Hospital, Baltimore, Maryland

I. INTRODUCTION

Carbohydrate malabsorption may occur in a variety of conditions affecting the infant (Table 1). Malabsorption of sugar is most commonly associated with injury of the small bowel mucosa. Other causes of carbohydrate malabsorption in infants include immaturity or congenital absence of enzymatic or transport processes needed to assimilate sugars.

Protein hydrolysate-containing formulas may be appropriate in treating a number of these conditions by virtue of their sugar composition alone, or because their protein, fat, *and* sugar content represent the most easily digestible mix of macronutrients for the condition being treated. For example, infants with severe nonspecific injury of the absorptive surface impairing assimilation of protein and sugars may require a hydrolyzed protein, disaccharide-free formula to avoid diarrhea and recover or maintain nutritional status. Similarly, infants with cow milk protein-sensitive enteropathy and associated villous injury may require a hydrolyzed protein lactose-free feeding.

This chapter will review the normal physiology of carbohydrate digestion and absorption, the pathophysiology of sugar absorption with emphasis on conditions where a protein hydrolysate formula might be indicated, current diagnostic techniques for the identification of carbohydrate malabsorption, and therapeutic strategies for the infant who malabsorbs sugar.

Table 1 Examples of Conditions Associated with
Carbohydrate Malabsorption

Primary
  Glucose-galactose malabsorption
  Congenital lactase deficiency
  Sucrase-isomaltase deficiency
Ontogenetic
  Lactase deficiency of the premature infant
Secondary
  Cow's milk- and soy protein-sensitive enteropathy
  Gluten-sensitive enteropathy
  Giardia lamblia infestation
  Contaminated small bowel syndrome
  Rotavirus infection

II. PHYSIOLOGY OF CARBOHYDRATE DIGESTION AND ABSORPTION

Carbohydrates represent 35-50% of the calories contained in infant formulas. The infant ingests sugars primarily as the disaccharides lactose and sucrose, and as starch. Infants receiving fruits, soft drinks, and honey receive additional sugar as fructose. Small amounts of nondigestible carbohydrates are ingested as cellulose.

Since carbohydrates must cross the mucosa in monosaccharide form as glucose, galactose, and fructose, all ingested sugars require reduction to their hexose components prior to absorption and transport by the enterocyte (Fig. 1) (1). Lactase and sucrase are carbohydrases with active hydrolytic sites at the brush-border surface of the small intestinal absorptive cell (2,3). These enzymes hydrolyze the dietary disaccharides lactose and sucrose, respectively, to their constituent monosaccharides. Lactose is the disaccharide present in cow's milk protein-containing formulas and breast milk. This sugar is split by lactase to glucose and galactose. Lactase activity is the rate-limiting step in the digestion and absorption of lactose (4). That is to say, release of glucose and galactose proceeds at a rate insufficient to give maximal rates of active transport. In contrast, brush-border sucrase is present in excess relative to the rate of absorption of its constituent hexoses, glucose and fructose. The relative difference in "reserves" of lactase and sucrase is generally offered as the basis for the clinical observation that lactose malabsorption is more likely than sucrose malabsorption following mucosal injury (1).

Starches are polymers of glucose which initially require hydrolysis in the intestinal lumen to shorter glucose chains by salivary and pancreatic amylase. The

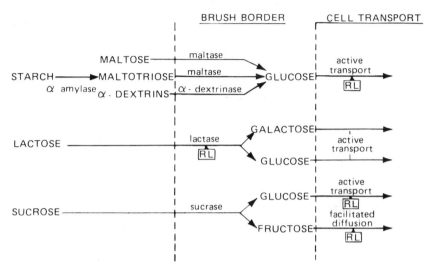

Figure 1 Schematic diagram of starch, lactose, and sucrose absorption. RL indicates the rate-limiting step in the overall digestion and absorption of the dietary sugar. (Modified from Ref. 1, with permission of the publisher.)

residual chains are then cleaved to free glucose by brush-border sucrose-alpha-dextrinase and glucoamylase (5).

Monosaccharides released by the action of intraluminal and surface hydrolysis require specific transport mechanisms for entry into the intestinal absorptive cell and subsequent exit into the intercellular spaces. Glucose and galactose share a common active transport mechanism. Affinity of these monosaccharides to the carrier is enhanced by simultaneous binding of sodium to the transporter (6). Fructose is absorbed by an independent transport mechanism, and absorption of this sugar appears to occur by facilitated diffusion (1,7).

III. CONSEQUENCES OF CARBOHYDRATE MALDIGESTION AND MALABSORPTION

Dietary sugars escaping small bowel absorption cause fairly typical symptoms and signs in the infant. These include watery diarrhea, abdominal distention, and flatulence. These manifestations can be understood when the pathophysiology of carbohydrate malabsorption is considered. Mechanisms associated with carbohydrate malabsorption are illustrated in Figure 2, using lactose malabsorption

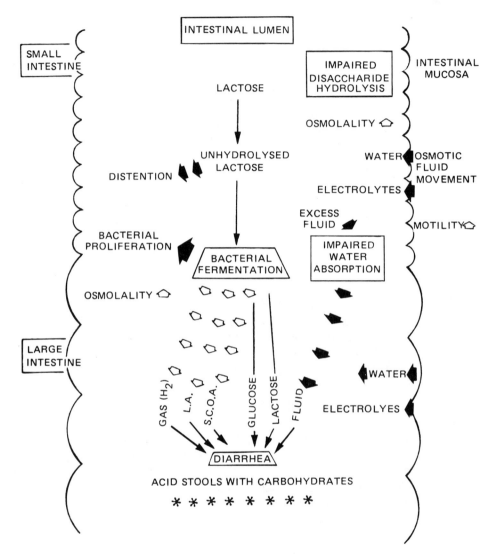

Figure 2 Mechanisms responsible for diarrhea and gas production in infants with sugar malabsorption, using lactose malabsorption as an example. (From Ref. 8, reproduced with permission of the publisher.)

as an example (8). Unabsorbed sugars in the lumen of the small bowel exert significant osmotic pressure, resulting in secretion of fluid and electrolytes (9). Carbohydrates escaping absorption may also stimulate proliferation of a colonic-type flora in the upper bowel which contributes to the osmotic load by further impairing sugar digestion and absorption (10).

The increased volume of water reaching the colon from the small intestine is sustained and augmented by the osmotic effect of malabsorbed sugars, a portion of which reaches the feces, and by production of osmotically active short-chain organic acids by bacteria. However, lactic and other acids resulting from fermentation of sugar by colonic organisms are largely absorbed (11). Thus, bacterial metabolism of dietary sugars to osmotically active but absorbable products in the form of organic acids reduces the fecal water volume which would otherwise result from malabsorbed carbohydrate (12-14). The degree to which the colonic flora ameliorate the fluid loss attributable to osmotically active sugar in the colon of the infant is unknown.

The bacterial processes which lead to the production of short-chain organic acids also result in production of hydrogen and carbon dioxide (15). Production of these gases causes the flatulence commonly observed in infants with carbohydrate malabsorption, and contributes to their abdominal distention.

Malabsorption of sugars may have serious metabolic consequences. Since fermentation of carbohydrate by bacteria results in generation of an excess of hydrogen ions and organic acids, metabolic acidosis may ensue. The presence of organic acids stimulates bicarbonate secretion to neutralize intraluminal contents, and it is also possible that absorption of organic acids produced by intestinal bacteria may result in a systemic acidosis (16).

IV. DISORDERS OF CARBOHYDRATE ABSORPTION

Malabsorption of carbohydrates in infancy may occur in primary, ontogenetic, or secondary form. Primary or congenital forms of carbohydrate malabsorption include glucose-galactose malabsorption, congenital lactase deficiency, and congenital sucrase-isomaltase deficiency. Glucose-galactose malabsorption is a rare autosomal recessive disorder characterized by an inability to transport monosaccharides in the intestine and kidney tubules (17). Fortunately, fructose absorption is normal, permitting carbohydrates in the diet in this form. Glucose-galactose malabsorption presents with diarrhea at birth if the infant is fed any standard formula or breast milk.

Similarly, congenital lactase deficiency presents at birth with diarrhea if the infant is fed a lactose-containing formula (18). This disorder is extremely rare, and there are very few patients with unequivocal evidence of absent lactase activity at birth. Congenital lactase deficiency must not be confused with primary or adult-onset lactase deficiency, a condition which occurs sometime following weaning, and, is thus an entity not seen in infancy.

Congenital sucrase-isomaltase deficiency is somewhat more common, particularly among Greenland Eskimos in whom the incidence approaches 10% (19). This disorder presents with diarrhea upon introduction of sucrose-containing formula or foods such as fruits to the infant.

The ontogenetic form of carbohydrate malabsorption occurs due to functional immaturity of the infant's digestive system. Fetal development of intestinal lactase occurs relatively late in gestation and some very premature infants may not be able to hydrolyze the amount of lactose in human milk or lactose-containing formulas (16,20). Unlike primary forms of carbohydrate malabsorption, lactose malabsorption in the premature infant is transient. Similarly, starch maldigestion in infancy due to immaturity of pancreatic amylase secretion is transient and does not appear to be an important clinical condition, perhaps due to compensatory hydrolysis of starch by salivary amylase and brush-border glucoamylase (21).

In contrast, malabsorption of sugars secondary to a variety of disorders which affect the intestinal mucosa is extremely common in infancy. Insufficient surface absorptive area will impair sugar absorption due to inadequate exposure of carbohydrates to enzymatic and transport mechanisms. Thus, the infant with short bowel is likely to malabsorb sugars (22). Clinically important sugar malabsorption may occur when the brush border is injured by microbial organisms including viruses, parasites, and bacteria. Rotavirus infection is commonly associated with transient intolerance to lactose (23). Similarly, significant *Giardia lamblia* infestation can result in secondary carbohydrate malabsorption. Contamination of the upper small bowel by bacteria also induces diarrhea through interference with intestinal transport processes as well as degradation of the brush-border enzymes (10). Injury to the small bowel mucosa leading to carbohydrate malabsorption may also be induced by dietary factors. The infant who has celiac disease may be intolerant to lactose for a number of weeks after gluten is removed from the diet (24). Lactose absorption recovers as the mucosal injury heals.

V. RELATIONSHIP OF PROTEIN SENSITIVITY AND CARBOHYDRATE MALABSORPTION

Exposure of a cow milk or soy protein-sensitive infant to offending proteins will result in carbohydrate malabsorption. Powell (25) demonstrated prompt development of carbohydrate malabsorption within 24 hours following oral challenge of milk- and/or soy-allergic infants with formulas containing these proteins. The infants had no evidence of sugar malabsorption immediately prior to challenge. Further evidence of the association between dietary protein-induced enteropathy and sugar malabsorption is provided by Walker-Smith (26), who demonstrated in a series of infants recovering from acute gastroenteritis that feeding of breast milk containing 7% lactose did not induce diarrhea, whereas cow milk feeding containing identical amounts of lactose caused a recurrence of diarrhea accompanied by sugar in the stool.

These observations can readily be understood in view of the mucosal injury associated with cow milk- or soy protein-induced enteropathy (27–29). Numerous investigators have demonstrated reduction in disaccharidase activity following small intestinal mucosal damage due to protein sensitivity (26,30–32). Depletion of disaccharidase activity may not be limited to lactase, but may also include brush-border amylase and sucrase activity. Impairment of monosaccharide absorption in some infants with cow milk protein-sensitive enteropathy has also been reported (31,33). Failure to absorb hexoses may be mediated by severe mucosal injury, or by concomitant small bowel bacterial overgrowth which affects glucose transport.

Sufficient data do not exist to accurately establish recovery for normal carbohydrate absorption in infants recovering from protein-mediated injury of the small bowel. Rate of recovery of disaccharidase activity after intestinal injury is variable after this or any other insult, may occur over weeks to months, and may not necessarily parallel histologic recovery of the absorptive surface (34).

VI. DIAGNOSIS OF CARBOHYDRATE MALABSORPTION

How does one identify sugar malabsorption, and assess recovery of absorptive capacity? The fate of malabsorbed carbohydrates reaching the colon forms the basis for screening tests designed to demonstrate sugar malabsorption. These tests include reducing sugars in the stool, fecal pH measurements, and the breath hydrogen test.

A. Sugar in Feces

Tests for reducing sugars in the stool are based on excretion of carbohydrate in the feces (35). The test is performed by placing a small amount of fecal material in a test tube. The stool is then diluted with twice its volume of water and 15 drops of the resulting suspension are placed in a second test tube together with a Clinitest tablet. The resulting color is compared with the chart provided in the Clinitest kit for testing of urine. Positive results are considered to be $\geq$ 0.5%. A result of 0.25% is considered equivocal. Sucrose is not a reducing sugar. Consequently, an accurate test for sucrose malabsorption requires the use of 1 N hydrochloric acid instead of water, followed by brief boiling. Validity of sugar detection in stool requires the presence of the suspected sugar in the infant's diet.

B. Fecal pH

Production of organic acids by bacterial fermentation forms the basis for utilizing fecal pH measurements as a screening test for sugar malabsorption (35).

Validity of this test, like the Clinitest, requires the presence of the suspected offending sugar in the infant's diet. The fecal pH test is performed by dipping Nitrazine paper into the most liquid part of a fresh stool. The resulting color of the paper is compared with the chart provided. A fecal pH $\leq$ 5.5 is considered abnormal.

C. Breath Hydrogen Test

The most accurate noninvasive test currently available for identifying carbohydrate malabsorption is the H_2 breath test following administration of a sugar load (36–38). H_2 in breath results when carbohydrate escaping small bowel absorption is fermented by colonic bacteria. A portion of the H_2 produced is absorbed into the portal circulation and excreted in breath. The substrate for the test is chosen according to the function being assessed. For example lactose is the substrate used when lactose malabsorption is suspected. The test is commonly performed after an overnight fast, but fasting may be shortened in the smaller infant. A baseline sample of expired air is obtained followed by administration of an oral load of the test sugar, usually 2 g/kg with a maximum of 50 g as 20% solution. In infants less than 6 months, this author generally recommends a 10% solution to reduce the osmolality. Doses and concentration should also be reduced when severe intolerance is suspected. A positive test is indicated by a $\geq$ 20 ppm rise above baseline. A rise of 10–20 ppm is equivocal unless there has been a steady rise in the H_2 concentration above the fasting value. Rises less than 10 ppm above the baseline are considered indicative of a negative test.

Previous evidence has indicated that the breath H_2 technique may be utilized using formula as a substrate (39). It is, therefore, feasible to incorporate breath hydrogen tests with the cow milk or soy protein challenge described by Powell (25) (see Chapter 10). Thus, the child with documented or suspected protein sensitivity and carbohydrate malabsorption can be studied for both acquisition of tolerance to the protein and resolution of carbohydrate malabsorption. We perform the test as described by Powell with 100 cc of the test formula. Samples of breath for H_2 determination are collected before and every 30 minutes for 3 hours following the administration of the formula challenge.

The breath H_2 test has largely replaced the oral tolerance test in which an oral load of a specific sugar is administered followed by frequent determinations of serum glucose. This test can be distorted by variations in gastric emptying and intermediary glucose metabolism. Krasilnikoff et al. (40) have reported a 30% false-positive rate for this test in infants. It should be noted that *unabsorbed sugar* cannot be measured by the tolerance test, whereas breath measurements directly address the clinical question: Is malabsorption occurring?

While small bowel biopsy with measurement of disaccharidase activity is helpful in assessing intestinal injury, the disaccharide assay itself may suffer from the fact that enzyme activity in a biopsy may not accurately reflect the capacity of the entire small bowel to absorb sugar (34). This is particularly true when lactose malabsorption results from mucosal injury due to a variety of causes.

VII. MANAGEMENT OF CARBOHYDRATE MALABSORPTION

Treatment of carbohydrate malabsorption in infancy requires removal of the offending sugar from the diet. Numerous proprietary formulas are available, permitting easy modification of the infant's carbohydrate intake (Table 2). The occasional infant with a *primary form* of carbohydrate malabsorption requires prolonged adherence to an appropriate diet. Infants with glucose-galactose malabsorption are treated by elimination of all dietary sugars with the exception of fructose. This is best accomplished by the use of a formula which is carbohydrate free to which fructose is added. Since no defect in protein digestion and absorption exists, a protein hydrolysate formula is not required. Similarly, infants with congenital sucrase-isomaltase deficiency require restriction of sucrose intake. They may be managed using a standard lactose-containing formula.

Transient or ontogenetic lactose malabsorption occurring with prematurity may be managed using formulas designed for prematures which provide a portion of the carbohydrate in the form of glucose polymers. These formulas include Enfamil Premature, Similac Special Care, and Preemie SMA. No more than 60% of the carbohydrate content of these formulas consists of lactose. While the carbohydrate content of generally available protein hydrolysate formulas, in-

Table 2 Examples of Formulas Useful for Infants with Carbohydrate Malabsorption

---

Mono- and disaccharide free
  Mead Johnson 3232A[a,b]
  Ross Carbohydrate Free
Glucose polymers
  Isomil SF
  Pregestimil[a,b]
  Prosobee
Sucrose containing
  Isomil[c]
  Nursoy
  Nutramigen[a,b]

---

[a]Contains small amounts of modified starch as stabilizer.
[b]Protein hydrolysate formulas.
[c]Contains 50 glucose polymers.

cluding Pregestimil and Nutramigen, is also lactose-free, there is otherwise no rationale for their use as a standard infant feeding in the well premature.

The design of protein hydrolysate formulas makes them particularly useful in a variety of conditions associated with *secondary* carbohydrate malabsorption. Protein hydrolysate formulas are lactose free, and are also available in sucrose and glucose polymer-free form. Choice of an appropriate formula depends on the degree to which carbohydrate absorption is impaired. On the basis of previously discussed considerations, impairment of absorption generally progresses in the order lactose/sucrose/glucose. The infant with injury severe enough to impair monosaccharide absorption requires a mono- and disaccharide-free formula. Formulas such as Ross Carbohydrate-Free (RCF), which contains soy protein, may be used unless the infant is thought to be soy protein sensitive or at risk for soy protein sensitization. When soy protein sensitization is a concern, a protein hydrolysate, mono- and disaccharide-free formula such as Mead Johnson 3232A is more suitable. In using these products, carbohydrate must initially be provided parenterally. Dextrose or glucose polymers may be added to the formula in increasing amounts as tolerance to monosaccharides improves. A similar approach is useful in infants with monosaccharide malabsorption due to bacterial overgrowth during the initial days of treatment with oral antibiotics.

If monosaccharide absorption is intact but disaccharidase activities are suppressed, a protein hydrolysate formula containing glucose polymers, like Pregestimil, is useful in conditions where intake of hydrolyzed protein is also indicated. Such conditions include the presence of sensitivity to both cow's milk and soy protein with an enteropathy extensive enough to decrease both lactase and sucrase activity. This formula may also be appropriate in conditions where the surface absorptive area is insufficient for hydrolysis of both intact proteins and disaccharides. Thus, the infant with a short gut may be successfully alimented with Pregestimil.

The infant who absorbs sucrose and requires a protein hydrolysate formula may receive a protein hydrolysate-sucrose-containing formula such as Nutramigen. If no indication exists for the use of protein hydrolysate in an infant who absorbs sucrose but malabsorbs lactose, a wide variety of lactose-free formulas are available to the infant at considerably lower cost. Virtually all soy protein-containing formulas are lactose free.

VIII. SUMMARY

It is generally agreed that carbohydrate is the nutrient most likely to influence tolerance to a particular infant formula. Carbohydrate digestion and absorption may be impaired in a wide variety of conditions affecting the gastrointestinal tract. Relatively simple, noninvasive office procedures are available to detect sugar malabsorption, and to identify those sugars that can and cannot be tolerated by a particular infant during a given time period. Accurate diagnoses should be made whenever possible so that appropriate choices can be made among the wide variety of proprietary formulas currently available for the infant who malabsorbs sugar.

REFERENCES

1. Gray, G. M. Intestinal disaccharidase deficiencies and glucose-galactose malabsorption. In: *The Metabolic Basis of Inherited Disease*, 5th edition. Stanbury, J. B., Wyngaarden, J. B., Frederickson, D. S., Goldstein, J. L., and Brown, M. S. (eds.). McGraw-Hill, New York, 1983, p. 1729-1742.
2. Miller, D., and Crane, R. K. The digestive function of the epithelium of the small intestine. II. Localization of disaccharide hydrolysis in the isolated brush border portion of intestinal epithelial cells. *Biochim. Biophys. Acta* 52, 293-298, 1961.
3. Dalhquist, A., and Borgstrom, B. Digestion and absorption of disaccharides in man. *Biochem. J.* 81, 411-418, 1961.
4. Gray, G. M., and Santiago, N. A. Disaccharide absorption in normal and diseased human intestine. *Gastroenterology* 51, 489-498, 1966.
5. Gray, G. M., Lally, B. C., and Conklin, K. A. Action of intestinal sucrase-isomaltase and its free monomers on an α-limit dextrin. *J. Biol. Chem.* 254, 6038-6043, 1979.
6. Crane, R. K. Hypothesis for mechanisms of intestinal active transport of sugars. *Fed. Proc.* 21, 891-895, 1962.
7. Gray, G. M., and Ingelfinger, F. J. Intestinal absorption of sucrose in man; interrelation of hydrolysis and monosaccharide product absorption. *J. Clin. Invest.* 45, 388-398, 1966.
8. Lifshitz, F. Carbohydrate problems in paediatric gastroenterology. *Clinics Gastroenterol.* 6, 415-429, 1977.
9. Launialia, K. The effect of unabsorbed sucrose and mannitol on the small intestinal flow rate and mean transit time. *Scand. J. Gastroenterol.* 39, 665-671, 1968.
10. Perman, J. A. Carbohydrate intolerance and the enteric microflora. In: *Carbohydrate Intolerance in Infancy*, Lifshitz, F. (ed.). Marcel Dekker, New York, 1982, p. 137-152.
11. Ruppin, H., Bar-Meir, S., Soergel, K. H., Wood, C. M., and Schmitt, M. G., Jr. Absorption of short chain fatty acids by the colon. *Gastroenterology* 78, 1500-1507, 1980.
12. Bond, J. H., Jr., and Levitt, M. D. Fate of soluble carbohydrate in the colon of rats and man. *J. Clin. Invest.* 57, 1158-1164, 1976.
13. Bond, J. H., and Levitt, M. D. Quantitative measurement of lactose absorption. *Gastroenterology* 70, 1058-1062, 1976.
14. Bond, J. H., Currier, B. E., Buchwald, H., and Levitt, M. D. Colonic conservation of malabsorbed carbohydrate. *Gastroenterology* 78, 444-447, 1980.
15. Newcomer, A. D., McGill, D. B., Thomas, P. J., and Hofman, A. F. Prospec-

tive comparison of indirect methods for detecting lactase deficiency. *N. Engl. J. Med.* 293, 1232-1236, 1975.

16. Lifshitz, F., Diaz-Benussen, S., Martinez-Garza, V., Abdo-Bassols, F., and Diaz de Castillo, E. Influence of disaccharides on the development of systemic acidosis in the premature infant. *Pediatr. Res.* 5, 213-225, 1971.

17. Elsas, L. J., Hillman, R. E., Patterson, J. H., and Rosenberg, L. E. Renal and intestinal hexose transport in familial glucose-galactose malabsorption. *J. Clin. Invest.* 49, 576-585, 1970.

18. Lifshitz, F. Congenital lactase deficiency. *J. Pediatr.* 69, 229-237, 1966.

19. McNair, A., Gudmand-Hoyer, E., Jarnum, S., and Orrild, L. Sucrose malabsorption in Greenland. *Br. Med. J.* 2, 19-21, 1972.

20. MacLean, Jr., W. C., Fink, B. B. Lactose malabsorption by premature infants: Magnitude and clinical significance. *J. Pediatr.* 97, 383-388, 1970.

21. Lee, P. C. Alternate pathways in starch digestion. In: *Carbohydrate Intolerance in Infancy*, Lifshitz, F. (ed.). Marcel Dekker, New York, 1982, p. 223-233.

22. Bury, K. D. Carbohydrate digestion and absorption after massive resection of the small intestine. *Surg. Gynecol. Obstet.* 135, 177-187, 1972.

23. Schreiber, D. S., Trier, J. S., and Blacklow, N. R. Recent advances in viral gastroenteritis. *Gastroenterology* 73, 174-183, 1977.

24. Katz, A. J., and Falchuk, Z. M. Current concepts in gluten sensitive enteropathy (celiac sprue). *Pediatr. Clin. North Am.* 22, 767-786, 1975.

25. Powell, G. K. Milk- and soy-induced enterocolitis of infancy. *J. Pediatr.* 93, 553-560, 1978.

26. Walker-Smith, J. A. Interrelationship between cow's milk protein intolerance and lactose intolerance. In: *Carbohydrate Intolerance in Infancy*, Lifshitz, F. (ed.). Marcel Dekker, New York, 1982, p. 155-171.

27. Shiner, M., Ballard, J., Brook, C. G. D., and Herman, S. Intestinal biopsy in the diagnosis of cow's milk protein intolerance without acute symptoms. *Lancet* II, 1060-1063, 1975.

28. Ament, M. E., and Rubin, C. E. Soy protein -another cause of the flat intestinal lesion. *Gastroenterology* 62, 227-234, 1972.

29. Kuitunen, P., Visakorpi, J. K., Savilahti, E., and Pelkonen, P. Malabsorption syndrome with cow's milk intolerance: Clinical findings and course in 54 cases. *Arch. Dis. Child.* 50, 351-356, 1975.

30. Poley, J. R., Bhatia, M., and Welsh, J. D. Disaccharidase deficiency in infants with cow's milk protein intolerance. *Digestion* 17, 97-107, 1978.

31. Iyngkaran, N., Abdin, Z., Davis, K., Boey, C. G., Prathap, K., Yadav, M., Lam, S. K., and Puthucheary, S. D. Acquired carbohydrate intolerance and cow milk protein-sensitive enteropathy in young infants. *J. Pediatr.* 95, 373-378, 1979.

32. Maluenda, C., Phillips, A. D., Briddon, A., and Walker-Smith, J. A. Quantitative analysis of small intestinal mucosa in cow's milk protein intolerance (cow's milk allergy). The American College of Allergists Third International Food Allergy Symposium, 1980.

33. Goel, K., Lifshitz, F., Khan, E., and Teichberg, S. Monosaccharide intolerance and soy-protein hypersensitivity in an infant with diarrhea. *J. Pediatr.* 93, 617-19, 1978.
34. Harrison, M., and Walker-Smith, J. A. Reinvestigation of lactose intolerant children: Lack of correlation between continuing lactose intolerance and small intestinal morphology, disaccharidase activity, and lactose tolerance tests. *Gut* 18, 48-52, 1977.
35. Silverman, A., and Roy, C. C. *Pediatric Clinical Gastroenterology.* C. V. Mosby, St. Louis, 1983, p. 893.
36. Barr, R. G., Perman, J. A., Schoeller, D. A., and Watkins, J. B. Breath tests in pediatric gastrointestinal disorders: New diagnostic opportunities. *Pediatrics* 62, 393-401, 1978.
37. Perman, J. A., Barr, R. G., and Watkins, J. B. Sucrose malabsorption in children: Noninvasive diagnosis by interval breath hydrogen determination. *J. Pediatr.* 93, 17-22, 1978.
38. Barr, R. G., Watkins, J. B., and Perman, J. A. Mucosal function and breath hydrogen excretion: Comparative studies in the clinical evaluation of children with nonspecific abdominal complaints. *Pediatrics* 68, 526-533, 1981.
39. Solomons, N. W., Garcia-Ibanez, R., and Viteri, F. E. Hydrogen breath test of lactose absorption in adults: The application of physiological doses and whole cow's milk sources. *Am. J. Clin. Mutr.* 33, 545-554, 1980.
40. Krasilnikoff, P. A., Gudmand-Hoyer, E., and Moltke, H. H. Diagnostic value of disaccharide tolerance tests in children. *Acta Paediatr. Scand.* 64, 693-698, 1975.
41. Gray, G. M. Progress in gastroenterology. Carbohydrate digestion and absorption. *Gastroenterology* 58, 96–107, 1970.

12

Fat Malabsorption

Jon A. Vanderhoof
University of Nebraska, Omaha, Nebraska

I. INTRODUCTION

Fat constitutes approximately 40% of the calorie intake in the average American diet; comparable levels of fat are also included in most infant formulas (1). Most dietary fat is present in the form of triglycerides or triacylglycerols, formed from three fatty-acid chains on a glycerol backbone. Besides triglycerides, other dietary lipids include phospholipids and cholesterol as well as fat-soluble vitamins and certain other sterols. As much as 90% of dietary triglycerides are the long-chain variety, usually 16 or 18 carbon chains with varying degrees of saturation, and the remaining 10% are medium-chain triglycerides, usually with carbon chains ranging from 6 to 12 (2).

Lipids are relatively insoluble in water, a property that creates major problems in digestion and absorption in the aqueous environment of the intestinal lumen. For this reason, bile acids, 24C carboxylic acids derived from cholesterol metabolism, are required to solubilize lipids in the aqueous phase of the gut lumen (3).

Malabsorption of fat may occur in many situations. As digestion and absorption of fat is a multistage process, depending on the disease process involved, malabsorption of fat may be impaired at one or more different stages. Appropriate therapy for fat malabsorption is generally dependent upon the specific stage affected.

II. LIPOLYSIS

The first stage of fat absorption is that of digestion or lipolysis. Each triglyceride, more properly called triacylglycerol, must be hydrolyzed to two fatty acids and one 2-monoglyceride (4). Hydrolysis occurs primarily by pancreatic lipase at the one and three positions leaving monoglycerides, some diglycerides, and free-fatty acids (FFA). Dietary phospholipids are comparably hydrolyzed, primarily by phospholipase (5). Pancreatic colipase is also required in this process, and facilitates lipase action by binding to bile salt lipid surfaces and improving the interaction of lipase with triglyceride. Bile salts themselves facilitate the activity of pancreatic lipase, which functions well at the intraduodenal pH 6-6.5 (6-8).

Release of cholecystokinin (CCK) from duodenal epithelium occurs primarily in response to lipid and protein in the duodenal lumen, and stimulates pancreatic secretion, gallbladder contraction, and simultaneous relaxation of the sphincter of Oddi. This maximizes efficiency of hydrolysis by providing adequate concentration of enzyme, bile salt, buffer, and cofactor for mixing in the duodenum.

The major clinical problem observed in this stage is pancreatic insufficiency. In the pediatric age group, this most often results from cystic fibrosis, as 90% of children with cystic fibrosis have pancreatic insufficiency (9-11). Other causes include Shwachman syndrome (pancreatic insufficiency with neutropenia). During infancy when pancreatic function is diminished, substantial hydrolysis may occur in the stomach due to gastric and salivary lipase activity, and may account for 15-20% of total lipid hydrolysis (11-16). Preterm infants, therefore, have a relative degree of pancreatic insufficiency, as do term infants although to a lesser degree (17,18).

Therapy for pancreatic insufficiency consists of oral pancreatic enzyme supplementation. Enteric-coated oral preparations are preferable because they resist inactivation in the acid pH of the stomach. Enzymes should be administered to the patient during feedings to optimize mixing with enteric contents (9,19).

As small preterm infants have partial pancreatic insufficiency, special formulas are available to meet their specific needs. A portion of the fat in these formulas is provided as medium-chain triglyceride, which does not require hydrolysis for absorption (20).

III. MICELLAR SOLUBILIZATION AND
PENETRATION OF THE UNSTIRRED LAYER

The second phase of fat absorption is micellar solubilization, largely a function of bile salts. Trihydroxy or dihydroxy bile acids are synthesized in the liver and subsequently conjugated with either taurine or glycine (3). A full 80% of bile acids are primary, including cholic acid and chenodeoxycholic acid. The remaining 20% are produced through the metabolic action of bacteria, forming deoxycholic acid from cholic acid and lithocholic acid from chenodeoxycholic acid.

Bile salts are capable of solubilizing lipids because of their amphiphilic properties (3). These molecules have both a hydrophobic and a hydrophilic end. The final end products of lipase action aggregate with the bile salts with hydrophilic portions of molecules facing the water interface and hydrophobic ends facing the interior lipid molecules. The end result is a disc-shaped, water soluble, mixed bile layer micelle containing fatty acids, monoglycerides, phospholipids, cholesterol, and fat-soluble vitamins (A, D, E, and K).

The overall rate-limiting step of lipid absorption is diffusion through the unstirred water layer, the stagnant fluid layer immediately adjacent to the epithelial surface (21). Long-chain monoglycerides and fatty acids, because of their poor solubility, penetrate the unstirred layer poorly unless incorporated into micelles. The major function of the bile acid micelle, therefore, is to permit water-insoluble lipids to penetrate the unstirred layer (22-27).

The complexity of the small intestinal mucosal membrane, because of the villi and microvilli, substantially increase the ratio of the effective surface area of the membrane to the area of the interface between the unstirred water layer and the bulk phase of the intestinal lumen. Solubilized molecules must first penetrate the relatively small area of the unstirred water layer before reaching a vastly greater mucosal surface area. It is estimated that the ratio of effective surface area of the unstirred water layer to the underlying brush-border membrane is at least 1 to 500 (24,27).

The efficacy of bile salt functions in lipid absorption is primarily dependent upon bile salt concentration (28-32). Micelles do not form unless bile salt concentration reaches a state known as critical micellar concentration. Subsequently, complex interrelationships exist between the lipid concentration, micelle size, and ease of diffusion across the unstirred water layer. The net result is at least a 100-fold increase in diffusibility of long-chain fatty acids, monoglycerides, and cholesterol in the presence of adequate bile acid concentration (33).

Once the unstirred water layer is traversed, the micelle must pass through the mucus coat overlying the surface of the brush-border membrane. This layer is less than 1% of the thickness of the unstirred water layer (34). Once the micelle has reached the lipid bilayer brush-border membrane, lipid contents of the micelle are released and bile salts remain within the intestinal lumen to reform other micelles until they are finally reabsorbed in the distal ileum.

Fat malabsorption due to decreased intraluminal bile acid concentration may result from either liver disease or small bowel disease. Liver disease may cause bile acid deficiency either because of decreased production or decreased excretion. In infants, excretory problems include neonatal cholangiopathic disorders such as neonatal hepatitis and biliary atresia, and, less commonly, disorders such as choledochal cyst and congenital intrahepatic biliary hypoplasia (35-40). In older children, chronic active hepatitis, alpha$_1$-antitrypsin disease, cystic fibrosis, and other hepatic disorders may cause bile acid deficiency. Patients on long-term parenteral nutrition, especially small infants, often develop cholestasis. Physiologic bile acid insufficiency may occur in preterm infants resulting in some degree of fat malabsorption (41).

Impaired bile salt reabsorption due to small intestinal disease may likewise deplete the bile acid pool. This usually occurs either because of ileal resection or small bowel bacterial overgrowth (42-44). Patients with Crohn's disease or neonates with necrotizing enterocolitis are likely to undergo ileal resection. Normally, most bile acids are reabsorbed in the terminal ileum, removed from portal blood by the liver, and resected into the bowel, a process known as enterohepatic circulation. Interruption of this process will limit the bile acid concentration to that which can be synthesized in the liver. Because of the liver's limited capacity for synthesis, ileal resection patients often develop bile acid insufficiency. In adults, less than 100 cm of terminal ileal resection does not result in steatorrhea, because increased hepatic synthesis of bile salt can compensate for increased fecal loss, maintaining critical micellar concentration of bile salts in the jejunum. Once greater than 100 cm of ileum has been resected, the maximal increase in hepatic synthesis of bile acids can no longer compensate for increased fecal excretion. In infants and children, proportionally smaller degrees of ileal resection are likely to result in fat malabsorption. Steatorrhea may also result from disorders which cause ileal disease in the absence of resection, such as Crohn's disease.

Small bowel bacterial overgrowth can produce bile acid insufficiency as bacteria deconjugate glycine and taurine from the bile acid molecule, preventing reabsorption (45-47). Bacterial overgrowth may occur in small bowel motility disorders, which increase transit time, and with anatomic strictures such as occur in Crohn's disease or postoperative patients. Patients with short bowel syndrome frequently have bacterial overgrowth, especially after resection of the ileocecal valve. In addition to bile salt malabsorption, massive bacterial overgrowth may cause vitamin B_{12} deficiency resulting in megaloblastic anemia (48).

Cyclic broad-spectrum antimicrobial therapy is often beneficial in the treatment of bacterial overgrowth. Documentation is best obtained through an appropriately collected sterile aspirate of the proximal small intestine, and subsequent identification of the bacterial content. Bacterial counts exceeding 10^5 organisms/ml in the jejunum are generally considered abnormal. Hydrogen breath tests following a glucose or lactulose load may be utilized as a relatively sensitive screening test (49,50). Periodically, a 7-10 day course of broad-spectrum antibiotics such as clindamycin, metronidazole, chloramphenicol, or tetracycline may be necessary. The interval between treatment courses varies greatly; patients may require retreatment after only a few weeks or after several months. Surgical correction of strictures or other anatomic abnormalities may be helpful in many patients. Repeat culture, or evaluation of the degree of steatorrhea, vitamin B_{12} absorption, or breath hydrogen excretion may serve as an indication of successful therapy.

In the absence of bile acids, only about one-third of dietary triglycerides and a small percentage of fatty acids are absorbed. Cholesterol and fat-soluble vitamins, however, are almost totally malabsorbed. If not correctable by elimination of bacterial overgrowth, therapy for bile salt insufficiency consists of decreasing dietary long-chain fats. Because medium-chain triglycerides are less dependent upon bile acids for absorption, substituting a major percentage of dietary long-chain fats with either medium-chain triglycerides or carbohydrates may be helpful (51). Therapeutic administration of exogenous bile is rarely beneficial. While this may increase intraluminal bile acid concentration, the dosages required will usually result in severe diarrhea because of excess bile acid in the colon, which causes fluid secretion. Short bowel syndrome patients are also commonly treated with cholestyramine, a resin which nonspecifically binds bile acids, preventing secretory diarrhea. This practice unfortunately may further enhance bile acid malabsorption and exacerbate bile acid deficiency, resulting in increased fat malabsorption.

Fat-soluble vitamins (A, D, E, and K) are lipids and, therefore, are malabsorbed along with other dietary lipids in patients with steatorrhea. It is usually necessary to administer additional fat-soluble vitamins in these cases. In the case of severe malabsorption, either parenteral or water-soluble oral forms may be needed to maintain adequate serum and tissue levels. Unlike water-soluble vitamins, fat-soluble vitamins are stored in large quantities in the body, and deficiency states may develop slowly.

Medium-chain triglycerides are an important therapeutic modality in the treatment of patients with bile acid deficiency (51). Since administration of exogenous bile often results in intolerable diarrhea, substitution of dietary fat with medium-chain triglycerides may be required to improve fat absorption. Medium-chain triglycerides constitute a mixture of triacylglycerols with fatty acids of chain lengths of C6 to C12, the majority of which are C8, and a smaller percentage C10 (52,53). Owing to their small molecular weight, medium-chain triglycerides are more rapidly hydrolyzed by pancreatic lipase. Hydrolysis of medium-chain triglycerides is rapid and complete; absorption occurs mainly as free-fatty acids rather than mono or diacylglycerols. In the event pancreatic lipase activity is inadequate, a large percentage of medium-chain triglycerides can be absorbed as triacylglycerols.

Medium-chain triglycerides are rapidly oxidized following absorption, producing ketone bodies and supplying a quick source of energy. Oxidation of fatty acids in the liver and utilization of ketone bodies in the extrahepatic tissue provide the major means for metabolism. Recent evidence obtained from studies in rats suggests that medium-chain triglycerides result in less than expected gains in body weight and fat content, most likely due to differences in metabolism or absorption. Substituting long-chain triglycerides with medium-chain triglycerides in preterm infant formulas likewise results in increased total fat absorption, but this does not necessarily translate into improved weight gain, growth, or nutritional status (54,55).

IV. MUCOSAL UPTAKE AND TRANSPORT

Once the major barrier to lipid absorption, the unstirred layer, has been traversed, the lipolytic products pass from the micellar phase into the mucosal cell by a poorly understood process. The mucosal surface membrane itself is a mostly lipid structure in a dynamic state. The length of fatty acids composing the membrane, the degree of unsaturation, and the type of lipids all contribute to the relative fluidity or rigidity of the membrane (56). All of these factors may influence lipid absorption. Most evidence indicates that lipids are absorbed through the mucosal membrane by passive diffusion. However, some data suggests that the uptake of fatty acids across the membrane may be adversely affected by removal of sodium, and that fatty acid uptake is a saturable process exhibiting competitive inhibition (57). Similar evidence has been obtained in studies of cholesterol absorption.

Many disorders which cause damage to the epithelial surface of the proximal small intestine can impair mucosal uptake. Examples include acute viral enteritis, milk and soy protein intolerance with small bowel mucosal injury, celiac sprue, and intestinal stasis syndrome. In each instance, substitution of some dietary long-chain triglycerides with medium-chain triglycerides will result in enhanced fat absorption. Replacement of some fat with carbohydrate is also occasionally helpful, although generalized mucosal diseases also impair carbohydrate and protein absorption.

Most long-chain triglycerides reach the enterocyte in the form of 2-monoacylglycerol and unesterified fatty acids. Once inside the enterocyte, they are immediately resynthesized to triacylglycerols. Two separate enzymatic pathways appear to be involved in this process, both located in the endoplasmic reticulum. Once synthesized, lipid molecules accumulate and coalesce to form lipid droplets within the confines of the smooth endoplasmic reticulum. As the triacylglycerols migrate through the endoplasmic reticular system, newly synthesized lipoproteins are added to begin chylomicron formation. These substances are then transported to the Golgi apparatus within the microtubular system where glycosylation occurs, attaching a carbohydrate moiety to the molecule to form a glycoprotein. The particles then enter the Golgi apparatus where they are packaged into secretory vesicles. Further glycosylation may also occur within the Golgi complex. Triglycerides and esterified cholesterol are now stabilized within a central core formed by more polar molecules including apoproteins, phospholipids, free cholesterol, and some diglycerides. The outer structure of chylomicron then likely fuses with the basolateral membrane of the enterocyte and the content is released into the lamina propria to be carried to the lacteals.

The rate-limiting steps for this process are probably final assembly within the Golgi cells and exocytosis. Microtubules are likely to be important in the intracellular movement of the secretory vesicles from the Golgi apparatus to the basolateral membrane (2).

Abetalipoproteinemia is an example of a disorder in which transport of lipid through the enterocyte is specifically impaired. These patients are unable to synthesize apoprotein B, making chylomicron formation impossible. The clinical syndrome is characterized by failure to thrive after the first year of life, diarrhea, abdominal distention, and subsequent progressive loss of muscle strength, neurological symptoms including ataxia, and the appearance of abnormal red blood cells known as acanthocytes. These patients have decreased serum levels of cholesterol and triglyceride, and serum lipoprotein electrophoretic pattern demonstrates near absence of beta lipoproteins (58). Histologically, enterocytes are engorged with lipid droplets. Additional patients have been reported with similar histological findings, but normal levels of serum apoprotein B, and appear to have a defect in chylomicron secretion (59). In both cases, restricting dietary long-chain fat, and if necessary, supplementation with medium-chain triglycerides is useful in the treatment of the disorder. As in most fat malabsorption syndromes, additional exogenous fat-soluble vitamins must often be administered.

Once chylomicron synthesis has been completed in the Golgi, the secretory vesicles containing chylomicrons migrate through the cytoplasm to the basolateral membrane where they fuse with the lateral plasmalemma. They are then extruded through exocytosis from the secretory vesicles into the lateral intercellular spaces and pass through gaps in the basement membrane. Chylomicrons then diffuse through the lamina propria gaining access to lymphatic channels through gaps between adjacent endothelial cells and are carried through mesenteric lymph channels into the blood stream.

Once chylomicrons have left the enterocyte, disorders which impair lymphatic flow such as intestinal lymphangiectasia may impair fat absorption. Lymphangiectasia may be primary or secondary, and lymphatic compression may occur in a variety of disorders including congestive heart failure, constrictive pericarditis, and cirrhosis. Any disorder which causes inflammation of the mesentery, such as Crohn's disease, may also cause some degree of lymphangiectasis.

Patients with intestinal lymphangiectasia develop ruptured mucosal lacteals which leak lymph into the lumen, resulting in protein and fat loss. Patients typically develop hypoproteinemia, hypogammaglobulinemia, and lymphocytopenia as well as steatorrhea (60). Small bowel biopsy in such patients usually demonstrates widely dilated lacteals within the villi. Because the disease may be patchy, small bowel biopsies are occasionally normal. Some patients with this disorder may be diagnosed endoscopically, as multiple white punctate lesions may be seen in the proximal duodenum, and direct biopsy under visualization will allow histologic confirmation of the diagnosis (61).

Unless lymphatic obstruction is a secondary disorder amenable to medical or surgical therapy, management must be aimed at reducing intestinal lymphatic pressure by reducing long-chain fats in the diet. Although substituting long-chain with medium-chain triglycerides is frequently recommended, this form of dietary management is often unsuccessful. Use of elemental diets very low in total fat content, such as Vivonex*, may be better tolerated in the refractory patient, although administration by continuous enteral infusion is occasionally necessary because of the poor palatability of the diet.

V. APPROACH TO THE PATIENT

From the practical standpoint, it is best to approach the patient with fat malabsorption by considering the pathophysiology involved. However, treatment modalities are somewhat limited. Specific forms of therapy include administration of exogenous pancreatic lipase, useful in patients with pancreatic insufficiency, administration of exogenous bile, rarely beneficial, often exacerbating bile acid-induced diarrhea, and administration of antibiotics in a cyclical fashion, are often helpful in patients with bacterial stasis syndrome. These treatment modalities are specific for certain disorders. However, the dietary substitution with medium-chain triglycerides is useful in a variety of different disorders affecting multiple stages of fat absorption. Likewise, increasing the ratio of carbohydrate and protein to fats in a diet may be useful. In making such adjustments, however, one must consider that disorders which cause fat malabsorption simply because of decreased or injured absorptive surface area may also cause protein and carbohydrate malabsorption. In such patients, supplementing oral intake with intermittent or continuous parenteral nutrition may be necessary.

Both preterm infant and therapeutic infant formulas are available which contain a large percentage of their calories in the form of medium-chain triglycerides. Perhaps the most commonly used medium-chain triglyceride-containing therapeutic formulas are Pregestimil† and Portagen.† Pregestimil is a protein hydrolysate diet designed for use in patients with decreased mucosal function or surface area. This formula is most useful in the treatment of intractable diarrhea of infancy and short bowel syndrome. The fat content of Pregestimil is 38% medium-chain triglycerides; the remainder is in the form of long-chain triglycerides. Portagen has a much higher percentage of medium-chain triglycerides, 85%, but is not a predigested formula, and its major use should be directed toward the treatment of disorders in which medium-chain triglycerides offer specific therapeutic benefit. Examples include intestinal lymphangiectasia, abetalipoproteinemia, and certain disorders of mucosal function in which carbohydrate and protein absorption appear to be relatively preserved. In addition, low

---

*Norwich Eaton Laboratories, Norwich, New York.
†Mead Johnson Laboratories, Evansville, Indiana.

fat elemental diets are available for use in adults, and can occasionally be used in children. Many are currently available, and most are protein hydrolysate based, although Vivonex has an amino acid base. In disorders such as intestinal lymphangiectasia when fat intake, especially long-chain fat intake, must be dramatically restricted, these formulas are useful. Unfortunately, it is possible that increased linoleic acid requirements of growing infants may not be met by these formulas.

VI. EVALUATION OF STEATORRHEA IN THE LABORATORY

The only accurate means of quantifying steatorrhea is determination of 72-hr fecal fat excretion, since almost all fat in the stool is derived from dietary sources. Measuring the fecal fat content is a reliable means of assessing fat malabsorption. However, the technique is cumbersome and samples are difficult to collect, especially in small infants and children.

Before attempting to assess fecal fat excretion, a patient should be placed on a normal diet containing at least 35% of its total calories as fat. This diet should preferably be initiated 5, but at least 2, days prior to the beginning of the test. During the 48 hr preceding the collection and throughout the collection period, total calorie intake must be carefully monitored and recorded. After the initial 48 hr, a 72-hr fecal sample must be obtained. Occasionally, these are obtained between nonabsorbable markers such as charcoal or carmine red.

There are multiple ways to collect stools. In older children, this is usually not a problem. In small children and infants, diapers may be turned inside out or lined with plastic wrap. Ostomy bags can be devised to fit around the anus. Total fat content may be determined titrimetrically or gravimetrically, and the percentage of total fat absorbed calculated to express the coefficient fat absorption, relating the percentage of daily fat excretion to the daily dietary fat intake. Healthy adults and children over 2 years of age absorb greater than 93% of their daily fat intake. Preterm infants may absorb only 60-75% and newborn infants a somewhat greater 80-85%.

Because of the cumbersome nature of assessing steatorrhea directly, numerous indirect tests have been devised in an attempt to screen patients who might need further assessment of fat absorption. None of the tests are totally adequate but some are helpful in evaluating patients with suspected steatorrhea, or in determining response to therapy in infants or children with steatorrheal disorders. Perhaps the simplest screening test is determination of microscopic fat in the stool. However, the Sudan stain for fecal fat is generally considered unreliable. Likewise, specific tests measuring an orally ingested lipid in the serum, such as Lipiodol or vitamin A, are likewise generally unreliable.

In patients with generalized mucosal disease, especially proximal disease such as celiac sprue, measurement of urinary xylose excretion in the older child and adult, or one-hour blood xylose levels after ingestion of an oral D-xylose load may be helpful in assessing the degree of mucosal injury. In some series, however, the test correlates poorly with intestinal biopsy results (62). Xylose is a pentose primarily absorbed by passive diffusion in the proximal small intestine. The percentage of absorption correlates to some degree with the severity and extent of injury in the small bowel, but the tests can be significantly affected by differences in intestinal transit time, gastric emptying, as well as the extent and location of the lesion.

Indirect assessment of fat absorption through measurement of nutrients in the serum which are lipid or lipid soluble are also used to screen for fat malabsorption, as long as one remembers that such studies are diet dependent. Most commonly used is the serum carotene determination. Carotene is a precursor to vitamin A and depends upon normal fat transport for absorption. Carotene levels drop rapidly when dietary intake is low, although vitamin A stores are substantial in the liver and levels remain normal for several months after dietary withdrawal. Carotene levels are useful as a screening test in patients with steatorrhea. Patients who do not eat green and yellow vegetables, however, are frequently deficient in beta-carotene, so the test is not useful in infants under 8 months of age not fed green and yellow vegetables or in patients on restricted diets.

Perhaps the most useful test in evaluating patients with steatorrhea is the small bowel biopsy. Peroral small bowel biopsy techniques have been utilized for several years. The suction biopsy apparatus remains the best technique for adequate sampling of the small bowel mucosa. Directable biopsy devices allow small bowel biopsies to be safely obtained on an outpatient basis in very few minutes (63). Endoscopic equipment also permits biopsy of the small intestine; however, specimens are usually inadequate because these instruments induce crushed artifact, biopsy only the most proximal small intestine, and obtain small tissue samples which are frequently inadequate for complete histological examination.

Small bowel biopsies provide a variety of information. Evaluation of mucosal detail, exclusion of specific disorders such as intestinal lymphangiectasia and abetalipoproteinemia, and determination of the severity and extent of mucosal inflammatory disease are all possible. Enzymatic assays of biopsy material for disaccharidase content can be utilized to correlate function with the degree of histologic injury. In the case of pancreatic disease, or bile salt deficiency, small bowel biopsy is of little value.

There are a variety of approaches to patients with steatorrhea. Screening tests should generally be performed initially to determine if steatorrhea is present. Serum carotene in children over 8 or 9 months of age is usually helpful provided that it is done fasting and only performed on children who have a normal dietary intake of green and yellow vegetables. If the serum carotene is low, steatorrhea should be suspected. Cystic fibrosis should be excluded by determination of sweat chloride. Other disorders suspected clinically should be excluded, but usually in the absence of cystic fibrosis or liver disease, small bowel mucosal disease is likely and a small bowel biopsy can then be performed. If the biopsy is normal, further assessment of pancreatic function and bile salt concentration may be necessary. Assessment of pancreatic enzyme function will require performance of a duodenal drainage procedure stimulating pancreatic secretion with secretin and cholecystokinin.

VII. SUMMARY

Fat absorption is a complex process characterized by many different stages. Malabsorption of fat may be caused by disorders which affect one or more of these stages. Therapy is most successful when directed at the specific cause of the absorptive defect. A variety of drugs, dietary manipulations, and special use formulas are available for treatment of these problems and are quite beneficial when utilized appropriately.

REFERENCES

1. Food and Nutrition Board, National Research Council. *Recommended Dietary Allowances.* Ninth Edition. National Academy of Sciences, Washington, D.C., 1980.
2. Friedman, H. I., and Nylund, B. Intestinal fat digestion, absorption, and transport. A review. *Am. J. Clin. Nutr.* 33, 1108-1139, 1980.
3. Hofmann, A. F., and Small, D. M. Detergent properties of bile salts: Correlation with physiological function. *Annu. Rev. Med.* 18, 333, 1967.
4. Kayden, H. J., Senior, J. R., and Mattson, F. H. The monoglyceride pathway of fat absorption in man. *J. Clin. Invest.* 46, 1695, 1967.
5. Borgstrom, B. Phospholipid absorption. In *Lipid Absorption: Biochemical and Clinical Aspects.* Rommell K., Goebell H., and Bohmer R. (eds.). University Park Press, Baltimore, 1971, pp. 65-70.
6. Borgstrom, B., and Erlanson, C. Pancreatic juice colipase: Physiological importance. *Biochim. Biophys. Acta.* 242, 509-513, 1971.
7. Borgstrom, B., and Erlanson, C. Pancreatic lipase and colipase. Interactions and effects of bile salts and other detergents. *Eur. J. Biochem.* 37, 60-68, 1973.
8. Verger, R., Rietsch, R., and Desnuelle, P. Effects of co-lipase on hydrolysis of monomolecular films by lipase. *J. Biol. Chem.* 252, 4319, 1977.
9. Vanderhoof, J. A. Nutritional and gastrointestinal problems in cystic fibrosis. *Pract. Gastroenterol.* 6, 40-44, 1982.
10. Kopel, F. B. Gastrointestinal manifestations of cystic fibrosis. *Gastroenterology* 62, 483-491, 1972.
11. Shwachman, H. Gastrointestinal manifestations of cystic fibrosis. *Pediatr. Clin. North Am.* 22, 787-805, 1975.

12. Plucinski, T. M., Hamosh, M., and Hamosh, P. Fat digestion in rat: Role of lingual lipase. *Fed. Proc.* 37, 700, 1978.

13. Borgstrom, B., Dahlquist, A., Lundh, G., and Sjovall, J. Studies of intestinal digestion and absorption in the human. *J. Clin. Invest.* 36, 1521-1536, 1957.

14. Cohen, M., Morgan, G. R. G., and Hofmann, A. F. Lipolytic activity of human gastric and duodenal juice against medium- and long-chain triglycerides. *Gastroenterology* 60, 1-15, 1971.

15. Hamosh, M., Klaevemen, H. L., Wolf, R. O., and Scow, R. O. Pharyngeal lipase and digestion of dietary triglyceride in man. *J. Clin. Invest.* 55, 908-913, 1975.

16. Hamosh, M., Sivasubramanian, K. N., Salzman-Mann, C., and Hamosh, P. Fat digestion in the stomach of premature infants. *J. Pediatr.* 93, 674-682, 1978.

17. Hadorn, B., Zoppi, G., Shmerling, D. H., Prader, A., McIntyre, I., and Anderson, C. M. Quantitative assessment of exocrine pancreatic function in infants and children. *J. Pediatr.* 73, 39-50, 1968.

18. Lebenthal, E., and Lee, P. C. Development of functional response in human exocrine pancreas. *Pediatrics* 66, 556-560, 1980.

19. Regan, P. T., Malagelada, J-R., DiMagno, E. P., Glanzman, S. L., and Go, V. L. W. Comparative effects of antacids, cimetidine and enteric coating on the therapeutic response to oral enzymes in severe pancreatic insufficiency. *N. Engl. J. Med.* 297, 854-858, 1977.

20. Greenberger, N. J., and Skillman, T. G. Medium-chain triglycerides. Physiologic considerations and clinical implications. *N. Engl. J. Med.* 280, 1045, 1969.

21. Thomson, A. B. R. Intestinal absorption of lipids: Influence of the unstirred water layer and bile acid micelle. In *Disturbances in Lipid and Lipoprotein Metabolism.* Dietschy, J. M., Gotto, A. M., Jr., and Ontko, J. A. (eds.). American Physiological Society, Bethesda, 1978, pp. 29-55.

22. Dietschy, J. M., Sallee, V. L., and Wilson, F. A. Unstirred water layers and absorption across the intestinal mucosa. *Gastroenterology* 61, 932-934, 1971.

23. Dietschy, J. M. Mechanisms of bile acid and fatty acid absorption across the unstirred water layer and brush border of the intestine. *Helv. Med. Acta.* 37, 89-102, 1973.

24. Westergaard, H., and Dietschy, J. M. Delineation of dimensions and permeability characteristics of the two major diffusion barriers to passive mucosal uptake in rabbit intestine. *J. Clin. Invest.* 54, 718-732, 1971.

25. Winne, D. Unstirred layer thickness in perfused rat jejunum in vivo. *Experientia* 1278-1279, 1976.

26. Read, N. W., Barber, D. C., Levin, R. J., and Holdsworth, C. D. Unstirred layer and kinetics of electrogenic absorption in the human jejunum in situ. *Gut* 18, 865-876, 1977.

27. Wilson, F. A., and Dietschy, J. M. The intestinal unstirred layer: Its surface area and effect on active transport kinetics. *Biochim. Biophys. Acta.* 363, 112-126, 1974.

28. Carey, M. C., and Small, D. M. Micelle formation by bile salts. *Arch. Intern. Med.* 130, 506-527, 1972.

29. Carey, M. C., and Small, D. M. Micelle formation by bile salts. Physical, chemical and thermodynamic considerations. *Arch. Intern. Med.* 130, 506-527, 1972.

30. Hofmann, A. F. Molecular association in fat digestion. Interaction in bulk of monolein, oleic acid and sodium oleate with dilute, micellar bile salts solutions. *Adv. Chem.* 84, 53-66, 1968.

31. Hofmann, A. F., and Borgstrom, B. The intraluminal phase of fat digestion in man: The lipid content of the micellar and oil phases of intestinal content obtained during fat digestion and absorption. *J. Clin. Invest.* 43, 247-257, 1964.

32. Hofmann, A. F., Thistle, J. L., Klein, P. D., Szczepanik, P. A., and Yu, P. Y. S. Chemotherapy for gallstone dissolution. II. Induced changes in bile composition and gallstone response. *JAMA* 239, 1138-1144, 1978.

33. Hofmann, A. F. Fat digestion: The interaction of lipid digestion products with micellar bile acid solutions. In *Lipid Absorption: Biochemical and Clinical Aspects.* Rommel K., Goebell H., and Bohmer R. (eds.). University Park Press, Baltimore, 1976, pp. 3-18.

34. Smithson, K. W., Millar, D. B., Jacobs, L. R., and Gray, G. M. Intestinal diffusion barrier: Unstirred water layer or membrane surface mucous coat? *Science* 214, 1241, 1981.

35. Cottrall, K., Cook, P. J. L., and Mowat, A. P. Neonatal hepatitis syndrome and alpha-1-antitrypsin deficiency. *Postgrad. Med. J.* 50, 435–439, 1974.

36. Odievre, M., Martin, J-P., Hadchouel, M., and Alagille, D. Alpha-1-antitrypsin deficiency and liver disease in children: Phenotypes, manifestations, and prognosis. *Pediatrics* 57, 226-231, 1976.

37. Sass-Kortsak, A. Management of young infants presenting with direct-reacting hyperbilirubinemia. *Pediatr. Clin. North Am.* 21, 777-799, 1974.

38. Alagille, D. Clinical aspects of neonatal hepatitis. *Am. J. Dis. Child.* 123, 287-291, 1972.

39. Aagenaes, O., Matlary, A., Elgjo, K., Munthie, E., and Fagerhol, M. Neonatal cholestasis in alpha-1-antitrypsin deficient children. *Acta Pediatr. Scand.* 61, 632-642, 1972.

40. Vanderhoof, J. A., and Antonson, D. L. Neonatal hepatitis and biliary atresia. In *Practice of Pediatrics.* Kelly V. C. G. (ed.). Harper and Row, Philadelphia, 1982.

41. Watkins, J. B., Szczepanik, P., Gould, J. B., Klein, P., and Lester, R. Bile salt metabolism in the human premature infant, preliminary observations of pool size and synthesis rate following prenatal administration of dexamethasone and phenobarbital. *Gastroenterology* 69, 706-713, 1975.

42. Rosenberg, I. H., Hardison, W. G., and Bull, D. M. Abnormal bile-salt patterns and intestinal bacterial overgrowth associated with malabsorption. *N. Engl. J. Med.* 276, 1391, 1967.

43. Donaldson, R. M., Jr. Studies on the pathogenesis of steatorrhea in the blind loop syndrome. *J. Clin. Invest.* 44, 1815, 1965.

44. Gray, Gary M. Maldigestion and malabsorption: Clinical manifestations and specific diagnosis. In *Gastrointestinal Disease*, Third Edition. Sleisenger M. H., and Fordtran J. S. (eds.). W.B. Saunders Company, Philadelphia, 1983, pp. 229-256.

45. Gracey, M., Burke, V., Oshin, A., et al. Bacteria, bile salts and intestinal monosaccharide malabsorption. *Gut* 12, 683-692, 1971.

46. Hofmann, A. G., and Poley, J. R. Role of bile acid malabsorption in pathogenesis of diarrhea and steatorrhea in patients with ileal resection. I. Response to cholestyramine or replacement of dietary long-chain triglyceride by medium-chain triglyceride. *Gastroenterology* 62, 918-934, 1972.

47. Donaldson, R. M., Jr. Small bowel bacterial overgrowth. *Adv. Intern. Med.* 16, 191, 1970.

48. Badenoch, J., Bedford, P. O., and Evans, J. R. Massive diverticulosis of the small intestine with steatorrhea and megaloblastic anemia. *Q. J. Med.* 24, 321, 1955.

49. Metz, G., Cassull, M. A., Drasar, B. S., Jenkins, D. J. A., and Blendis, L. M. Breath-hydrogen test for small intestinal bacterial colonization. *Lancet* 1, 668, 1976.

50. Rhodes, J. M., Middleton, P., and Jewell, D. P. The lactulose hydrogen breath test as a diagnostic test for small-bowel bacterial overgrowth. *Scand. J. Gastroenterol.* 4, 333, 1979.

51. Hofmann, A. F., and Poley, J. R. Role of bile acid malabsorption in pathogenesis of diarrhea and steatorrhea in patients with ileal resection. I. Response to cholestyramine or replacement of dietary long chain triglyceride by medium chain triglyceride. *Gastroenterology* 62, 918-934, 1972.

52. Greenberger, N. J., and Skillman, T. G. Medium-chain triglycerides. Physiologic considerations and clinical implications. *N. Engl. J. Med.* 280, 1045-1057, 1969.

53. Bach, A. C., and Babayan, V. K. Medium-chain triglycerides: An update. *Am. J. Clin. Nutr.* 36, 950-962, 1982.

54. Okamoto, E., Muttart, C. R., Zucker, C. L., and Heird, W. C. Use of medium-chain triglycerides in feeding the low-birth-weight infant. *Am. J. Dis. Child.* 136, 428-431, 1982.

55. Geliebter, A., Torbay, N., Bracco, E. G., Hashim, S. A., and Van Itallie, T. B. Overfeeding with medium-chain triglyceride diet results in diminished deposition of fat. *Am. J. Clin. Nutr.* 37, 1-4, 1983.

56. Chapman, D. Properties of cell membranes and penetration by lipid molecules. In *Lipid Absorption: Biochemical and Clinical Aspects*. Rommel K., Goebell, H., and Bohmer, R. (eds.). University Park Press, Baltimore, 1976, pp. 37-47.

57. Thomson, A. B. R., and Dietschy, J. M. Intestinal lipid absorption: Major extracellular and intracellular events. In *Physiology of the Gastrointestinal Tract*. Johnson, L. R. (ed.). Raven Press, New York, 1981, pp. 1147-1220.

58. Azibi, E., Zaidman, J. L., Eschar, J., and Szeinberg, A. Abetalipoproteinemia treated with parenteral and oral vitamins A and E and with medium chain triglycerides. *Acta Paediatr. Scand.* 67, 797-801, 1978.

59. Roy, C. C., Sniderman, A., Deckelbaum, R., Letarte, J., Brochu, P., Weber, A., Morin, C. L., and Justine, J.-P. Normal concentrations of serum and increased intestinal apo B with failure of chylomicron secretion: A new disorder of lipid transport (abstr.) *Pediatr. Res.* 16, 175A, 1982.
60. Vardy, P. A., Lebenthal, E., and Shwachman, H. Intestinal lymphangiectasis: A reappraisal. *Pediatrics* 55, 842-851, 1975.
61. Antonson, D. L. Personal communication.
62. Christie, D. L. Use of the one-hour blood xylose test as an indicator of small bowel disease. *J. Pediatr.* 92, 725, 1978.
63. Vanderhoof, J. A., Hunt, L. I., Antonson, D. L. A rapid procedure for small intestinal biopsy in infants and children. *Gastroenterology* 80, 938-941, 1981.

13

Dietary Management of Postinfectious Chronic Diarrhea in Malnourished Infants

Ulysses Fagundes-Neto
Escola Paulista de Medicina, São Paulo, Brazil

Fima Lifshitz
Cornell University Medical College, New York, and North Shore University Hospital, Manhasset, New York

Angel Cordano
Mead Johnson Nutritional Division, Evansville, Indiana

I. INTRODUCTION

Acute diarrhea is the major cause of death in infancy in developing countries and is the main factor inducing malnutrition. Estimates of 1 billion episodes of diarrhea and 4.6 million deaths in infants under 5 years of age were reported in 1980 in third world countries (1). During the first year of life, children in India have an average of 5 to 6 episodes of diarrhea per year (2). Diarrhea may lead to losses of fluids and electrolytes with intravascular depletion of water and electrolytes of variable degrees. Hypovolemic shock and death may rapidly ensue if fluids and electrolytes are not replaced. Diarrhea also increases the risk of malnutrition by a variety of mechanisms reviewed in detail elsewhere (3,4).

It is well known that some enteropathogenic microorganisms are capable of inducing functional and morphologic alterations in the small bowel, contributing to intestinal malabsorption of nutrients. The adherent strains of *Escherichia coli* and rotavirus, for example, may provoke severe mucosal injury leading to chronic diarrhea and nutrient malabsorption (5,6). Several authors have reported complications such as disaccharidase deficiencies with disaccharide intolerance, particularly of lactose (7); but, at times carbohydrate malabsorption involving all dietary sugars occurs with the development of acquired monosaccharide intolerance (8). These patients may have severe alterations of intestinal morphology (9) and bacterial proliferation in the upper portions of the small bowel (10,

11). Bacterial proliferation, particularly of anaerobes such as Bacteroides, induce 7-alpha-dehydroxylation and deconjugation of bile salts (12,13). Free bile salts in the small intestine may cause disruption of the intestinal mucosa, thereby altering the barrier of permeability and allowing the penetration of intact macromolecules (14). There may be potentially antigenic proteins absorbed, leading to cow's milk protein and soybean protein sensitivity (15,16). The above-mentioned factors present in patients with gastroenteritis may lead to malabsorption of dietary nutrients, aggravation of the nutritional status, and persistence of diarrhea.

In this chapter, we describe some of the factors of environmental contamination in a city slum (*favela*) in São Paulo, Brazil, which may account for the high incidence of diarrhea in infancy in transitional societies. We also describe some of the pertinent clinical aspects and intestinal alterations of these infants who also develop postinfectious chronic diarrhea. Finally, we present some data regarding the dietary management of such patients. Here we point out the great dilemma that impoverished, malnourished individuals face. The best care and dietary treatment of chronic diarrhea for these patients is the most expensive one. They require intense nutritional rehabilitation with special formulas and/or total parenteral nutrition (TPN). Therefore, we emphasize the need to prevent the vicious cycle of diarrhea and malnutrition by attacking it at its roots; that is, improving the environmental conditions where these infants live and encouraging the use of breastfeeding.

II. THE HAZARDOUS EFFECTS OF ENVIRONMENTAL CONTAMINATION ON SLUM AREA INFANTS

Several studies have demonstrated a lower incidence of diarrhea in breastfed infants during the first months of life (17,18). This may be due to the protective immune factors present in breast milk, such as leukocytes, specific immunoglobulins, and nonspecific anti-infectious factors. However, an equal, if not more important protective feature of exclusive breastfeeding is that these infants avoid ingesting contaminated foods. Poor socioeconomic conditions, illiteracy, poor sanitation and sewage systems, and lack of a safe water supply are but a few causal factors of the prevalence of diarrhea and malnutrition in the developing world. It is estimated that 78% of the rural population in the third world lacks a clean water supply and 85% have no adequate sewage and other excreta disposal facilities. This situation is even more serious in the large urban cities of developing countries where poverty belts surround the big cities.

During the last decades, there has been a massive migration from the rural areas toward the large urban centers throughout the world. Brazil has suffered this phenomenon in a very intensive way. The population in the urban areas, as compared with the rural sections of the country, has increased from 36% in

1950, to 45% in 1960, and 56% in 1970. Presently, it is estimated that the urban population has risen to 70% of the entire population. This population is settled in many urban centers throughout the country, principally in crowded slums around the large cities.

São Paulo, the most important industrial city in Latin America, is also the largest Brazilian city, with 15 million inhabitants (Greater São Paulo). During the 1970s, São Paulo's general population increased 43.3%, the rate of people living in the slums grew 684%. This migratory mass is comprised of low income families with practically no professional skills. They came to the urban areas with the illusion of finding better living conditions. The abrupt change in the distribution of the Brazilian population within its territory brought with it numerous problems in settling the new migrants. The large urban centers had insufficient infrastructural conditions to adequately accommodate the newcomers. The three most basic living conditions could not be supplied: housing, water supply, and sewage.

In a recent study performed by Dr. Fagundes-Neto and his co-workers (19, 20), an assessment was made of the social and economic conditions of a slum population. The nutritional status of children under 10 years of age living in a favela community was measured by anthropometry, and the level of environmental contamination was tested by performing stool cultures and parasitologic analysis.

This study was conducted in the Cidade Leonor slum which was formed about 30 years ago on the outskirts of São Paulo. This favela has changed drastically in the last 15 years, reaching its present severely overcrowded condition. The estimated population is 3700 inhabitants, of which 1200 are children under 10 years of age. The *barracos* were built along a stream that crosses the slum, in an area of about 100 meters, making irregular contours in the slum borders. The barracos vary in size and material used for their construction, but the great majority are made out of wood, measuring about 3 x 4 m. The structure of the barracos is wood derived from leftovers of the construction phase of regular city buildings (concrete forms, protection walls, etc.). Barracos are normally one single room, two rooms at the most. There is no sewage system, although sometimes a collective water supply as well as electricity can be found.

The survey indicated that 74.6% of the population came from the rural areas of North and Northeast regions of Brazil, the poorest in the country. They had a very low level of education, 75% of the childrens' parents were illiterate. The monthly average family income was lower than US$135 in 58.7% of the population and the income per capita was as low as US$35/month in 72.1%. The average number of people per barraco was 5.33, thus, each person occupied a mean area of 2 square meters.

Breastfeeding was not usual in this community. Information on the practice of breastfeeding was available for 520 children; 176 (33.9%) had never received

Table 1 Parasites Isolated in the Stools of the Children Living in Cidade
Leonor Slum

Ascaris lumbricoides	9
Ascaris lumbricoides + Trichocephalus trichiurus	14
Ascaris lumbricoides + Trichocephalus trichiurus + Giardia lamblia	8
Ascaris lumbricoides + Trichocephalus trichiurus +	
Giardia lamblia + Hymenolepsis nana	1
Ascaris lumbricoides + Giardia lamblia + Hymenolepsis nana	1
Ascaris lumbricoides + Giardia lamblia	5
Ascaris lumbricoides + Trichocephalus trichiurus +	
Cisto Giardia lamblia	2
Ascaris lumbricoides + Hymenolepsis nana	3
Ovos *Ascaris lumbricoides*	5
Ovos *Ascaris lumbricoides* + Cisto *Giardia lamblia*	1
Ovos *Ascaris lumbricoides* + Ovos Anciolostomideos +	
Ovos *Trichocephalus trichiurus*	1
Cisto *Giardia lamblia*	5
Giardia lamblia	3
Giardia lamblia + Hymenolepsis nana	1
Enterobius vermicularis + Trichocephalus trichiurus	1
Trichocephalus trichiurus	8
Hymenolepsis nana	5
Tenia solium + Giardia lamblia	1
Negatives	9

the benefits of breastfeeding, 150 (28.8%) were breastfed for less than 1 month
of life. Forty-five (8.6%) were breastfed for less than 2 months, 40 (7.7%) were
breastfed for less than 3 months of life. Only 109 (21.0%) were breastfed for
longer than 3 months of life. This practice is in marked contrast with the cul-
tural habits of the same population living in rural centers before migration.
There, breastfeeding is an unusual practice at times extending beyond the first
year of life.

The evaluation of the nutritional status of children living in this favela by the
Seoane and Latham criteria (21) showed the following results: 43.1% were well
nourished, 24.6% had acute malnutrition, 19.0% had nutritional dwarfism, 9.2%
exhibited chronic progressive malnutrition and 4.1% had chronic malnutrition
in recovery. In contrast, the average birth weight for favela children was 3150 g
distributed as follows: 8.8% had birth weight lower than 2500 g, 32.1% had
birth weight between 2500 and 3000 g, and 59.1% of the children had birth
weight over 3000 g.

The search for ova and parasites in the stools of these children revealed impressive rates of parasitosis; all but 9 of them had two or more parasites in their stools (Table 1). The microbiologic survey of the stools of children under 5 years of age also showed a high frequency of various enteropathogenic bacteria and rotavirus isolated from the stools of children living in this favela (Table 2). The random examination of 224 infants less than 2 years of age, living in the favela revealed that almost one-half of them (107) were sick with diarrhea at any given time. There were frequent enteropathogenic microorganisms (56.7%) isolated from children with diarrhea, but there were also frequent pathogenic bacteria found (32.5%) in children without diarrhea ($p < 0.05$ chi square test).

The high rate of diarrhea in these infants is not surprising due to the prevalent contamination with parasites and enteropathogenic organisms. The lack of apparent disease in the slum infants who had no diarrhea despite the presence of similar stool pathogens is of interest. How such living conditions with such high prevalence of infection permits the existence of infants with apparent normal nutrition and no diarrhea needs to be studied further. However, this study of a slum community did characterize the deleterious effects of the environment on most children. The important factors that make these children prone to acquire repeated intestinal infections at an early stage of life are: unfavorable environmental conditions, high levels of fecal contamination, low socioeconomic levels with poor living conditions, and the low frequency of breastfeeding. As seen, the combination of these negative influences of the environment are often associated with diarrhea and malnutrition.

III. CHRONIC POSTINFECTIOUS DIARRHEA IN INFANCY

Chronic postinfectious diarrhea is extremely frequent in underdeveloped countries. As mentioned above, this is due to a variety of factors pertaining to the unfavorable sanitary, social, and economic conditions that affect most of the population. The result is chronic, repeated infections, chronic diarrhea, and malnutrition.

Chronic postinfectious diarrhea in infancy is a clinical entity currently referred to by various terms. Avery et al. (22) in 1968, coined the term *intractable diarrhea*. Lifshitz et al. in 1970 described it as monosaccharide intolerance (8), and subsequently Hyman et al., in 1971, introduced the term *protracted diarrhea* (23). Schwachman et al. (24), in 1973, described severe morphological changes of the small bowel in a group of patients with chronic postinfectious diarrhea and emphasized the reversibility of the lesions after parenteral feeding (25). In 1977, Larcher et al. (26) reported the largest series of patients with chronic postinfectious diarrhea, with special emphasis on the etiology of the process and dietary measures.

Table 2 Presence of Enteropathogenic Bacteria and Rotavirus in the Stools of Children Living in Cidade Leonor Slum

	Diarrhea								No diarrhea							
	0-11 months n=(28)		12-23 months n=(55)		≥24 months n=(24)		Total n=(107)		0-11 months n=(20)		12-23 months n=(50)		≥24 months n=(47)		Total n=(117)	
Enteropathogen	No.	%	No.	%	No.	%	No.	%	No.	%	No.	%	No.	%	No.	%
EPEC[b]	1	3.6	2	3.6	1	4.2	4	3.7	1	5.0	5	10.0	0	0.0	6	5.1
E. coli invasive	1	3.6	7	12.7	3	12.5	11	10.3	0	0.0	0	0.0	5	10.6	5	4.3
E. coli enterotoxigenic	1	3.6	6	10.9	0	0.0	7	6.5	2	10.0	1	2.0	3	6.4	6	5.1
Shigella	2	7.1	3	5.5	2	8.3	7	6.5	0	0.0	1	2.0	3	6.4	4	3.4
Salmonella	0	0.0	1	1.8	0	0.0	1	0.9	0	0.0	2	4.0	0	0.0	2	1.7
Yersinia enterocolitica	0	0.0	0	0.0	1	4.2	1	0.9	0	0.0	0	0.0	0	0.0	0	0.0
Campylobacter	3	10.7	4	7.3	3	12.5	10	9.3	3	15.0	2	4.0	3	6.4	8	6.8
Rotavirus	2	7.1	0	0.0	0	0.0	2	1.9	0	0.0	1	2.0	1	2.1	2	1.7
Mixed infections	2	7.1	3	5.5	2	8.3	7	6.5	1	5.0	1	2.0	3	6.4	5	4.3
Total	12	42.9	26	47.3	12	50.0	50	46.7	7	35.0	13	26.0	18	38.3	38	32.5

[a] n = number of children.
[b] Enteropathogenic E. coli.

Here we review the ultrastructural abnormalities found in the intestinal mucosa of malnourished infants with chronic postinfectious diarrhea and the possible implications of food intolerance in the genesis of diarrhea perpetuation. We also report our findings on the response to dietary treatment of such patients. These studies were carried out in the Pediatric Gastroenterology ward of Hospital São Paulo (Escola Paulista de Medicina) in São Paulo, Brazil. In all of these patients, chronic diarrhea followed gastroenteritis and lasted for more than 2 weeks. All patients were less than 1 year of age, and had significant impairment of their nutritional status. The mortality rate of this group of patients was 12.5%; 2 patients died of bronchopneumonia and/or sepsis due to a variety of organisms, i.e., *Staphylococcus aureus* or *Salmonella.* These patients had a course which is similar to the one described many years ago in patients with postinfectious gastroenteritis in Mexico (7,8). Often they did not tolerate lactose and at times there was intolerance to other carbohydrates and proteins (i.e., cow's milk and soy protein).

A. Intestinal Ultrastructural Alterations

Ultrastructural examination of intestinal biopsies from patients with postinfectious chronic diarrhea revealed a spectrum of alterations in the jejunal absorptive epithelium. Studies of cells in the middle third of villi showed enterocytes that ranged from normal to mildly, moderately, and severely damaged (Figs. 1 and 4). These altered epithelial cells were seen at focal sites. The changes varied from patient to patient, all of whom had active postinfectious diarrhea at the time of study. There appeared to be no simple relation between the severity of the morphologic damage observed and the clinical evolution of diarrhea. Clearly, this variation could in part be due to the focal nature of the structural changes in a "patchy" distribution of the lesions in the mucosa.

Some of the alterations in epithelial cells included; (a) a tendency to form tufts (twinning) of microvilli (Fig. 2), (b) blunting of microvilli (Fig. 3), and (c) severe destruction of the absorptive epithelial cell surface including loss of microvilli and vesiculation of intracytoplasmic organelles (Fig. 4). The microvilli were shortened and reduced in number, some areas were completely deprived of microvilli, while others had microvilli that were grouped and completely fused. The intracytoplasmic organelles also presented severe alterations, especially the mitochondria, that were diffusely swollen. The mitochondrial cristae lost the normal structural organization. The endoplasmic reticulum was also swollen, and free ribosomes scattered throughout the cytoplasm could be identified. Endocytotic activity was increased with a considerably increased number of multivesicular bodies.

The ultrastructural abnormalities described in our patients may reflect the existence of numerous well known alterations in the microecology of the small intestine of infants with chronic postinfectious diarrhea (27). Special emphasis

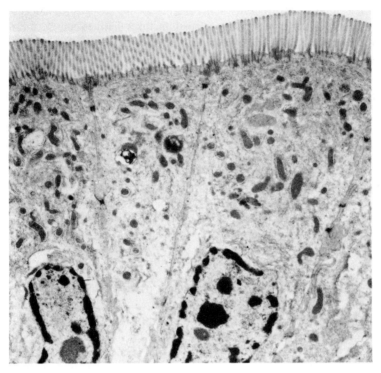

Figure 1 Electron micrograph of one absorptive epithelium from a patient with postinfectious chronic diarrhea, showing cells with normal morphology.

should be placed on the considerably increased number of multivesicular bodies frequently observed in most of the specimens of the small intestine obtained from our patients. This may indicate the existence of a significant absorption of potentially antigenic macromolecules by endocytosis. Furthermore, other alterations described here, such as shortening and destruction of the microvilli, or even lesions of the intracytoplasmic organelles, may cause the occurrence of the functional alterations observed in this group of patients leading to or contributing to chronic diarrhea. However, more studies need to be done to elucidate why some malnourished patients with postinfectious chronic diarrhea have a normal histological and ultrastructural organization. The reason for the lack of a strict correlation between clinical status and the degree of structural damage needs to be detailed further.

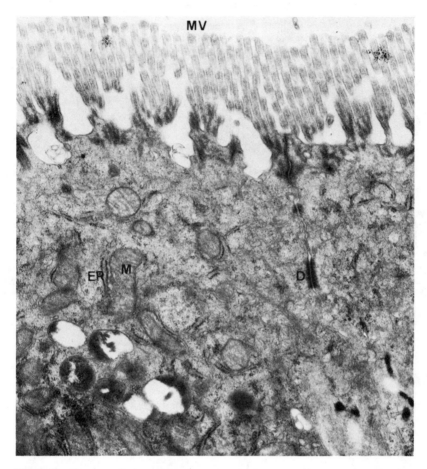

Figure 2 Portion of the absorptive epithelial surface from another infant with postinfectious chronic diarrhea that shows a mild cellular abnormality. Note the tufted or "twinned" microvilli (MV) at the apical mucosal surface. Mitochondria are unaltered (M), endoplasmic reticulum (ER), desmosome (D).

B. Response to Dietary Management of Malnourished Infants with Postinfectious Chronic Diarrhea

The cause of chronic diarrhea following gastroenteritis is ill defined, although it is characterized by nutritional deterioration of the patient and the presence of intestinal malabsorption and various degrees of intestinal mucosal damage. It is

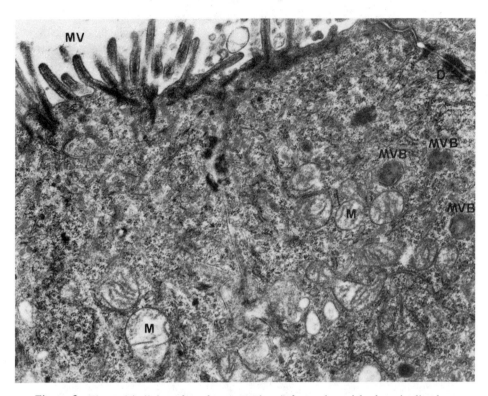

Figure 3 The epithelial surface from another infant, also with chronic diarrhea in which there is blunting of microvilli (MV) and the presence of apparently increased numbers of multivesicular bodies (MVB). Mitochondria M, desmosome D.

a well known clinical observation that infants with gastroenteritis who do not improve rapidly may deteriorate as the diarrhea persists and becomes chronic (7). These patients may develop further alterations in the absorption of carbohydrates, and at times monosaccharide intolerance may ensue (8), requiring the elimination of all carbohydrates from the diet before recovery can be achieved. Often the elimination of all feedings is needed. These patients only improve when total parenteral nutrition is administered (22–26). With improved technology of total parenteral nutrition, mortality associated with chronic diarrhea in infancy has been reduced to minimal levels of 10% in many specialized highly advanced technological centers (28). However, in most places throughout the world where this condition is prevalent, this form of therapy is still very expensive and risky for treatment of the malnourished infant with postinfectious chronic diarrhea.

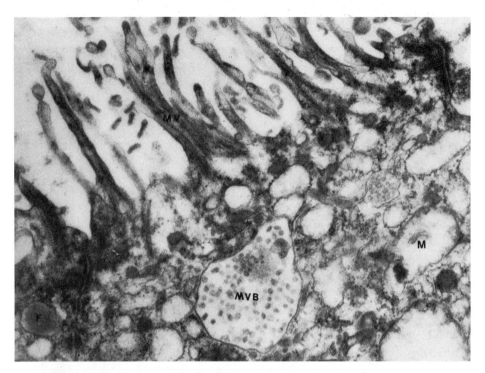

Figure 4 Severely damaged absorptive epithelial cell surface from another infant with chronic diarrhea. Note the absence of microvilli and associated membranous debris. The cytoplasmic compartments are extensively vacuolated and a damaged mitochondrion is at M. A large multivesicular body is at MVB.

The proper selection of specific formulas for treatment of such patients may thus alleviate and decrease the need for total parenteral nutrition in most instances. For years we have advocated the elimination of lactose and other specific carbohydrates for the treatment of infants with diarrhea (29). This recommendation was based on our observations of the presence of frequent lactose intolerance (7), which was confirmed by many other authors (30,31), requiring lactose-free diets before recovery. At times, these patients require disaccharide, glucose polymer, or carbohydrate-free diets before recovery (8,32). However, the appropriate means of feeding infants with chronic diarrhea have been predominantly tested by individual experiences and trial-and-error practices with various feeding regimens or several different modes of administration (28). There is a lack of controlled prospective studies to ascertain the most appropriate nutrients to be used in formulas for feeding infants with chronic postinfectious diarrhea.

We carried out a prospective study in the Escola Paulista de Medicina, São Paulo, Brazil to ascertain the acceptance and tolerance of 29 infants with chronic diarrhea following gastroenteritis to various feedings. These were similar milk formulas which varied only in the dietary protein content, all being lactose and disaccharide free. In these patients the use of a formula with protein hydrolysate and glucose polymers was found to be superior for treatment as compared with the response to feedings of other formulas containing the same carbohydrate with soy or casein base.

All infants studied were less than 9 months of age and had protein calorie malnutrition of various degrees. Diarrhea was chronic in all, and it followed a postinfectious process without improvement until admission to the hospital. During this time the patients were given cow's milk and/or cow's milk formula of various strengths. Diarrhea and other infections had been the cause of prior hospitalizations in most of these patients. Some of the details of the ultrastructural assessment of the mucosa of the small intestine of these patients were described above.

All patients persisted with diarrhea after admission to the hospital while being treated by traditional means of feeding: 1/2 to 2/3 strength cow's milk formula as recommended by the World Health Organization (WHO) (33). Additionally, in all patients there was evidence of lactose intolerance with excretion of acid stools and reducing substances. Selection for dietary treatment is described below.

The patients were divided into three groups at random, and each was initially fed a different formula. The three formulas were made by Mead Johnson, all contained similar concentrations of carbohydrate, fat, protein, minerals, and vitamins. The carbohydrate was 7% corn syrup solids and the protein was either 2.5% hydrolyzed casein, casein, or soy protein isolate. The formula was started as a full-strength substance, quantities sufficient to provide 70 kcal/kg of body weight. The patients who tolerated the formula as determined by improved consistency, decreased number of stools, and the cessation of excretion of acid feces and/or carbohydrates in the stools were given increased quantities of the formula as tolerated until full recovery was obtained. The formula was maintained for a minimum of 2 weeks of normal stools and normal growth. At this point, cow's milk formula was reintroduced to the diet and its tolerance tested.

Those patients who did not tolerate the initial assigned formula were introduced to another formula as shown in Figure 5. The duration of the formula trial varied in accordance with the evolution of the patient and severity of diarrhea while being fed any one of these formulas.

The response to treatment with the protein hydrolysate formula was impressive when given as the initial treatment after milk (Fig. 5). All but one of the 10 patients given this formula to treat the postinfectious chronic diarrhea and lactose intolerance rapidly improved.

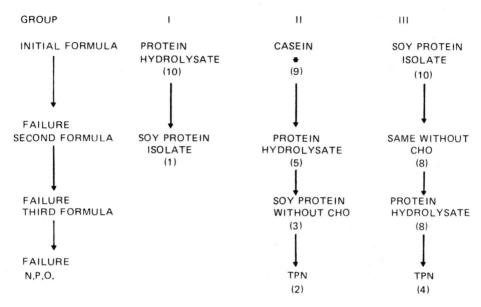

Figure 5 The response to dietary treatment of malnourished infants with post-infectious chronic diarrhea. All formulas were initially fed full strength to provide 70 kcal/kg per day. Gradual increments to a maximum of 120 kcal/kg per day were given as tolerated. The carbohydrate of the formulas was glucose polymers at 7% except in the casein formula*. Only patients who failed to improve were shown in relation to the feeding which was tolerated after the previous formula employed. All patients had evidence of lactose intolerance before being treated with any one of these formulas. I. Pregestimil; II. Portagen; III. 3280. N.P.O.: nothing by os. TPN: Total parenteral nutrition. All Mead Johnson formulas. Exact composition available upon request.

The response to soy isolate formula and casein formula treatments was much less effective than the protein hydrolysate (Fig. 5). Only 2 out of 10 of the patients treated with soy and 4 of 10 of the casein-treated patients responded well. All others continued diarrhea as long as these diets were given. Even after the carbohydrate was eliminated from the diet and soy isolate without glucose polymers was fed, the patients continued with diarrhea. When these formulas were discontinued and substituted by protein hydrolysate formula, there was recovery of some of the patients (Fig. 5). However, there were many patients who continued with diarrhea and deteriorated to the point of requiring total parenteral nutrition before recovery. Thus, protein hydrolysates following treatment failure was less effective than when given as the initial treatment.

IV. CONCLUSIONS

We have further evidence that there is frequent lactose intolerance and cow's milk intolerance in postinfectious chronic diarrhea of infants who are malnourished. This is evident even when cow's milk is diluted. This observation is in agreement with previous observations (30) and casts doubts on the recommendation by the WHO and many pediatricians who continue to recommend diluted cow's milk formulas as the initial refeeding of infants with diarrhea (33). It is clear from our studies that the response of patients with postinfectious chronic diarrhea varied in accordance to the initial dietary treatment given.

The general clinical impression of the superior efficacy of protein hydrolysate formula with glucose polymers for the treatment of the above-mentioned infants was confirmed in this prospective study. Protein hydrolysate formula was found to be most impressive when given to the patients as the initial dietary treatment after milk. Only one failure occurred when this formula was the initial feeding treatment. This patient had intolerance to glucose polymers and responded to elimination of all dietary carbohydrates. Intolerance to this carbohydrate was also encountered in a previous study of ours with an incidence of 10–30% in infants with diarrhea and malnutrition (32). However, when the patients were given other dietary treatments after cow's milk and had dietary failures, protein hydrolysate formula was not as effective. The high incidence of poor response to soy protein isolate formula is of interest. In a previous study in a similar patient population, we found that other soy products with or without glucose polymers were generally better accepted and more useful to treat these types of patients (32). Only one-third of them failed to improve. This was due to glucose polymer intolerance and not to any apparent protein intolerance. In contrast, in this study even those given a carbohydrate-free soy isolate product failed to improve. Moreover, there was a high rate of protein hydrolysate failures (4/8) in patients who were previously fed the soy formula. The high rate of nonresponders to protein hydrolysate treatment with development to intolerance to all foodstuffs requiring TPN following soy treatment is of interest and requires further study.

Nutritional rehabilitation is the most important therapeutic modality for chronic diarrhea of infancy (34,35). It is now generally agreed that feedings must be offered to all patients with diarrhea as long as the stool losses are not massive and whenever there are no specific complications that preclude feedings (i.e., ileus). Oral intake should be attempted even in those patients who vomit. Breast feedings are ideal for feeding infants, even those with diarrhea. Only rare instances of chronic diarrhea postgastroenteritis in infancy have been encountered in infants who are breast fed (36), although we now recognize that antigens may be passed through breast milk with clinical consequences (37).

However, there is controversy regarding the feeding of choice for refeeding infants with diarrhea when the patient is not fortunate enough to be breastfed. In the treatment of the patients with postinfectious chronic diarrhea, the elimination from the diet of all the many ingredients which are not tolerated by the patient is needed, yet the patients must be provided with an adequate dietary intake to allow for recovery of diarrhea and eventually nutritional rehabilitation. Often total parenteral nutrition may be the only way to keep the patient alive (22-26); more often this is a useful therapeutic supplement which should be used with caution while the infant is able to ingest appropriate calories by mouth. The use of continuous enteral feedings improves tolerance and may allow for a faster recovery (28). However, the selection of the appropriate formula for these patients is still the most important consideration. The use of a protein hydrolysate glucose polymer-containing formula seemed to be the most effective for the dietary treatment of malnourished infants with postinfectious chronic diarrhea. This formula meets general sound principles for treatment of these infants in consideration of the pathophysiology and alterations in intestinal function usually found in these patients (34,35). However, our recommendations for this special dietary formula for infants with chronic diarrhea who are not breastfed pose a number of interesting considerations. Lactose-free formulas and special cow's milk substitutes are generally less available and are more expensive where they may be needed most and where they are least affordable. Nonetheless, this cost has to be viewed in relation to the possible benefits derived from appropriate, prompt nutritional treatment of the infant with chronic diarrhea and malnutrition. The rapid rehabilitation and recovery of the patient may save the cost of treatment of life-threatening complications and prolonged hospitalization of these desperately ill patients. However, we are still concerned that when these patients return to their contaminated living environment they may present again with the same problems.

REFERENCES

1. Merson, M. H. The global problem of acute diarrhoeal diseases and the WHO diarrhoeal diseases control programme. International Symposium on Bacterial Diarrheal Diseases, Osaka, 1982.
2. Nazer, H. Acute diarrhoea in the developing world. *J. Trop. Pediatr.* 28, 1-4, 1982.
3. Lifshitz, F., Teichberg, S., and Wapnir, R. A. Malnutrition and the intestine. In *Nutrition and Child Health Perspectives for the 1980's*. Nichols, B., and Tsang, R. (eds.). Alan R. Liss Inc., New York, 1981, pp. 1-24.
4. Lifshitz, F. The effect of diarrhea on infant nutrition. In *Gastrointestinal Development and Infant Nutrition*. Lebenthal, E. (ed.). Raven Press, New York, 1981, pp. 1003-1011.

5. Fagundes-Neto, U., Patricio, F. R. S., Wehba, J., Reis, M. H. L., Gianotti, O. F., and Trabulsi, L. R. An *Escherichia coli* strain that causes diarrhea by invasion of the small intestine mucosa and induces monosaccharide intolerance. *Arg. Gastroenterol.* 116, 205-208, 1979.

6. Sack, D. A., Roads, M., Molla, A., Molla, M., and Wahed, A. Carbohydrate malabsorption in infants with rotavirus diarrhea. *Am. J. Clin. Nutr.* 36, 1112-1118, 1982.

7. Lifshitz, F., Coello-Ramirez, P., and Gutierrez-Topete, G. Carbohydrate intolerance in infants with diarrhea. *J. Pediatr.* 79, 760-767, 1971.

8. Lifshitz, F., Coello-Ramirez, P., and Gutierrez-Topete, G. Monosaccharide intolerance and hypoglycemia in infants with diarrhea. In Clinical Course of 23 Infants. *J. Pediatr.* 77, 595-603, 1970.

9. Toccalino, H., and O'Donnell, J. O. Tecnica para la introduction de la sonda-capsula de Crosby en ninos. *Rev. Hosp. Ninos de Buenos Aires* 12, 29-30, 1962.

10. Fagundes-Neto, U., Reis, M. H. L., Wehba, J., Silvestrini, W. S., and Trabulsi, L. R. Small bowel bacterial flora in normal and in children with acute diarrhea. *Arg. Gastroenterol.* 17(2), 103-108, 1980.

11. Fagundes-Neto, U., Toccalino, H., and Dujovney, F. Stool bacterial aerobic overgrowth in the small intestine of children with acute diarrhea. *Acta Paediatr. Scand.* 65, 609–615, 1976.

12. Gracey, M., Burke, V., Oshin, A., Barker, J., and Glagow, E. Bacteria, bile salts, and intestinal monosaccharide malabsorption. *Gut* 12, 683-692, 1971.

13. Lifshitz, F. The enteric flora in childhood disease—diarrhea. *Am. J. Clin. Nutr.* 30, 1811-1818, 1977.

14. Fagundes-Neto, U., Teichberg, S., Bayne, M. A., Morton, B., and Lifshitz, F. Bile salt-enhanced rat jejunal absorption of a macromolecular tracer. *Lab Invest.* 44, 18-26, 1981.

15. Goel, K., Lifshitz, F., Kahn, E., and Teichberg, S. Monosaccharide intolerance and soy-protein hypersensitivity in an infant with diarrhea. *J. Pediatr.* 93, 617-619, 1978.

16. Iyngkaran, J., Abdin, Z., Davis, K., Boey, C. G., Prathap, M. B., Yadav, M., Lam, S. K., and Puthucheary, S. D. Acquired carbohydrate intolerance and cow's milk protein sensitive enteropathy in young infants. *J. Pediatr.* 95, 373-377, 1979.

17. Mata, L. Breast-feeding: Main promoter of infant health. *Am. J. Clin. Nutr.* 31, 2058-2065, 1978.

18. Taylor, B., Wadsworth, J., Golding, J., and Butler, N. Breast-feeding, bronchitis, and admissions for lower-respiratory illness and gastroenteritis during the first five years. *Lancet* II, 1227-1229, 1982.

19. Kallas, M. R. E., and Fagundes-Neto, U. Evaluation of the nutritional status of children from slums in Sao Paulo, Brazil (to be published).

20. Torres-Lleras, A., and Fagundes-Neto, U. Microbiologic research in acute diarrhea in children from slums in Sao Paulo, Brazil (to be published).

21. Seoane, N., and Latham, M. C. Nutritional anthropometry in the identification of malnutrition in childhood. *J. Trop. Pediatr.* 17, 98-104, 1971.

22. Avery, G. B., Villavicencio, O., Lilly, J. R., and Randolph, J. G. Intractable diarrhea in early infancy. *Pediatrics* 41, 712-722, 1968.
23. Hyman, C. J., Reiter, J., Rodnan, J., and Drash, A. L. Parenteral and oral alimentation in the treatment of the nonspecific protracted diarrheal syndrome of infancy. *J. Pediatr.* 78, 17-29, 1971.
24. Schwachman, H., Lloyd-Still, J. D., Khaw, K. T., and Antonowicz, I. Protracted diarrhea of infancy treated by intravenous alimentation. II-Studies of small intestinal biopsy results. *Am. J. Dis. Child.* 125, 365-368, 1973.
25. Lloyd-Still, J. D., Schwachman, H., and Filler, R. M. Protracted diarrhea of infancy treated by intravenous alimentation. I-Clinical studies of 16 infants. *Am. J. Dis. Child.* 125, 358-364, 1973.
26. Larcher, V. F., Shepherd, R., Francis, D. E. M., and Harries, J. T. Protracted diarrhea in infancy. Analysis of 82 cases with particular reference to diagnosis and management. *Arch. Dis. Child.* 52, 597-605, 1977.
27. Teichberg, S., Fagundes-Neto, U., Baynes, M. A., and Lifshitz, F. Jejunal macromolecular absorption and bile salt deconjugation in protein-energy malnourished rats. *Am. J. Clin. Nutr.* 34, 1281-1291, 1981.
28. Greene, H. L., McCabe, D. R., and Merenstein, G. P. Protracted diarrhea and malnutrition in infancy: Changes in intestinal morphology and disaccharidase activities during treatment with total parenteral intravenous nutrition or oral elemental diets. *J. Pediatr.* 87, 695–704, 1975.
29. Lifshitz, F. Malabsorption syndrome and intestinal disaccharide deficiencies. In: *Current Pediatric Therapy*, 6th ed. Gellis, S., and Kagan, B. M. (eds.). W.B. Saunders Co., Philadelphia, London, Toronto, 1973, p. 236.
30. Chandrasekaran, R., Kumar, V., Walia, B. N. S., and Moorthy, B. Carbohydrate intolerance in infants with acute diarrhoea and its complications. *Acta Paediatr. Scand.* 64, 483–488, 1975.
31. Kumar, V., Chandrasekaran, R., and Bhaskar, R. Carbohydrate intolerance associated with acute gastroenteritis. *Clin. Pediatr.* 16, 1123-1127, 1977.
32. Fagundes-Neto, V., Viarro, T., and Lifshitz, F. Tolerance to glucose polymers in malnourished infants with diarrhea and disaccharide intolerance. 41, 228-234, 1985.
33. World Health Organization: *Control of Diarrheal Disease. A Manual for the Treatment of Acute Diarrhea*. World Health Organization, Geneva, 1984, Rev. 1.
34. Lifshitz, F. Theoretical and practical considerations in the nutritional management of diarrhea in childhood. In *Advances in Pediatric Gastroenterology and Nutrition*. Lebenthal, E. (ed.). Excerpta Medica, Hong Kong, 1984, pp. 108-119.
35. Lifshitz, F. Nutrition in chronic diarrhea of infancy. In: *Nutrition of the Sick Infant.* Stern, L. (ed.). 11th Nestle Nutrition Workshop. Raven Press, New York, 1985, in press.
36. Goel, K., Lifshitz, F., Kahn, E., and Teichberg, S. Monosaccharide intolerance and soy protein intolerance and soy protein hypersensitivity in an infant with diarrhea. *J. Pediatr.* 93, 617–619, 1978.
37. Lothe, L., Lindberg, T., and Jacobsson, I. Cow's milk formula as a cause of infantile colic; a double blind study. *J. Pediatr.* 70, 7-10, 1982.

14

Comparison of Protein Hydrolysates and Elemental Diets in the Intractable Diarrhea Syndrome of Infancy

John D. Lloyd-Still
Northwestern University Medical School and Children's Memorial Hospital, Chicago, Illinois

Alice E. Smith
Children's Memorial Hospital and University of Illinois, Chicago, Illinois

Deborah K. Sullivan
University of Illinois, Chicago, Illinois

Roberta A. Cooper
Children's Memorial Hospital, Chicago, Illinois

I. INTRODUCTION

In 1975, Sherman et al. (1) pioneered the use of the elemental diet Vivonex (Norwich Eaton) by constant intragastric infusion in our institution, and concluded that the majority (89%) of infants with intractable diarrhea could be managed by the oral route. Because elemental diets such as Vivonex are deficient in essential fatty acids for infants, they are not suitable for long-term usage, and these infants are usually weaned on to some other nutritionally complete formula such as Nutramigen or Pregestimil (Mead Johnson).

At present it is still unclear whether the technique of constant infusion intragastric administration, or the elemental diet, or the combination of the two is the most important factor in the recovery of these infants. Therefore, a study was devised to compare Vivonex and Pregestimil regimens in the treatment of intractable diarrhea syndrome (IDS) in terms of (a) therapeutic effectiveness, (b) duration of hospitalization, and (c) cost effectiveness.

II. METHODS

A. Study Protocol

In 1983, a protocol adapted from Sherman et al. (1) was devised, and parents of all infants less than 2 years of age having intractable diarrhea of greater than 2 weeks duration and who had failed conventional therapy, were asked to sign the informed consent form after the study protocol had been explained. Participants were randomly assigned to receive either Vivonex or Pregestimil when enteral refeeding was started. The enteral formula regimens were matched calorie for calorie and millimeter for millimeter starting at 50 ml/kg per day and advancing to 165 ml/kg per day over 3 days. Concentration was increased from 5 calories per 30 ml to 20 calories per 30 ml over 3 days as determined on tolerance (according to stool volume and presence of reducing sugars).

Baseline data included average age of onset (months), age of admission, number of formula changes, length of hospitalization, duration of central total parenteral nutrition (TPN), and peripheral parenteral nutrition (PPN), days on intravenous lipids, and duration of oral alimentation. Other parameters collected included anthropometric [weight, height, weight/height (% ideal), triceps skin fold (TSF), mid-arm muscle circumference (MAMC), mid-arm muscle area (MAMA), and fat area], nutritional (complete blood count, protein, and albumin), and absorptive (D-xylose, stool trypsin, Schillings test, sweat electrolytes, radiological investigations, and intestinal biopsies).

Statistical evaluation was performed utilizing (a) Paired t-test comparing initial and final values of weight, albumin, protein, TSF, MAMC, MAMA, fat area, and weight/height (% ideal) within each formula. (b) Two sample t-tests comparing all parameters between formulas. (c) Analysis of variance on weight gain adjusted for length of stay (using length of stay as covariate because of significant differences between the two formulas). (d) Analysis of variance on albumin, protein, TSF, MAMC, MAMA, fat area, and weight/height ratio gain per day adjusted for days on the protocol.

Resources included a special nutritional laboratory modeled after the pharmacy's intravenous mixture room for the compounding and distribution of specialty formulas; a unit of use formula distribution system for the daily dispensing of individually labeled products; a patient profiling system for the documentation of specialty formula dispensed to the patient, and for the collection and organization of clinical data from medical work rounds and medical records. Information on anticipated changes in medical treatment and formula regimens was obtained from the rounding program with the medical residents. A microcomputer software system was used for the nutrient analysis of individual enteral intake and the calculation and monitoring of individual intravenous hyperalimentation. The Pharmacy/Clinical Dietetics program included professional staff coverage of each nursing unit for the dispensing and monitoring of drug and nutritional therapy.

B. Retrospective Analysis

Data obtained by our study protocol was compared with data of retrospective analysis of the clinical records and investigations of 29 infants with IDS seen at Children's Memorial between 1980 and 1982. Clinical and laboratory parameters similar to those of the prospective group were monitored except that anthropometric measurements only included height, weight, and weight/height (% ideal).

III. RESULTS

Comparisons of the two enteral products (Vivonex and Pregestimil) in the prospective protocol are shown in Tables 1 and 2. Clinical findings were similar for both groups and included low anthropometrics, hypoalbuminemia, and secondary monosaccharide intolerance. Paired t-test comparisons (pre and post values for each formula) showed more significant increases with Vivonex (5 parameters) than Pregestimil (2 parameters). Both formulas produced significant weight/height changes. The pre- and postalbumin levels in patients treated with Pregestimil increased significantly ($p < .022$) despite a shorter duration on the protocol (13.1 days).

Table 2 shows the results of two sample t-tests between the two formulas. Parameters such as age of onset, age of admission, weight on admission, discharge weight, and various absorptive and anthropometric measurements were similar. The length of stay averaged 25.6 days for Pregestimil compared to 57.8 for Vivonex, although the p value was borderline at .06. The duration on the protocol with Pregestimil (13.1 days) compared to Vivonex (37.5 days) was significantly less ($p < .04$).

Figure 1 shows some of the findings when the retrospective group (29 patients) was compared to the first 13 patients from the prospective group (Vivonex and Pregestimil combined). Clinical findings were similar for both groups,

Table 1 Paired t-Test Results Comparing Pre- and Post Values for Various Parameters During the Protocol with Pregestimil and Vivonex (See Sect. II.A for Abbreviations)

Change in	Pregestimil	Vivonex
Weight	NS	$p < .011$
Albumin	$p < 0.22$	NS
Protein	NS	$p < .042$
TSF	NS	$p < .039$
MAMC	NS	NS
MAMA	NS	NS
Fat area	NS	$p < .033$
Wt/Ht (% ideal)	$p < .018$	$p < .013$

NS: not significant.

Table 2 Results of Two Sample t Tests Comparing Various
Parameters in Pregestimil and Vivonex Groups

	Pregestimil	Vivonex
Number	7	9
Age onset (mos.)	7.6	4.9
Age admission (mos.)	8.4	5.8
Length of stay (days)	25.6	57.8
Days on peripheral (PPN)[d]	3.3	8.1
Days on central (TPN)	6.8	20.6
Days on protocol	13.1[a]	37.5
Admission weight (kg)	6.45	5.15
Discharge weight (kg)	6.7	6.6
Initial albumin (g/dl)	2.8	3.0
Final albumin (g/dl)	3.5	3.2
Initial wt/ht (% ideal)	90.1[c]	78.8
Final wt/ht (% ideal)	107.6[b]	93.4

[a]$p < .05$.
[b]$p < .03$.
[c]$p < .01$.
[d]Hyperalimentation.
Initial and final total protein, TSF, MAMC, MAMA, and fat
area showed no significant differences.

and included low anthropometrics, hypoalbuminemia, and secondary monosaccharide intolerance. Use of the protocol resulted in 31% fewer days per admission ($\overline{X}$ savings 22 days), and 28% and 55% savings in TPN and PPN, respectively
per patient (2). Average charge savings per protocol patient was $14,564 ($\overline{X}$
savings $9592 base room rate, $2530 TPN charges, and $2422 PPN charges).
Extension of the protocol to 16 patients confirmed these findings with similar
reductions in average length of hospitalization and cost effectiveness.

IV. DISCUSSION

There is still controversy concerning the optimal nutritional therapy for acute
attacks of chronic inflammatory bowel disease (Crohn's disease and ulcerative
colitis) in adults. The traditional approach with total bowel rest, corticosteroids,
and intravenous hyperalimentation corrects the nutritional deficits, but in a controlled trial (3), intravenous hyperalimentation was shown to have no primary
therapeutic effect in acute colitis, with an equal number of patients ultimately
requiring surgery. By contrast, in Crohn's disease, elemental diets can have a
primary role in the therapy of an acute attack. When patients with acute exacer-

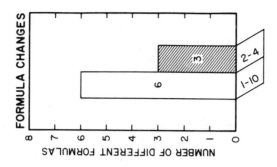

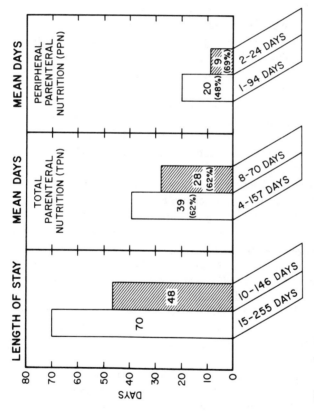

Figure 1 Comparison between the retrospective group (n = 29) and the prospective group (Vivonex and Pregestimil combined n = 13). Data from Ref. 2.

bations of Crohn's disease were randomized to receive either prednisone 0.75 mg/kg per day or an elemental diet (Vivonex) as their sole therapy for 4 weeks, assessment at 4 and 12 weeks showed that the patients treated with the elemental diet had improved as much as and, by some criteria, more than the steroid-treated group (4).

There are a number of theoretical physiologic advantages of enteral over intravenous feeding (5). Animal studies have shown that luminal nutrition is needed to maintain the structural and functional integrity of the small intestine. Intravenously fed rats had lower gut weight, decreased mucosal thickness, and less mucosal protein, deoxyribonucleic acid, and disaccharidase activity than orally fed control rats (6). After jejunostomy, intravenously fed dogs showed no functional adaptation and had decreased villous height of the recovering ileum compared with orally fed dogs that developed functional adaptation and increased villous height (7). These morphologic changes are thought to be mediated by humoral factors. Further advantages of the enteral technique were demonstrated by Parker et al. (8) when they compared constant intragastric infusion with intermitent oral feeding in IDS and demonstrated that the continuous enteral method resulted in a decrease in fecal weight, steatorrhea, nitrogen, calcium, and zinc loss, and a significant increase in the enteral balance of the major nutrients.

Recently Orenstein (9) performed a prospective, randomized study comparing enteral and parenteral therapy in IDS, and found that enteral therapy produced comparable correction of malnutrition to TPN with better correction of malabsorption, shorter hospitalization, and fewer complications. There were only 4 patients in each of her severe groups. The majority of our patients with IDS were older and had severe secretory diarrhea unresponsive to oral therapy, and required a central line. However, we agree that early use of enteral alimentation is indicated and is frequently advantageous.

The choice of formula for enteral feeding in IDS is still being debated. Sherman et al. (1) compared standard and high nitrogen Vivonex and performed metabolic studies with measurement of serum and urine amino acid profiles, nitrogen balance, glucose, electrolytes, acid base status, proteins, liver function, and lipoprotein electrophoresis. The high nitrogen Vivonex was found to cause elevation in amino acids and blood urea nitrogen and was not recommended.

Our data show that establishment of a protocol in the therapy of IDS resulted in reduction in length of stay with resultant savings in cost. When the Vivonex and Pregestimil groups were compared on the protocol, few significant differences were demonstrated, and both regimens produced clinical improvement. The documentation of the effectiveness of Pregestimil compared to Vivonex in this study makes Pregestimil the therapy of choice in IDS because it is a nutritionally complete formula, whereas Vivonex is deficient in essential fatty acid content for infants. In addition, patients treated with Vivonex still have to be weaned on to another formula, thus taking longer to achieve effective therapy.

V. SUMMARY

Comparison of a protein hydrolysate formula (Pregestimil) and an elemental diet (Vivonex) in infants with intractable diarrhea showed similar findings in therapeutic effectiveness. Establishment of a protocol for the treatment of intractable diarrhea of infancy reduced the length of hospitalization by one third with resultant cost effectiveness.

REFERENCES

1. Sherman, J. O., Hamly, C., and Khachadurian, A. K. Use of an oral elemental diet in infants with severe intractable diarrhea. *J. Pediatr.* 86, 518-523, 1975.
2. Smith, A. E., Powers, C. A., Cooper, R. A., and Lloyd-Still, J. D. Improved nutritional management reduces length of hospitalization in intractable diarrhea (Abstr.). The American Dietetic Association 67th Annual Meeting, Washington, D.C., 1984, pp. 53-54.
3. Dickinson, R. J., Ashton, M. G., Axon, A. T. R., Smith, R. C., Yeung, C. K., and Hill, G. L. Controlled trial of intravenous hyperalimentation and total bowel rest as an adjunct to the routine therapy of acute colitis. *Gastroenterology* 79, 1199-1204, 1980.
4. Morain, C. O., Segal, A. W., and Levi, A. J. Elemental diet as primary treatment of acute Crohn's disease: A controlled trial. *Br. Med. J.* 288, 1859-1862, 1984.
5. Heymsfield, S. B., Bethel, R. A., Ansley, J. D., Nixon, D. L., and Rudman, D. Enteral hyperalimentation: An alternative to central venous hyperalimentation. *Ann. Intern. Med.* 90, 63-71, 1979.
6. Levine, G. M., Deren, J. J., Steiger, E., and Zinno, R. Role of oral intake in maintenance of gut mass and disaccharidase activity. *Gastroenterology* 67, 975-982, 1974.
7. Feldman, E. J., Dowling, R. H., McNaughton, J., and Peters, T. J. Effects of oral versus intravenous nutrition on intestinal adaptation after small bowel resection in the dog. *Gastroenterology* 70, 712-719, 1976.
8. Parker, P., Stroop, S., and Greene, H. A controlled comparison on continuous versus intermittent feeding in the treatment of infants with intestinal disease. *J. Pediatr.* 99, 360-364, 1981.
9. Orenstein, S. R. Intractable diarrhea of infancy (IDI): Prospective, randomized study of enteral vs. parenteral therapy. *Pediatr. Res.* 19, 229A, 1985.

15

The Use of Continuous Nasogastric Feeding in Malabsorption Syndromes of Infancy

Harry L. Greene
Vanderbilt University Medical Center, Nashville, Tennessee

I. INTRODUCTION

Nasogastric feeding has been used widely for many years for the nutritional management of patients unable to consume adequate calories orally. There has been a renewed interest in the use of nasogastric or nasoenteric feeding during the past decade due to improvements in formulas and equipment for nutrient delivery. When oral feedings are not possible, nasoenteric feedings, when tolerated, have been found to be more efficacious, safe, and cost effective than parenteral feedings.

There are specific medical conditions for which nasoenteric feedings are preferred over other routes of nutrient administration; these are listed in Table 1. Protracted diarrhea with malnutrition and short bowel syndrome are two conditions commonly requiring nasogastric feedings. In both conditions, the question often asked is, "Should the feedings be given continuously or intermittently?" A study was therefore designed to answer this question. The study compares the two methods of enteral feeding in two groups of infants with impaired intestinal absorption.

Table 1 Conditions in Which a Trial of Tube Feeding May be Warranted, Based On Past Reports of Efficacy

---

Anorexia/weight loss associated with chronic illness
Pancreatic insufficiency
Short bowel syndrome
Gastroesophageal reflux[a]
Inborn errors of metabolism such as glycogen storage disease type I and III
Prematurity
Protracted diarrhea and malnutrition
Crohn's disease
Neurological disease with subsequent inability to swallow or high likelihood of
  aspiration
Anorexia nervosa
Cystic fibrosis associated with malnutrition

---

[a]If no improvement occurs within 10 days, further use of tube feedings probably will not be helpful.

II. METHODS

A. Patients

Informed consent was obtained from the parents or guardians of all children who served as subjects of the investigation. Two groups of patients were selected: The first (Group A) consisted of 11 patients with protracted diarrhea and malnutrition, and the second (Group B) consisted of 4 patients with chronic malabsorption as a result of extensive bowel resection. The patients in Group A were less than 6 months of age and had clinical evidence of malnutrition (1). Their weights were less than the third percentile for age, and serum albumin concentrations were between 2.3 and 3.1 g/dl. All had acute onset of diarrhea three to six weeks prior to the study; despite formula changes and transient intravenous administration of fluids, the diarrhea had not resolved. All except one had substantial enteric fluid losses (30-64 ml/kg) during the first 24 hours of hospitalization despite a lack of oral intake. Small bowel biopsy specimens showed moderate-to-severe morphologic abnormalities (villus to crypt ratio < 3 to 1, substantial infiltrate of plasma cells and lymphocytes), and disaccharidase activities (lactase, sucrase, and maltase) were below the normal range.

In Group B, patient 1 was 3 months of age and had approximately 21 cm of small bowel. Patient 2 was 7 months of age and had approximately 30 cm of small bowel. Patient 3 was 5 months of age and had approximately 25 cm of small bowel. Patient 4 was 8 months of age and had 20 cm of small bowel.

B. Study Protocol

Prior to beginning oral or intragastric feedings, patients in both groups received 3-10 days of fluids intravenously to correct water, mineral, and vitamin imbalances, as well as to provide minimal energy-protein intake. The intravenous fluids contained glucose (9 mg/dl), crystalline amino acids (2.5 g/dl), and vitamins with minerals (plus 4 mg zinc/liter) (2). Fluids were given intravenously during the period of no enteral feedings and at any other time of excessive intestinal losses.

The study in Group A patients consisted of three periods of three days each. At the end of each period there was one day with no enteral feedings, to minimize carryover effects from one treatment to the next. Because the intestinal anatomy might not have been uniformly altered, we felt it important to use each patient as his/her own control. However, since the study lasted approximately 12 days there was likely to be some improvement in anatomy and physiology by the latter part of the study. For this reason, the sequence of periods was randomized so that three infants received continuous intragastric feedings first, three received oral bolus feedings first, and three were given no enteral feeding first. Bolus feedings consisted of orally administered feedings, 120 kcal/kg per day of expected weight for height, divided into equal volumes and given at 4-hour intervals. The continuous feeding consisted of the same volume of formula per 24 hours.

Patients in both groups had all stools examined for the presence of reducing sugars. This was performed at the bedside, by nurses using the Clinitest method (3).

C. Dietary Formula

The formula was mixed locally using Portagen (Mead Johnson) as the base and adding additional ingredients to achieve the desired mixture of carbohydrate, fat, protein, and minerals. The content of the formula was as follows: protein, 9% of calories, equally divided between hydrolyzed and nonhydrolyzed casein; fat, 46% of calories, one-third vegetable oil and two-thirds medium-chain triglycerides (MCT); carbohydrate, 45% of calories, four-fifths dextrins and one-fifth sucrose; calcium 45.5 mg/dl; zinc 0.5 mg/dl; and copper 0.05 mg/dl. Other minerals were adjusted to meet the required daily allowance (RDA), and vitamins were added to provide 150% of RDA at an intake of 150 ml/kg per day. The osmolality was between 280 and 293 mOsm/kg at 20 kcal/oz.

Hydrolyzed casein was used because previous studies had demonstrated that infants with protracted diarrhea and malnutrition showed low pancreatic trypsin activity in duodenal fluids, and MCT were used because the infants also showed low lipase activity in duodenal fluid.

D. Measurements

Daily weights were monitored and mean weight changes recorded for each of the three-day periods. Fecal samples were collected separate from urine for 72-hour periods. Fecal collections from each of the 72-hour periods were weighed and blended to obtain a homogenous mixture. Aliquots of the stool mixture were assayed for their content of fat (9), nitrogen (10), calcium (11), zinc, and copper (12). To ensure consistency in the formula mixture, the same measurments were also made on the formula.

III. RESULTS

A. Group A

During continuous enteral feeding, weight gain was 152 ± 14 g; during bolus feeding a net loss of 119 ± 24 g occurred; and while NPO (on intravenous fluids)

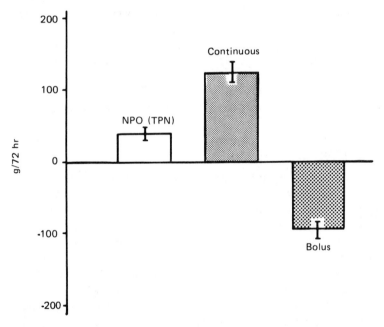

Figure 1 Changes in weight in protracted diarrhea seen during the three treatment periods. NPO = No enteric feedings; continuous = continuous nasoenteric tube feeding; bolus = intermittent feeds of equal feedings given at four intervals to match the 24-hour volume of continuous feedings.

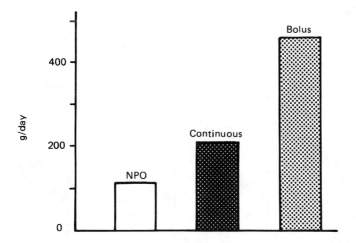

Figure 2 Fecal output in protracted diarrhea during the three treatment periods. Bolus feedings caused a significant ($p < 0.001$) increase in fecal losses compared to both other treatment regimens. There was a slight difference ($p < 0.05$) between the period of NPO and continuous regimen.

a net gain of 62 ± 6.6 g occurred (Fig. 1). The mean daily weight gain during continuous infusion was not different from that seen during treatment with intravenous fluids, although there was a significant increase in weight ($p < 0.001$) with the continuous infusion when compared to the bolus feeding. The fecal weight was significantly greater ($p < 0.001$) during the period of bolus feeding (Fig. 2). Daily fecal weight was not significantly different during the periods of total parenteral nutrition (TPN) alone and continuous infusion feeding.

Enteral intake, fecal losses, and the net enteral balance of nutrients and minerals during the three study periods are shown in Figures 3 and 4. The enteral balance of nutrients was determined by the difference between enteral intake and fecal losses during the periods of bolus and continuous feedings, and by fecal losses only during the period of TPN alone. Net balance was not determined, since urine measurements and the amount of nutrients and minerals received intravenously were not determined. Bolus feedings resulted in significantly greater daily fecal losses and less daily enteral retention of all nutrients and minerals than did continuous infusion. During the periods of bolus feedings the patients were actually in negative balance for zinc, calcium, and copper. In fact, enteral balance of zinc and calcium was more negative during bolus feeding than when the patients received no enteral feeding at all.

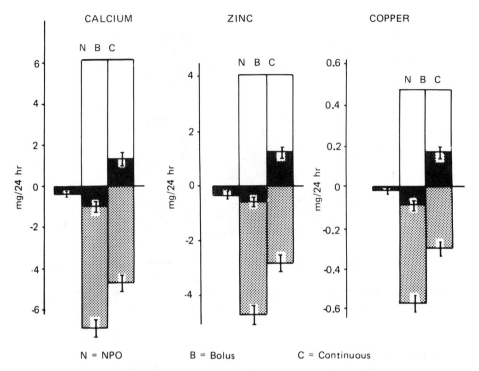

Figure 3 Enteric mineral balance in protracted diarrhea during the three study periods. N = no enteric feedings; B = bolus feedings; C = continuous nasoenteric tube feedings.   Open bars above the zero axis indicate total enteric intake.   The lightly shaded bars below the zero axis indicate fecal output. The darkly shaded bars indicate net balance. Both no feeding and bolus feeding protocols resulted in negative balances of all minerals, whereas continuous feeding resulted in positive balance.

B. Group B

During continuous infusion, patients with short bowel syndrome, as a whole, demonstrated maximum weight gain ($p < 0.02$). During bolus feeding Patient 1 lost weight, whereas Patients 2, 3, and 4 gained weight to a lesser degree than with continuous feeding.

Percent absorption of fat, nitrogen and calcium during the two study periods are shown in Figure 5. With the exception of fecal fat in Patient 2, greater fecal losses and less enteral retention of all nutrients occurred with bolus feedings in all patients.

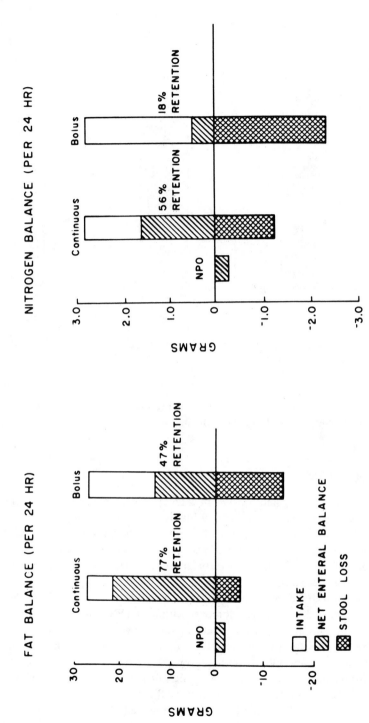

Figure 4 Enteric fat and nitrogen balance indicates significantly more ($p < 0.002$) retention with continuous as compared to bolus feeding. The bars below zero axis indicate fecal losses and hatched bars above zero axis indicate net retention.

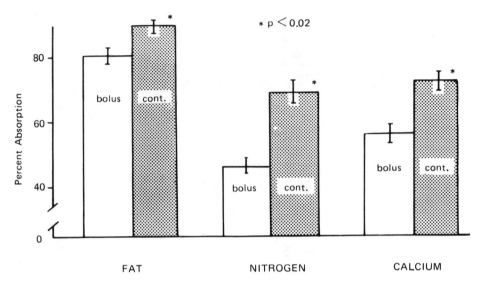

Figure 5 Comparison of nutrient absorption for fat, nitrogen, and calcium absorption in children with short bowel syndrome.

Patients in both groups had 2+ to 4+ reducing substances in stool while receiving bolus feedings, and 0 to 1+ reducing substances while receiving continuous feedings.

IV. DISCUSSION

Protracted diarrhea and malabsorption in infancy is common in several of the urban underprivileged areas of the United States and in developing countries of the world. If allowed to persist, it usually leads to malnutrition and associated abnormalities in intestinal morphology. In some instances enteral feedings of any type are not well tolerated and TPN through a central venous catheter is necessary in order to achieve positive nutrient balance. Although such procedures may be life-saving, metabolic or catheter-induced complications make alternative methods of feeding desirable (4). Moreover, although TPN alone may result in adequate weight gain and partial recovery of small bowel morphology, enteral nutrients are required for a complete return of bowel function (1,5,6). In addition, the ability of some infants with protracted diarrhea and malnutrition to tolerate cautious early feedings of an elemental diet make the concept of prolonged "bowel rest" in these infants debatable (7,8).

In spite of the potential benefits of the "predigested" formulas in the feeding of such infants, some tolerate them poorly (1,9). We have noted that some infants continue to have voluminous, watery stools shortly after nipple feedings, possibly caused by the high osmotic load in most hydrolyzed formulas. In addition, gastric distention from the bolus feeding may promote the mass movement of bowel contents toward the rectum (gastrocolic reflex) (10). We hypothesized that the effects of the gastrocolic reflex could be partially or completely negated by changing from intermittent bolus feedings to continous feedings. To test our hypothesis, enteral retention of nutrients and minerals was studied in infants with bowel disease who could be fed with either oral bolus feedings or in a continuous manner.

Our results indicate that continuous intragastric feedings result in significantly greater energy, protein, and mineral absorption than intermittent bolus feedings of the same formula. The positive fat and nitrogen retention which occurred with the continuous feedings was associated with a mean daily weight gain of almost two ounces, whereas the poor retention of fat and nitrogen seen with bolus feedings resulted in approximately one ounce of daily weight loss. The large losses of fat and nitrogen were positively correlated with fecal weight, as has been previously described (11).

Although the net enteral mineral balance was negative without enteral intake, the net enteral losses of zinc and calcium were greater when bolus feedings were given. This finding indicates that a net secretion of these minerals was induced by the bolus feedings, and suggests that bolus feedings could actually favor more rapid development of mineral depletion. The presence of stool reducing sugar may act as an osmotic agent to increase water and mineral excretion. This finding correlates well with that of Ghishan et al. (12) who demonstrated that perfusion of infant rat intestine with slightly hypertonic solutions of mannitol caused net secretion of calcium, magnesium, and zinc. The reason(s) for the noted differences between the two feeding regimens is not entirely clear, but may relate to the gastrocolic reflex and possibly to an osmotic effect of unabsorbed carbohydrate. Although the study formula was nearly isotonic, the presence of carbohydrate in the stool would promote excess water and mineral loss. The continuous infusion resulted in a marked diminution in reducing sugars present in the stool and, therefore, in less water and mineral losses. In addition, the continuous infusion should have caused less distention of the stomach and small intestine and less mass propulsion of enteric contents.

This finding that continuous feeding could improve nutrient and mineral retention in infants with protracted diarrhea and malnutrition suggested that infants with other types of bowel disease might also benefit from this method of feeding. This hypothesis was tested in four patients with markedly decreased absorptive surface area as a result of surgical removal of more than 60% of the small intestine. All infants showed improvements in nutrient absorption with continuous feeding when compared to bolus feeding. One of the infants with the greatest degree of bowel compromise (Patient 1) had the most impressive response.

Our findings indicate that infants with chronic diarrhea and malnutrition or with short bowel syndrome are often able to tolerate continuous intragastric feeding when intermittent bolus feeding results in continuing diarrhea and nutritional deterioration. The use of this technique should provide adequate nutritional support and may either avoid or shorten the use of TPN in these patients. The findings further suggest that patients with other causes of malabsorption may benefit from continuous enteral feeding. We have found this particularly useful in management of malnourished children with cystic fibrosis and other conditions associated with malnutrition (13).

Our observations indicate that when comparing formulas of different nutritional composition in patients prone to malabsorption, the method of formula delivery should be standardized as to the volume given with each feeding as well as the frequency of feeding. Most "therapeutic" formulas are designed to improve absorption in patients with underlying digestive disease, and such infants may respond most favorably to the formula if it is given as a continuous infusion.

ACKNOWLEDGMENTS

Supported in part by NIH CNRU Grant NIADDKD AM No. 26657-05 and unrestricted funds from Bristol-Myers.

REFERENCES

1. Greene, H. L., McCabe, D. R., and Merenstein, G. B. Protracted diarrhea and malnutrition in infancy: Changes in intestinal morphology and disaccharidase during treatment with total intravenous nutrition and elemental diets. *J. Pediatr.* 87, 695, 1975.
2. Meng, H. C., Stahlman, M. T., Ohen, A., Dolonski, E. A. Caldwell, M. D., and O'Neill, J. A. The use of a crystalline amino acid mixture for parenteral nutrition in low-birth-weight infants. *Pediatrics* 59, 699, 1977.
3. Anderson, C. M., and Burke, V. Disorders of carbohydrate digestion and absorption. In: *Pediatric Gastroenterology*, Anderson, C. M., and Burke, V. (eds). Blackwell Scientific Publishers, London, 1975, p. 201.
4. Heird, W. C., and Winter, R. W. Total parenteral nutrition: The state of the art. *J. Pediatr.* 86, 2, 1975.
5. Williamson, R. C. N. Intestinal adaption, structural, functional and cytokinetic changes I. *N. Engl. J. Med.* 298, 1393, 1978.
6. Williamson, R. C. N. Intestinal adaption, structural, functional and cytokinetic changes II. *N. Engl. J. Med.* 298, 1444, 1978.
7. MacLean, W. C., DeRomana, G. L., Massa, E., and Graham, G. G. Nutritional management of chronic diarrhea and malnutrition: Primary reliance on oral feeding. *J. Pediatr.* 97, 316, 1980.

8. Larcher, V. F., Shepperd, R., Francis, D. E. M., and Harries, J. T. Protracted diarrhoea in infancy. *Arch. Dis. Child.* 52, 597, 1977.

9. Walker, W. A., and Isselbacher, K. J. Uptake and transport of macromolecules by the intestine-possible role in clinical disorders. *Gastroenterology* 67, 531, 1974.

10. Guyton, A. C. Movement of food through the alimentary tract. In: *Textbook of Medical Physiology*, Guyton, A. C. (ed.). W. B. Saunders Company, Philadelphia, 1976, p. 850.

11. Viteri, F. E., and Schneider, R. E. Gastrointestinal alteration in protein calorie malnutrition. *Med. Clin. North Am.* 58(6), 1487, 1974.

12. Ghishan, F. K., Parker, P. H., and Helinek, G. Intestinal maturation: Effect of luminal osmolality on net mineral secretion. *Pediatr. Res.* 15, 985–990, 1981.

13. Courtney, M. E., Greene, H. L., Donald, W. D., Dunn, G. D., and Hutchison, A. Nocturnal tube feeding in cystic fibrosis (CF). *Pediatr. Res.* 17, 186 A, 1983.

16

Feeding of the Premature Infant

Narmer F. Galeano and Claude C. Roy
Hôpital Sainte-Justine and Université de Montréal, Montréal, Québec, Canada

I. INTRODUCTION

The last 15 years have seen a rapid increase in rates of survival and improved outcome of low-birth-weight (LBW) infants. Intensive medical care and technological advances have played a significant role in these improvements (1,2). A better understanding of nutrient needs and the coming of age of parenteral nutrition have undoubtedly decreased morbidity and mortality. However our knowledge still remains very sketchy as to when, what, and how to feed LBW neonates. The purpose of this chapter is to reflect on these uncertainties and to discuss the relative merits of human milk and formulas.

Low-birth-weight neonates are particularly vulnerable to malnutrition. Several factors need to be taken into account when planning the nutritional care of prematures.

1. Small LBW infants have very limited protein and energy reserves. If starved, their approximate life expectancy is 7 days (3,4). A 1.0 kg infant has only 10 g of stored fat compared to 400 g in the term neonate (5). Thus there is an urgent need to establish an adequate nutrient intake. Furthermore, nutrients must provide not only for energy and replacement of tissue but also for rapid growth involving an increase in size of organs and substantial changes in body composition.
2. The ratio of surface area to body weight is exceptionally high, thus nutritional requirements are increased.

3. The capacity to tolerate, absorb, and metabolize nutrients is functionally limited. Reduced gastric capacity, impaired digestive phase and metabolic immaturity are factors which limit achievable growth.

II. WHAT IS OPTIMAL GROWTH?

The central difficulty in describing the optimal food for prematures is our lack of knowledge of their nutrient requirements. In the case of the term infant, requirements have been determined by the study of the composition and volumes of human milk consumed by thriving infants. This approach has not been possible in the case of LBW infants since they do not thrive on banked human milk. Current recommendations of the Committee on Nutrition of the American Academy of Pediatrics (AAP) define the optimal diet for the LBW infant as one that supports a rate of growth close to that of the third trimester of intrauterine life without imposing stress on the developing metabolic or excretory systems (6). A further goal that has many adherents is to mimic not only the in utero rate of growth, but also the same tissue accretion rate or quality of growth (7-9). There is currently no definite evidence that such goals are correct. The optimal rate of growth is variable from one baby to another and is affected by genetic growth potential and the degree of gastrointestinal and metabolic maturity (10).

III. ESTIMATED ENERGY AND NUTRIENT NEEDS

Estimates of nutrient requirements of the premature have been made by assessing in utero accretion rates and the chemical composition of the "reference fetus" (11). Even if the nutrient needs for growth calculated in this manner were fully satisfactory, the proportion of these needs for nongrowth (dermal, urinary, and gastrointestinal losses) is very high. These are only rough estimates as they are drawn from several different studies performed in a small number of babies. Although the estimates in Table 1 remain imprecise, they constitute useful guidelines. Advisable intakes of nutrients listed correspond to an arbitrary increase of 10% above estimated requirements. Recommended energy intake is based on estimation of total fetal caloric requirements for metabolic expenditures and accretion of new tissue. The total caloric requirement of the human fetus has been estimated at 90 to 100 kcal/kg per day by Battaglia and Simmons (14).

In recent years, energy needs and the partitioning of energy utilization have been determined by a few groups using calorimetric measurements (12,15-17). Although energy intakes differed significantly, resting metabolic rates were quite comparable and close to the basal metabolic rate estimated in fetuses (14). Stool and urinary losses as well as energy used for physical activity correlated well with energy intakes. These studies carried out in healthy LBW infants remind us of the need for flexibility since nongrowth expenditures are extremely variable. The current AAP recommendation for energy intake is 130 kcal/kg per day (6).

IV. HUMAN MILK AND THE LOW-BIRTH-WEIGHT INFANT

A. Banked Human Milk

The initial indication that LBW infants do not thrive on banked human milk was published in 1947 (18). Results of carefully designed studies of human milk or formulas based on cow's milk with a variable protein content (whey:casein of 18:82 or 60:40) suggest that human milk was more suitable (19). Other investigators observed that weight gain was less on human milk, but they concluded from amino acid patterns, blood ammonia, urea, and acid-base studies that the potential "metabolic price" of using artificial formulas was excessive (20).

The nutritional inadequacies of human milk in terms of growth rate and protein intake were pointed out (21) and subsequently verified by several clinical studies (22-24). The evidence is now clear that pooled human milk is inadequate in terms of energy, protein, sodium, calcium, and phosphorus to allow the prematurely born infant to grow and retain these nutrients at a rate similar to that which would occur in the intrauterine environment (25).

Table 1 Estimated Requirements and Recommended Intakes of Energy[a] and Nutrients[b] in Premature Infants

Birth weight	Estimated requirements (per day)		Recommended daily intake (per kg)	
	800-1200 g	1200-1800 g	800-1200 g	1200-1800 g
Energy (kcal/kg)	120	120	130	130
Protein (g)	3.64	4.78	4.0	3.5
Sodium (mEq)	3.22	4.08	3.5	3.0
Potassium (mEq)	2.52	3.45	2.5	2.3
Calcium (mEq)	188	251	210	185
Phosphorus (mg)	126	171	140	123
Magnesium (mg)	8.7	11.7	10	8.5

[a]From the AAP Committee on Nutrition (6) and Sinclair et al. (12).
[b]Modified from Ziegler et al. (13).

B. Preterm Milk

In the controversy as to whether a mother's milk is appropriate for her LBW infant, the possibility that the composition of the milk of a mother giving birth before term might differ from that of pooled human milk was overlooked until recently.

In the past few years, several reports have attracted attention to the fact that milk from mothers who deliver before term contains higher concentrations of energy, protein, fat, and sodium (26-28), but a lower concentration of lactose (28) (Table 2). However, the higher concentration of macronutrients has been subject to controversy (30). It could not be documented in some studies (31,32) and was related to a lower volume output in others (33,34). The degree of prematurity appears to be an important variable. The advantages of preterm milk in terms of macronutrient composition and energy are largely limited to very preterm milk (26–31 weeks) (35). Furthermore, considerable variability of preterm milk composition between mothers delivering prematurely (34) and in the same mother over time (35) are shortcomings which need to be contended with before making a general statement on the suitability of preterm milk with regard to protein content.

Despite these potential drawbacks, studies with both pooled preterm human milk (36) and the LBW's own mother's milk (27,37) have shown growth rates comparable to those achieved by "preemies" fed premature formulas and the retention of nutrients at a rate similar to those which would occur in the intrauterine environment. However, a multicenter trial showed that 15 LBWs weighing less than 1200 g each exhibited weight gains which were significantly lower than those fed preterm formulas and similar to the group given banked human

Table 2 Human Milk: Term vs. Preterm[a]

Constituents (per dl)	Term		Preterm	
	Early milk[b]	Mature milk[c]	Early milk	Mature milk
Energy (kcal)	59 ± 6	62 ± 2	71 ± 8	70 ± 9
Proteins (g)	1.7 ± 0.18	1.29 ± 0.09	1.86 ± 0.19	1.41 ± 0.08
Lipids (g)	2.9 ± 0.73	3.05 ± 0.25	4.14 ± 1.01	4.09 ± 0.79
Lactose (g)	5.98 ± 0.73	6.51 ± 0.56	5.55 ± 0.35	5.97 ± 0.35
Sodium (mEq)	1.4	1.1	2.04	1.23
Phosphorus (mg)	15	13	15	15
Calcium (mg)	29	26	30	28

[a]Modified from Anderson (29).
[b]Early milk: 8-11 days of lactation.
[c]Mature milk: 26-29 days of lactation.

milk (23). These observations were recently confirmed by another group who found no advantage of preterm milk over mature donor milk (38). On the other hand, calcium and phosphorus levels (36,37) along with trace elements copper, zinc, and iron (39) were judged to be inadequate in preterm milk.

Mineral-deficient bone disease has frequently been observed in LBW infants although this is usually subclinical. It has been associated with low intakes of calcium and phosphorus as well as with inadequate concentrations of biologically active vitamin D facilitating the uptake of these two minerals (40). Formula manufacturers have developed mineral fortification mixtures (Natural Care or Enfamil Human Milk Fortifier) to be mixed with the LBS infant's own mother's milk. Although adequate absorption and subsequent metabolism of vitamin D has been shown (41) it is advisable to continue the current recommendation to provide 400 IU of vitamin D daily to breast-fed infants (42).

Although preterm human milk is not the perfect food in view of the variability in its protein concentration and its nutrient deficiencies there are good reasons to suggest that of the choices presently available it may be the best (5) because of nonnutrient factors such as anti-infective properties and easier digestibility (43). The "insufficient milk syndrome" is a frequent problem in mothers giving birth prematurely. The lack of contact between the mother and her infant, a poor sucking reflex, and low prolactin levels (44) are some of the factors responsible for unsuccessful breast feeding in prematures. When supplementation is necessary, it should be done with a premature formula rather than with banked human milk as the latter regimen leads to impaired growth (23).

V. FORMULAS FOR LOW-BIRTH-WEIGHT INFANTS

A better understanding of the macronutrient needs as well as of the requirements for minerals and vitamins of premature infants has led to the development of formulas specially designed for the LBW infant during the first few months of life. The composition of these formulas (Table 3) has also taken into consideration the limited capacity of the LBW infant to tolerate large loads of proteins and solutes as well as its impaired digestive phase for proteins, fat, and carbohydrates.

A. Quantity and Quality of Proteins

As pointed out recently, no prototype exists for feeding preterm infants (13). One approach has been to minimize stress to the immature metabolic system with diets that allow less rapid growth while the other has been to achieve more rapid growth rates by increasing the energy and the protein concentration of formulas. Current AAP recommendation is for 2.25-5 g/kg per day–but, on the basis of protein synthesis and turnover studies, it was found that increasing the protein intake from 4.3 to 5.1 g/kg per day resulted in no significant change in protein turnover (45). The figure of 3-4 g/kg per day proposed by Ziegler and

Table 3 Composition of Special Premature Formulas

Per dl	Enfamil 68 kcal	Enfamil Premature 81 kcal	SMA Preemie 81 kcal	Similac 68 kcal	Similac Special Care 81 kcal
Protein (g)	2	2.4	2.0	1.8	2.2
whey:casein	60:40	60:40	60:40	60:40	60:40
Fat (g)	3.4	4.1	4.4	3.7	4.4
MCT % ($\leqslant$C12)	40	40	27.5	50	50
LCT % ($>$C12)	60	60	72.5	50	50
Carbohydrate (g)	7.4	8.9	8.6	7.2	8.6
Lactose %	40	40	50	50	50
Glucose polymers %	60	60	50	50	50
Minerals					
Calcium (mg)	79	95	75	121	144
Phosphorus (mg)	40	48	40	60	72
Magnesium (mg)	7.1	8.5	7	8.3	10
Sodium (mEq)	1.1	1.4	1.4	1.4	1.7
Potassium (mEq)	1.9	2.3	1.9	2.4	2.9
Chloride (mEq)	1.6	1.9	1.5	1.7	2.0
Zinc (μg)	690	810	500	1000	1200
Copper (μg)	63	76	70	170	200
Vitamins					
A (IU)	210	254	320	462	550
D (IU)	42	51	51	101	120
E (IU)	1.32	1.6	1.5	2.5	3
C (mg)	5.7	6.9	7	25	30
B_1 (μg)	50	60	80	170	200
B_2 (μg)	60	70	130	420	500
Niacin (mg)	0.85	1.0	0.63	3.4	4
B_6 (μg)	41.3	47.6	50	170	200
B_{12} (μg)	0.21	0.25	0.2	0.37	0.45
Folic acid (μg)	20	24	10	25	30
K_1 (μg)	6.3	7.6	7	8.3	10
Osmolality mOsm/kg water	244	300	268	240	300

co-workers (13) is currently accepted. Recent studies have shown that a growth rate approaching that of the third-intrauterine trimester without imposing stress on developing metabolic and excretory systems (6) is achievable with these levels of protein intake.

Räihä and co-workers (20) were the first to point out that protein quality might also be a factor in metabolic stress of very small infants. They showed that whey-predominant (60:40) formulas have metabolic advantages over casein-predominant (20:80) formulas. However their advantage with regard to nitrogen retention and growth remains debatable. On the same energy intake, both the amount and the quality of the nitrogen source determines the extent of nitrogen retention. Our recent study showed that the whey:casein ratio had little influence on nitrogen retention and growth in LBW infants fed large energy (150 kcal/kg per day) and nitrogen intakes (4.3 g/kg per day). However, both nitrogen retention and growth were adversely affected when a 20:80 whey:casein iso-caloric formula of lower biologic quality providing 3.5 g/kg per day of proteins was fed (46). Protein hydrolysate formula was of no advantage in the healthy low-birth-weight newborn and should be reserved for those infants with specific gastrointestinal alterations (46).

In designing feeding regimens for LBW infants, it is important to remember that energy utilization for growth is remarkably sensitive to the quantity of protein in the diet and is inefficiently used when protein intake in relation to energy is inadequate (47). At a high energy intake, a protein source of lower quality fed in large amounts is unlikely to affect nitrogen retention and growth. Therefore, protein requirements should be thought of in terms of protein:energy ratios rather than in absolute terms. The ratio of 2.7 (protein intake/100 kcal) proposed in 1981 appears to be a reasonable figure (13).

B. Lipid Source

Fat is a major source of energy to the young infant and comprises 40 to 50% of the total calories present in human milk and most milk formulas. Lipids are not only a vital source of energy and of linoleic acid, but also the vehicle for fat-soluble vitamins. Linoleic acid cannot be synthesized de novo and is essential for growth and integrity of membranes as well of brain structural lipids. The AAP Committee on Nutrition recommends that in full-term infants linoleate should account for at least 2.7% of total calories (48).

The digestive phase of fat absorption is impaired in the LBW infant. As a result, a significant proportion of calories is lost in the stools. This is due to a low activity of pancreatic lipase and esterase (49) and impaired bile salt metabolism (50). Medium-chain triglycerides (MCT) are more easily hydrolyzed and, in view of their solubility, do not require micellar solubilization. Although the substitution of 80% of the long-chain triglyceride content by MCT is known to correct the coefficient of fat absorption to values of >95% (51,52), concerns have been expressed with regard to gastrointestinal tolerance and the potential danger of linoleic acid deficiency.

The MCT content of milks from various species is variable and accounts for more than two thirds of lipids in the rabbit. It is of interest to note that preterm human milk contains more MCT than term milk (35). In the hope of improving overall fat absorption, MCT made up of fatty acids with 12 or fewer carbons account for 27 to 50% of triglycerides in presently available premature formulas. The use of MCT in premature infant formulas has been questioned because no clear evidence has been found that the percentage of fat absorption is significantly better than with ordinary formulas which contain up to 20% of MCT (46,53, 54). Calcium absorption is reportedly ameliorated in preterm infants fed formulas with high concentrations of MCT (55); however, these observations could not be confirmed by another study (53). Experimentally, medium-chain triglycerides have recently been shown to stimulate hepatic gluconeogenesis by increasing the availability of glucose precursors such as lactate and alanine (56). It remains to be seen if, clinically, MCT could protect against hypoglycemia.

C. Carbohydrates

One third to one half of the energy needs of the newborn are met by carbohydrates present in human milk and formulas. The capacity of the newborn for digestion and absorption of carbohydrates is incompletely established at birth.

Although pancreatic amylase activity is practically absent at birth, salivary amylase is abundant and glucoamylase activity in the brush border of the small intestine is high (57,58). The latter has optimal hydrolytic activity against medium-chain length glucose polymers (5-9 units) with most of the molecular bonds being of the 1,4 variety and therefore with minimal branching.

A temporary malabsorption of lactose is well identified in neonates, particularly in preemies. Lactase activity is only 30% of that found in full-term neonates by 26-34 weeks of gestation. Most prematures have a positive lactose breath test, and it has been suggested that in some cases more than two thirds of ingested lactose reaches the colon (59). Although reducing substances are present in the stools of close to 50% of newborns on human milk or formula, their concentration rarely reaches 0.5% (Clinitest).

These findings have been taken into consideration for the design of premature formulas, which differ from full-term formulas in that 50% of lactose is replaced by medium-chain length glucose polymers. However, a recent study has shown no difference in terms of metabolizable energy derived from carbohydrates in response to the administration of a formula containing 100% lactose versus another with 50% lactose and 50% glucose oligopolymers (60). A further objection to a move away from lactose is in a recent paper comparing calcium uptake from a lactose to a sucrose/corn starch hydrolysate formula. The results show that the lactose-containing formula had distinct advantages with regard to calcium absorption and phosphorus retention (61). The only possible advantage of oligopolymers over lactose is that they contribute relatively less to the osmolality of the formulas in view of their higher molecular weight.

D. Micronutrients and Vitamins

1. Calcium, Phosphorus, and Vitamin D

In LBW infants fed formulas of composition similar to that of mature human milk, bone growth and mineralization is compromised. This is not surprising in view of the fact that the reference fetus has a daily increase of 129 mg of calcium at 28-29 weeks of gestation. In order to meet this fetal retention rate an intake of more than 210 mg/kg per day is necessary in 800-1200 g prematures (40).

A decade ago, oral calcium supplements added to common formulas were shown to be effective in mimicking the intrauterine accretion rate of calcium and improving bone mineralization (62). Formulas designed for prematures contain higher concentrations of calcium and phosphorus. They have been shown to increase the bone mineral content at the fetal rate (63,64). Another factor in bone metabolism in the small premature is a high vitamin D requirement shown by the development of rickets while on formulas containing only the usual 400 IU of vitamin D per liter (65). Currently available premature formulas contain somewhat higher concentrations of vitamin D (Table 3).

2. Vitamins E and C

Intakes of vitamins from available formulas are generally less than advisable because of the smaller amounts of formulas consumed. In addition, there is evidence of increased requirements.

Vitamin E. Requirements for α-tocopherol (vitamin E) are higher in the premature than in the term infant. The main reason is the poor absorption of vitamin E (66) and the greater fragility of their red cell membranes to hydrogen peroxide (67). It is therefore recommended that formulas fed to prematures should contain 0.7 IU of vitamin E (0.5 mg of α-tocopherol) per 100 kcal. In view of the well known relationship between vitamin E requirement and the intake of polyunsaturated fatty acids (PUFA), it is best to link the vitamin E intake to the intake of PUFA. In the premature formulas, concentrations of vitamin E vary between 1.5 and 2.5 IU/g of linoleic acid, a figure which is well above the AAP recommendation of 1.0 IU/g.

Vitamin C. Ascorbic acid enhances the activity of hepatic p-hydroxyphenylpyruvic acid oxidase and may decrease high tyrosine blood levels in LBW. Premature formulas provide variable amounts of vitamin C. Some fall short of the recommended intake of 60 mg/day while others provide ample amounts (13).

3. Trace Elements

The importance of trace elements such as iron, copper, zinc, and manganese of the neonate has been demonstrated in several species. Deficiencies of these essential nutrients may lead to high neonatal mortality, impaired immunocompetence (68), and abnormal development or poor growth. As the only food of the neonate is milk, its capacity to meet the trace-element needs are crucial. Of recent concern is the observation that the bioavailability of trace metals is profoundly affected by their competition for absorption and their interaction.

Iron. The preterm infant is born with low iron stores since most of the iron store is accumulated during the third trimester of gestation. There is evidence that iron acts as a catalyst in the oxidative destruction of the erythrocyte lipid membrane (69). However, vitamin E, by protecting the polyunsaturated fatty acid component of the lipid membrane from peroxidation, prevents to some extent the oxidant effect of iron. Because of the potential side effects of iron and the fact that iron therapy has no benefit on the physiologic anemia of prematurity (70), premature formulas are not supplemented with iron.

Zinc. It is apparent from several studies that zinc in formulas and in cow's milk is less bioavailable than zinc from human milk. Even with levels of 5.8 mg/liter of formula, plasma zinc values are significantly lower in formula-fed than in human milk-fed infants receiving only 1-3 mg/liter (71).

The fetal retention rate for zinc is 250 μg/kg per day in fetuses of 24-36 weeks of gestation growing along the fiftieth percentile (72). In LBW infants this retention rate could not be met even with human milk containing up to 454 μg/dl (73). Although premature formulas contain more than twice this amount there is as yet no evidence that a positive zinc balance is obtained.

Copper. Neonatal copper deficiency can present with neutropenia, osteoporosis, depigmentation of skin, and central nervous system abnormalities (74). Prematures are at greater risk of developing low serum copper levels (75).

Human milk and formulas have a relatively low copper content. However, in the former it is of high biological availability and can sustain normal plasma and hair concentration (76). It is well known that a high level of dietary zinc interferes with copper uptake (77). Of more significance with regard to premature formulas is the observation that a high calcium and phosphorous diet enhances the fecal sequestration of copper (78).

Copper accretion rate in utero between 24 and 36 weeks of gestation amounts to 51 μg/kg per day. This range of retention cannot be achieved by the amount of copper supplied by preterm milk (79) and, as a result, copper balances are negative. Therefore, close attention to the formula copper content is important. At this writing, there are large variations of copper content (60-200 μg/dl) in premature formulas. Copper balance studies need to be performed to find out if in utero accretion rates can be obtained.

E. Fluid Intake, Renal Solute Load, and Caloric Density

The water requirement of premature infants is determined by the amount of water lost from the body by various routes and the net amount retained during the synthesis of new tissues. The water intake provided should be the sum of the predicted losses using a volume for urine flow allowing excretion of the estimated renal solute load which will be well within the limits of the renal concentrating capacity (80).

A well-conducted randomized trial in prematures has shown that a high volume of water intake ($\overline{X}$: 169 ml/kg) led to a higher incidence of patent ductus arteriosus and necrotizing enterocolitis (NEC) than did a low volume ($\overline{X}$: 122 ml/kg) (80). Hyponatremia is well tolerated clinically, but it may lead to growth retardation (81) in LBW infants who, nevertheless, have a low capacity to excrete a high solute load in view of their limited capacity to concentrate urine. Formulas with a high caloric density (81 kcal/dl) have a somewhat higher osmolality but are still in the range of 300 mOsm/kg H_2O. However they provide a higher solute load through their increased concentration of proteins (4 mOsm/g of dietary protein). There is, therefore, less free water available for excretion of solutes. Furthermore, it has been shown that the daily intake of such formulas tends to be lower (82).

VI. RECOMMENDATIONS

Feeding preterm infants presents multiple challenges only now beginning to be faced. Preterm human milk supplemented with calcium and phosphorus meets most known requirements. However its compositional variability and the findings of some studies dampen one's enthusiasm for the recommendation that each mother provide human milk for her own LBW infant. Close monitoring of prematures fed by their own mothers is therefore in order.

Addition to human milk of commercial fortifiers containing significant amounts of protein, calcium, phosphorus, copper, and zinc is a promising approach (83) to correct for the mineral and nutrient shortcomings of preterm milk. Special premature formulas represent a significant advance and are strongly recommended for the routine feeding of LBW infants who do not have access to human milk. However, much still remains to be done on their long-term effects on morbidity, growth, and development.

ACKNOWLEDGMENT

This study was supported in part by the Medical Research Council of Canada and Mead Johnson & Company.

REFERENCES

1. Parreth, N., Kiely, J. L., Wallestein, S., Marcus, M., Pakter, J., and Susser, M. Newborn intensive care and neonatal mortality in low-birth weight infants. A population study. *N. Engl. J. Med.* 307, 149–155, 1982.

2. Williams, R. L., and Chen, P. M. Identifying the sources of the recent decline in perinatal mortality rates in California. *N. Engl. J. Med.* 306, 207-214, 1982.

3. Heird, W. C., Driscoll, J. N., Schullinger, J. N., Grebin, B., Winters, R. W. Intravenous alimentation in pediatric patients. *J. Pediatr.* 80, 351-372, 1972.

4. Widdowson, E. M. Growth and composition of the fetus and newborn. In *Biology of Gestation,* Vol. 2. Assali, N. S. (ed.). Academic Press, New York, 1968, pp. 1-49.

5. Anderson, G. A., and Bryan, M. H. Is the premature infant's own mother's milk best? *J. Pediatr. Gastroenterol. Nutr.* 1, 157-159, 1982.

6. Committee on Nutrition. American Academy of Pediatrics. Nutritional needs of low-birth-weight infants. *Pediatrics* 75, 976-986, 1985.

7. Putet, G., Senterre, J., Rigo, J., and Salle, B. Nutrient balance, energy utilization and composition of weight gain in very low birth weight infants fed pooled human milk or a preterm formula. *J. Pediatr.* 105, 79-85, 1984.

8. Chessex, P., Reichmann, B., Verelleu, G., Putet, G., Smith, J. M., Heim, T., and Swyer, P. Quality of growth in premature infants fed their own mother's milk. *J. Pediatr.* 102, 107-112, 1983.

9. Duffy, B., Gumm, T., Collinge, J., and Pencharz, P. The effect of varying protein quality and energy intake on the nitrogen metabolism of parenterally fed very low birth weight (<1600 g) infants. *Pediatr. Res.* 15, 1040-1044, 1981.

10. Stern, L. Early postnatal growth of low birth weight infants. What is optimal? *Acta Paediatr. Scand.* (Suppl) 296, 6-13, 1982.

11. Ziegler, E. E., O'Donnell, A. M., Nelson, S. E., and Fomon, S. J. Body composition of the reference fetus. *Growth* 40, 329-341, 1976.

12. Sinclair, J. C., Driscoll, J. M., Jr., Heird, W. C., and Winters, R. W. Supportive management of the sick neonate. *Pediatr. Clin. North Am.* 17, 863-893, 1970.

13. Ziegler, E. E., Biga, R. L., and Fomon, S. J. Nutritional requirements of the premature infant. In *Textbook of Pediatric Nutrition.* Suskind, R. M. (ed.). Raven Press, New York, 1981. pp. 29-39.

14. Battaglia, F. C., and Simmons, M. A. The low-birth weight infant. In *Human Growth,* Vol. 2. Falkner, F., and Tamer, J. M. (eds.). Plenum Press, New York, 1978, pp. 507-555.

15. Chessex, P., Reichmann, B. L., Berellen, G. L. E., Putet, G., Smith, J. M., Heim, T., and Swyer, P. Influence of postnatal age, energy intake and weight gain on energy metabolism in the very low-birth weight infant. *J. Pediatr.* 99, 761-766, 1981.

16. Brooke, O. G., Alvear, J., and Arnold, M. Energy retention, energy expenditure and growth in healthy immature infants. *Pediatr. Res.* 13, 215-220, 1979.

17. Gudinchet, F., Shutz, Y., Micheli, J. L., Stettler, E., and Jequier, E. Metabolic cost of growth in very low-birth weight infants. *Pediatr. Res.* 16, 1025-1030, 1982.

18. Gordon, J. H., Levine, S. J., and McNamara, H. Feeding of the premature infant: A comparison of human and cow's milk. *Am. J. Dis. Child.* 73, 442-452, 1947.

19. Sinclair, J. C. Energy metabolism and fetal development. In *Fetal Growth and Development.* Waisman, H. A., and Kerr, G. R. (eds.). McGraw-Hill, New York, 1970, pp. 187-204.

20. Räihä, N. C. R., Heinarren, K., Rassin, D. K., and Gaull, G. E. Milk protein quantity and quality in low birth weight infants: I. Metabolic responses and effects on growth. *Pediatrics* 57, 659-674, 1976.

21. Fomon, S. J., Ziegler, E. E., and Vasquez, H. D. Human milk and the small premature infant. *Am. J. Dis. Child.* 131, 463-467, 1977.

22. Davies, D. P. Adequacy of expressed breast milk for early growth of preterm infants. *Arch. Dis. Child.* 52, 296-301, 1977.

23. Lucas, A., Gore, S. M., Cole, T. J., Bamford, M. F., Dossetor, J. B. F., Barr, I., Dicarlo, L., Cork, S., and Lucas, P. J. Multicentre trial on feeding low birth weight infants: Effects of diet on early growth. *Arch. Dis. Child.* 59, 722-730, 1984.

24. Tyson, J. E., Lasky, R. E., Mize, C. E., Richards, C. J., Blair-Smith, N., Whyte, R., and Beer, A. E. Growth, metabolic response and development in very low-birth-weight infants fed banked human milk or enriched formula I. Neonatal findings. *J. Pediatr.* 103, 95-104, 1983.

25. Committee on Nutrition. American Academy of Pediatrics. On the feeding of supplemental foods to infants. *Pediatrics* 65, 1178-1181, 1980.

26. Atkinson, S. A., Bryan, M. H., and Anderson, G. H. Human milk differences in nitrogen concentration in milk from mothers of term and premature infants. *J. Pediatr.* 93, 67-69, 1978.

27. Atkinson, S. A., Bryan, H., and Anderson, H. Human milk feeding in premature infants: Protein, fat and carbohydrate balances in the first two weeks of life. *J. Pediatr.* 99, 617-624, 1981.

28. Anderson, G. H., Atkinson, S. A., and Bryan, M. H. Energy and macronutrient content of human milk during early lactation from mothers giving birth prematurely and at term. *Am. J. Clin. Nutr.* 34, 258-265, 1981.

29. Anderson, G. H. Human milk feeding. *Pediatr. Clin. North Am.* 32, 335-353, 1985.

30. Mc Lean, W. C., and Graham, G. G. Preterm milk. *Am. J. Clin. Nutr.* 34, 2331-2332, 1981.

31. Chan, G. M., Thomas, M. R., Parsons, M. H., Demkowicz, M. F., and Gervase, M. M. Preterm and term human milk composition and maternal dietary effects. *Clin. Res.* 28, 136A, 1981.

32. Anderson, D., Pittard, W., Shulman, P., Mitman, F., Merkatz, R., and Kerr, D. Comparative nutrient composition of human milk. *Pediatr. Res.* 15, 525, 1981.

33. Harzer, G., Hang, M., Dieterich, I., and Gentner, P. R. Changing patterns of human milk lipids in the course of the lactation and during the day. *Am. J. Clin. Nutr.* 37, 612-621, 1983.

34. Lucas, A., and Hudson, G. J. Preterm milk as a source of protein for low birth weight infants. *Arch. Dis. Child.* 59, 831-836, 1984.
35. Lepage, G., Collet, S., Bouglé, D., Kien, L. C., Lepage, D., Dallaire, L., Darling, P., and Roy, C. C. The composition of preterm milk in relation to the degree of prematurity. *Am. J. Clin. Nutr.* 40, 1042-1049, 1984.
36. Gross, S. J. Growth and biochemical response of preterm infants fed human milk or modified infant formula. *N. Engl. J. Med.* 308, 237-241, 1983.
37. Atkinson, S. A., Radde, I. C., and Anderson, G. H. Macromineral balances in premature infants fed their own mother's milk or formula. *J. Pediatr.* 102, 99-106, 1983.
38. Shanler, R. J., and Oh, W. Nitrogen and mineral balance in preterm infants fed human milk or formula. *J. Pediatr. Gastroenterol. Nutr.* 4, 214-219, 1985.
39. Mendelson, R. A., Bryan, M. H., and Anderson, G. H. Trace mineral balances in preterm infants fed their own mother's milk. *J. Pediatr. Gastroenterol. Nutr.* 2, 256-261, 1983.
40. Atkinson, S. A. Calcium and phosphorus requirements of low birth weight infants: A nutritional and endocrinological perspective. *Nutr. Rev.* 41, 69-78, 1983.
41. Salle, B. L., David, L., Glorieux, F. H., Delvin, E., Senterre, J., and Renaud, H. Early oral administration of vitamin D and its metabolites in premature neonates. Effect on mineral homeostasis. *Pediatr. Res.* 16, 75-78, 1982.
42. Committee on Nutrition. American Academy of Pediatrics. Vitamin and mineral supplement needs in normal children in the United States. *Pediatrics* 66, 1015-1021, 1980.
43. Fleischman, A. R., and Finberg, L. Breast milk for term and premature infants—optimal nutrition. *Semin. Perinatol.* 3, 397-405, 1979.
44. Ehrenkranz, A., and Ackerman, B. Effect of metoclopramide on faltering milk production by mothers of premature infants. *Pediatr. Res.* 19, 218A, 1985.
45. Pencharz, P. B., Masson, M., Desgranges, F., and Papageorgiou, A. Total-body protein turnover in human premature neonates: Effects of birth weight intrauterine nutritional status and diet. *Clin. Sci.* 61, 207-215, 1981.
46. Darling, P. Lepage, G., Tremblay, P., Collet, S., Kien, L. C., and Roy, C. C. Protein quality and quantity in preterm infants receiving the same energy intake. *Am. J. Dis. Child.* 139, 186-190, 1985.
47. Mac Lean, W. C., and Graham, G. G. The effect of level of protein intake in isoenergetic diets on energy utilization. *Am. J. Clin. Nutr.* 32, 1381-1387, 1979.
48. Barness, L. A. Infant feeding: Formula, solids. *Pediatr. Clin. North Am.* 32, 355-362, 1985.
49. Lebenthal, E., and Lee, P. C. Development of functional response in human exocrine pancreas. *Pediatrics* 66, 556-560, 1980.
50. Harries, J. T. Fat absorption in the newborn. *Acta Paediatr. Scand.* (Suppl) 299, 17-23, 1982.

51. Tantibhedhyangkul, P., and Hashim, S. A. Medium chain triglyceride feeding in premature infants: Effect on fat and nitrogen absorption. *Pediatrics* 55, 359-370, 1975.

52. Roy, C. C., Ste-Marie, M., Chartrand, L., Weber, A., Bard, H., and Doray, B. Correction of the malabsorption of the preterm infant with a medium chain triglyceride formula. *J. Pediatr.* 86, 446-450, 1975.

53. Huston, R. K., Reynolds, J. W., Jensen, C., and Buist, N. R. M. Nutrient and mineral retention and vitamin D absorption in low birth weight infants. The effect of medium chain triglycerides. *Pediatrics* 72, 44-48, 1983.

54. Okamoto, E., Muttart, C. R., Zucker, C. L., and Heird, W. C. Use of medium-chain triglycerides in feeding the low-birth-weight infant. *Am. J. Dis. Child.* 136, 428-431, 1982.

55. Roy, C. C., Lepage, G., Chartrand, L., and Fontaine, A. Early postnatal nutrition and later growth of low birth weight newborns. *Pediatr. Res.* 13, 407, 1979.

56. Pegorier, J. P., Leturque, A., Ferre, P., Turlan, P., and Girard, J. Effects of medium-chain triglyceride feeding on glucose homeostasis in the newborn rat. *Am. J. Physiol.* 244, E329-E344, 1983.

57. Lebenthal, E., and Lee, P. C. Glucoamylase and disaccharidase activities in normal subjects and in patients with mucosal injury of the small intestine. *J. Pediatr.* 97, 389-393, 1980.

58. Kerzner, B. Mucosal glucoamylase activity. *J. Pediatr.* 99, 338-339, 1981.

59. Mac Lean, W. C., Jr., and Fink, B. B. Lactose malabsorption by premature infants: Magnitude and clinical significance. *J. Pediatr.* 97, 316-323, 1980.

60. Kien, C. L., Summers, J. E., Stetina, J. S., Heimler, R., and Grausz, J. P. A method for assessing carbohydrate energy absorption and its application to premature infants. *Am. J. Clin. Nutr.* 36, 910-916, 1982.

61. Ziegler, E. E., and Fomon, S. J. Lactose enhances mineral absorption in infancy. *J. Pediatr. Gastroenterol. Nutr.* 2, 288-294, 1983.

62. Day, G. M., Chance, G. W., Radde, I. C., Reilly, B. J., Park, E., and Sheepers, J. Growth and mineral metabolism in very low birth weight infants. II. Effects of calcium supplementation on growth and divalent cations. *Pediatr. Res.* 9, 568-575, 1975.

63. Steichen, J. J., Gratton, T. L., and Tsang, R. C. Osteopenia of prematurity: The cause and possible treatment. *J. Pediatr.* 96, 528-534, 1980.

64. Greer, F. R., Steichen, J. J., and Tsang, R. C. Calcium and phosphate supplements in breast fed milk related rickets. *Am. J. Dis. Child.* 136, 581-583, 1982.

65. Lewin, P. K., Reid, M., Reilly, B. J., Swyer, P. R., and Fraser, D. Iatrogenic rickets in low birth weight infants. *J. Pediatr.* 78, 207-210, 1971.

66. Melhorn, D. K., and Gross, S. Vitamin E-dependent anemia in the premature infant: I. Relationships between gestational age and absorption of vitamin E. *J. Pediatr.* 79, 569-580, 1971.

67. Gross, S., and Melhorn, D. K. Vitamin E dependent anemia in the premature infant. *J. Pediatr.* 85, 753-759, 1974.

68. Chandra, R. K. Trace element regulation of immunity and infection. *J. Am. Coll. Nutr.* 4, 5-16, 1985.
69. Williams, M. L., Shott, R. J., O'Neal, P. L., and Oski, F. A. Role of dietary iron and fat on vitamin E deficiency anemia of infancy. *N. Engl. J. Med.* 292, 887-890, 1975.
70. Dallman, P. R. Iron, vitamin E and folate in the preterm infant. *J. Pediatr.* 85, 742-752, 1974.
71. Hambidge, K. M., Walravens, P. A., Casey, C. E., Brown, R. M., and Bender, C. Plasma zinc concentrations of breast-fed infants. *J. Pediatr.* 94, 607-608, 1979.
72. Shaw, J. C. L. Trace elements in the fetus and young infant: II. Copper, manganese, selenium and chromium. *Am. J. Dis. Child.* 134, 74-81, 1980.
73. Sann, L., Rigal, D., Galy, G., Bienvenu, F., and Bourgeois, J. Serum copper and zinc concentration in premature and small for date infants. *Pediatr. Res.* 14, 1040-1046, 1980.
74. Ashkenazi, A., Levin, S., Djaldetti, M., Fishel, E., and Benvenisti, D. The syndrome of neonatal copper deficiency. *Pediatrics* 52, 525-533, 1973.
75. Manser, J. I., Crawford, C. S., Tyrala, E. E., Bradsky, N. L., and Grover, W. D. Serum copper concentrations in sick and well preterm infants. *J. Pediatr.* 97, 795-799, 1980.
76. Solomon, N. W. Biochemical, metabolic and clinical role of copper in human nutrition. *J. Am. Coll. Nutr.* 4, 83-105, 1985.
77. Greger, J. L., Zaikis, S. C., Abernathy, R. P., Bennett, O. A., and Huffman, J. Zinc, nitrogen, copper, iron and manganese balance in adolescent females fed two levels of zinc. *J. Nutr.* 108, 1449-1456, 1978.
78. Snedecker, S. M., Smith, C. A., and Greger, J. L. Effect of dietary calcium and phosphorus on utilization of iron, copper and zinc by adult males. *J. Nutr.* 112, 136-143, 1982.
79. Mendelson, R. A., Anderson, G. H., and Bryan, M. H. Zinc, copper and iron content of milk from mothers of preterm and full term infants. *Early Hum. Dev.* 6, 145-151, 1982.
80. Bell, E. F., and Oh, W. Water requirements of premature newborn infants. *Acta Paediatr. Scand.* (Suppl) 305, 21-26, 1983.
81. Aperia, A., Broberger, O., and Zetterström, R. Implications of limitation of renal function for the nutrition of low birthweight infants. *Acta Paediatr. Scand.* (Suppl) 296, 49-51, 1982.
82. Brooke, O. G., and Kinsey, J. M. High energy feeding in small for gestation infants. *Arch. Dis. Child.* 60, 42-46, 1985.
83. Bromberger, P., Saunders, B., and Akins, M. Supplemented human milk effect on growth and serum biochemistries in pre-term infants. *Pediatr. Res.* 18, 191A, 1984.

17

Infantile Colic and the Role of Casein Hydrolysate Formulas

Brian W. C. Forsyth
Yale University School of Medicine and Yale-New Haven Hospital, New Haven, Connecticut

I. INTRODUCTION

Infantile colic is a common problem, affecting 10-20% of infants in the first few months of life (1-3). Although there is no single definition for infantile colic, the mainstay of the diagnosis is paroxysms of intense, inconsolable crying most commonly during the evening hours. During crying episodes the infant often draws his legs up to his abdomen and turns red. There is frequently abdominal distention and there may be increased flatus. For the infant there is apparent distress and possibly pain. For the parents, the inconsolable crying produces feelings of helplessness, frustration, decreased confidence in their own parenting abilities and, at times, anger. Despite the long history and high frequency of colic, and numerous articles in the pediatric and psychological literature on colic and excessive crying, there are few methodologically sound studies which assess the cause of colic and little is known (although there is much speculation) about the best way to manage this problem.

Pediatricians giving advice about colic tend to take one of two approaches: the first is based on the assumption that colic is an extreme form of crying behavior (Fig. 1) and that the associated symptoms are simply a part of this behavior. (The abdominal distention and excessive flatus are felt to be a result of air swallowing.) Colic is therefore managed with a behavioral approach. The second approach assumes that colic is a separate entity (Fig. 2) and that the excessive crying and other symptoms are all part of an adverse reaction to the

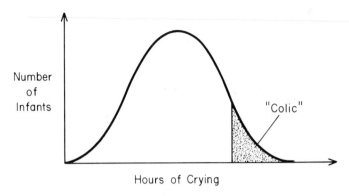

Figure 1   Colic as an extreme of crying behavior.

milk that the infant is taking. This theory is an old one and through the ages the cause of colic has been ascribed to numerous different components of the milk: "too rich, too weak, too hot, too cold, contains too much fat; too much carbohydrate or too much protein" (1). For several decades the most popular theory held that colic is a specific allergic reaction to the protein content of the milk (4,5). Another considered possibility is that colic is due to a partial malabsorption of lactose. These theories have led pediatricians to frequently recommend changing the formulas fed to these infants from a cow's milk to a soy protein or casein hydrolysate-based formula containing neither cow's milk protein nor lactose. In 1980 we conducted a study designed to assess what proportion of infants received a change of formula (6). We enrolled 174 healthy newborn infants who were receiving a cow's milk formula and who were to

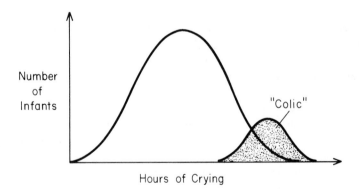

Figure 2   Colic as a separate pathological entity.

be followed by pediatricians in private practice. By four months of age, 26% of these infants had had their formula changed to a non-cow's milk formula. Usually, the change was to a soy protein formula rather than to a casein hydrolysate formula. Only 5% of the formula changes were to a casein hydrolysate formula. However, soy protein formulas, as well as cow's milk formulas, have been implicated in colic (7). In 1983, the Committee on Nutrition of the American Academy of Pediatrics recommended that soy protein formulas should not be used "in the routine management of colic" (8). The Committee noted that it is questionable whether soy protein formulas are less allergenic than cow's milk formulas and suggested that casein hydrolysate formulas are preferable for the management of allergy. Since colic is possibly an allergic phenomenon, this would imply that casein hydrolysate formulas would also be appropriate for the management of colic.

The aim of this chapter is to assess the evidence supporting the role of casein hydrolysate formulas in the management of colic. However, there are, in fact, no well-designed studies which have specifically looked at the effects of managing colic by changing the infant's formula to a casein hydrolysate formula. It is therefore necessary to review other studies that contribute to our knowledge of colic and the possible etiologic role played by milk. These studies are of three main types: (a) those that describe findings associated with colic that are inconsistent with theories of allergy or intolerance to milk; (b) studies that have looked for markers suggestive of allergy or intolerance to milk, and (c) studies that have looked for clinical improvement following the elimination of cow's milk from the diet.

II. TYPES OF STUDIES CONTRIBUTING TO OUR KNOWLEDGE OF COLIC AND THE POSSIBLE ETIOLOGIC ROLE OF MILK

A. Studies with Findings Inconsistent with Allergy or Intolerance to Milk

1. It is generally accepted that the prevalence of colic in breast- and formula-fed infants is equal (2,3), which would appear to be inconsistent with the theory that colic is a form of allergy. However, cow's milk protein ingested by a mother may pass in her breast milk to her baby (9-11). It still seems unlikely, however, that the prevalence, presentation, and duration of colic in breast- and formula-fed infants would be the same considering that the pathophysiology of the allergic response to the small amount of antigen present in breast milk is reported to be very different from that resulting from exposure to the large amount of antigen present in formulas (12-16). Other manifestations of cow's

milk protein allergy, such as vomiting or diarrhea, are much less common in infants taking breast milk than in infants taking cow's milk formulas.

2. In placebo-controlled trials designed to assess the efficacy of medications for the treatment of colic, the colic has resolved in more than half of the infants receiving the placebo (17,18). In one study conducted by O'Donovan and Bradstock (18), 84% of the subjects taking a placebo were reported to have a decrease in the symptoms of colic. This placebo response could be explained either by a change in the symptoms or, more likely, by a change in the perceptions of the parent and thus a change in the reporting of symptoms. This apparent response to a placebo makes it unlikely, however, that these infants had an allergy to their milk. This placebo response also demonstrates the need for proper blinding of studies designed to investigate the effect of changing an infant's milk formula.

3. Infantile colic tends to resolve at 10–12 weeks of age. While this is inconsistent with our present knowledge of allergy or intolerance, it is consistent with the pattern of normal crying behavior in which the amount of crying increases for the first 6 weeks of infancy, plateaus, and then decreases (19).

B. Studies Investigating Markers of Allergy or Intolerance to Milk

A possible way to demonstrate that colic is an allergic phenomenon is to identify markers of allergy in infants with colic. Such markers might include an increase in IgE, milk precipitins, immune complexes, and specific antibodies to milk proteins. Markers of intolerance to milk or malabsorption of lactose include the demonstration of acidic stools and reducing substances in the stools. There are, in fact, few studies that have attempted to demonstrate these markers in infants with colic. Harris et al. (20) demonstrated an increase of IgE plasma cells in the jejunal mucosa of 14 children. These children did not all have colic but were selected from a group of 100 infants who had a tentative diagnosis of milk allergy. The title ("Cow's milk allergy as a cause of infantile colic: immunofluorescent studies on jejunal mucosa") and results of this paper are misleading. Although the results may provide some information about milk allergy, they do not help determine the etiology of colic.

In a further study of markers of milk allergy and lactose intolerance, Liebman evaluated 56 infants with colic (21). He found no abnormality in quantitative IgE, radioallergosorbent tests (RAST) for cow's milk protein, and tests for stool pH and reducing substances, and was therefore unable to conclude that colic was caused by the milk. To date, no one has studied infants with colic using the breath hydrogen test, a more sensitive measure of lactose malabsorption.

C. Cow's Milk Elimination Studies

Because of the lack of a definitive diagnostic test implicating cow's milk as the cause of colic, it has been necessary to perform studies in which the results are determined by the response to the elimination of cow's milk from the diet. There are, however, a number of principles which have to be taken into account when performing this type of research.

1. "Blinding"

Because there is a potential for a placebo effect, the investigators and parents should be unaware of the changes being made. This is difficult to ensure when one type of formula smells and tastes very different from another. It is well known that parents often taste the milk before offering it to their infant. A good example of the need for blinding is demonstrated by the studies which have investigated the effects on breast-fed infants of their mothers taking cow's milk. Without blinding, a large proportion of mothers will report that their infant's colic improves when they themselves stop taking cow's milk and the colic returns when they again take cow's milk (9). Evans et al. used a research protocol in which the mothers were blinded to the type of milk they were taking (11). They were given soy-based formulas with vanilla flavoring added. On certain days cow's milk was added to the formula. In this study the symptoms of colic were not found to be related to the type of milk ingested by the mothers.

2. "Washout" Period

It is uncertain how long it takes before a change in diet will have an effect on the symptoms of colic. However, it has been reported that it may take more than 48 hours for the symptoms of milk allergy to become evident (22). This necessitates a "washout" period of at least 48 hours before the effects of the dietary change can be measured. In the majority of cow's milk elimination studies no reference is made to a "washout" period. In the study by Evans et al. (11), the "washout" period was only 24 hr. They measured the effects of the change between 24 and 48 hours after the alteration. There is therefore the potential for a carryover effect which may have biased the results and obscured a positive effect.

3. Definitions for Colic and Criteria for Improvement

Researchers need to identify definitions for colic and criteria for improvement. If, after a change of formula, a baby cries for 2-1/2 hours per day instead of 3 hours per day, would that baby still be considered to have colic or would that be considered a "cure"? No researchers have fully addressed this problem. Responses to formula changes are usually categorized as "improved," "the same," or "worse," thus allowing the results of a study to be determined by what may be small subjective changes.

4. Repeat Challenges

Because colic may resolve spontaneously, to confirm that improvement is, in fact, a response to the change of formula, a further challenge of cow's milk should be given. If, in response to this repeat challenge, the colic recurs, this would be evidence in favor of the cow's milk having had a role in causing the colic.

To date no research design has satisfied all of these principles. Earlier studies were simply reports of changing the diet without blinding and without rechallenging. More recent studies have tried to incorporate some, but not all of these principles into the research design. To illustrate the importance of these principles it is necessary to review some of the more recent studies in greater detail.

D. Review of Recent Studies of Infantile Colic

In the largest and most recently reported study involving the elimination of cow's milk formulas, Lothe et al. concluded that colic is frequently due to cow's milk (7). Sixty formula-fed infants between the ages of two weeks and three months were the subjects. The definition for colic was given as "paroxysmal abdominal pain" (which is a subjective impression), "severe crying for several hours per day," abdominal distention and "the wish to suck often." Subjects were given, in random order, a cow's milk formula for one week and a soy formula for one week. The formulas were not identified to the parents but the differences in appearance and taste make it unlikely that they were properly blinded. There were three outcome groups: those whose colic improved during both challenges (29%), those who were the same or worse with both challenges (53%), and those whose colic improved with the soy challenge but not with the cow's milk challenge (18%) (Table 1). Thus, from what was considered the blinded part of the study, only 18% of the subjects had colic that appeared to be related to the formula. However, the authors went on to report results based on further nonblinded formula changes: The 53% of infants whose colic was unchanged or worse while taking either formula were given Nutramigen (a casein hydrolysate formula) and in all of these infants the colic improved. Based on this nonblinded formula change the authors concluded that, in these infants, the colic was caused by both cow's milk and soy milk. Similarly, those 18% of infants who had colic on the cow's milk formula but not on the soy formula were given a nonblinded challenge with a cow's milk formula to ensure that symptoms returned and that the improvement was not due to a spontaneous resolution of symptoms. Although this study was reported as a double-blind study, the final results were arrived at using nonblinded changes of formula and are, therefore, less reliable. This study illustrates the point that not only should there be a rechallenge with a milk formula, but this rechallenge should also be blinded. This can be achieved by using a double-blind (both researchers and parents are blind), double cross-over design in which there is a change back to, or rechallenge with, the original formula. Very few studies have employed this research design. In Evans' study (11), in which they investigated the relationship between colic and the type of milk ingested by breast-feeding mothers,

Table 1 Summary of Study by Lothe et al. Investigating the Response of Infants with Colic to Changes of Formula (7)

"Blinded"			Percent of subjects with each pattern of response
Cow's milk formula	Soy formula	Nonblinded	
Improved	Improved		29%
Same or worse	Same or worse	Improved with casein formula	53%
Same or worse	Improved	Worse with cow's milk formula	18%

two different formulas were given to the mothers in randomized order each for three different periods. This design makes it likely that there were multiple cross-overs. This study demonstrated no association between the infants' colic and the ingestion of cow's milk by the mothers although, as noted previously, there are other faults with the design of the study.

In 1983 Jakobsson and Lindberg (23) reported a two-phase study investigating whether ingestion of cow's milk by mothers of breast-feeding infants was the cause of colic. The first phase was a nonblind study, in which 23 of 66 colicky infants (35%) had no colic when their mothers stopped taking cow's milk, but colic returned when their mothers resumed taking cow's milk. Sixteen of these 23 mother-infant pairs participated in the second, blinded phase of the study. The mothers were given, in random order, a challenge of cow's milk protein (whey protein) and a placebo (potato starch); each was given in capsules for a period of one day. The "washout" period was also only one day. Six infants were excluded from the final analysis because they did not have colic with either the challenge or placebo. Of the remaining 10 infants, 9 had colic with the challenge, but not with the placebo. These results certainly suggest that the symptoms of colic in some breast-feeding infants may be caused by the ingestion of cow's milk by their mothers. However, because only 10 of the original 66 infants were included in the final analysis, the conclusion that this is true for one third of breast-feeding infants is not well founded. Also, the investigators did not clearly define their criteria either for a diagnosis of colic or for improvement; therefore it is difficult to assess both the validity and generalizability of these results.

In a well-designed study, Barr et al. used a double-blind double cross-over design to test the hypothesis that increased crying is caused by a partial malabsorption of lactose (24). The subjects for this study were 17 normal, formula-feeding infants who did not have colic. They were given two different formulas; each formula was soy based but one contained added lactose and the other did not. The order of the formulas was alternated and each was given for two, 4-day periods. The breath hydrogen test was used to measure lactose malabsorption. Although the authors reported that breath hydrogen decreased during the course of the study as did the total daily duration of crying, they were unable to relate the duration of crying to the lactose content of the formulas, thus producing a somewhat confusing result. This might suggest that the amount of crying affects the amount of breath hydrogen excreted rather than the lactose content of the formula having an effect on the infant's crying.

E. Study in Progess of Infantile Colic

Because of the flaws and the contradictory results in previous studies, we are presently conducting a study in New Haven, Connecticut, to determine whether changing an infant's formula to a casein hydrolysate formula does, in fact, cure colic. This study is designed to satisfy the principles necessary to prevent erroneous conclusions. It is a double-blind, double cross-over design where, for each of four, 4-day periods, an infant receives either pure Nutramigen or a mixture of Nutramigen and a cow's milk formula. The presence of Nutramigen in each formula assures satisfactory blinding. Each infant receives two challenges of cow's milk formula, thus enabling us to detect those infants for whom the colic resolves spontaneously during the 16-day duration of the study. The first two days of each 4-day period will be excluded from the analysis, thus providing a satisfactory "washout" between formulas. In order to satisfy criteria for improvement, mothers are recording in a diary the time and duration of all crying episodes throughout each day, as well as documenting subjective impressions of colic. This diary is adapted from one developed by Barr, who showed a satisfactory correlation between the documented crying and the actual amount of crying recorded on a voice-activated tape recorder. It is hoped that this research will provide the conclusions necessary to recommend whether casein hydrolysate formulas have a role in the treatment of colic.

III. CONCLUSION

There are, as yet, no reported studies that definitively demonstrate that infantile colic is affected by the contents of milk ingested by the infant. The best study to date is that done by Jakobsson and Lindberg investigating breast-feeding infants (9), in which there are flaws. The most recent study investigating formula-fed infants has suggested that a change to a casein hydrolysate formula causes resolution of symptoms in all infants. However, in that study the change to a casein hydrolysate formula was not blind and a placebo effect cannot be ruled out; therefore these results should be interpreted with caution.

At the present time it is not known whether casein hydrolysate formulas truly have a role in the management of infantile colic. The results of more carefully designed, methodologically sound studies are needed before a definitive conclusion can be made.

REFERENCES

1. Illingworth, R. S. Three months' colic. *Arch. Dis. Child.* 29, 165–174, 1954.
2. Hide, D. W., and Guyer, B. M. Prevalence of infant colic. *Arch Dis. Child.* 57, 559–560, 1982.
3. Forsyth, B. W., Leventhal, J. M., and McCarthy, P. L. Mothers' perceptions of problems of feeding and crying behaviors. *Am. J. Dis. Child.* 139, 269–272, 1985.
4. Shannon, W. R. Colic in breast fed infants as a result of sensitization to foods in the mother's diet. *Arch. Pediatr.* 37, 756, 1921.
5. Speer, F. Colic and allergy. *Arch. Pediatr.* 75, 271–278, 1958.
6. Forsyth, B. W., McCarthy, P. L., and Leventhal, J. M. Problems of early infancy, formula changes and mothers' beliefs about their infants. *J. Pediatr.* 106, 1012–1017, 1985.
7. Lothe, L., Lindberg, T., and Jakobsson, I. Cow's milk formula as a cause of infantile colic. A double-blind study. *Pediatrics* 70, 7–10, 1982.
8. American Academy of Pediatrics, Committee on Nutrition: Soy-protein formulas: Recommendations for use in infant feeding. *Pediatrics* 72, 359–363, 1983.
9. Jakobsson, I., and Lindberg, T. Cow's milk as a cause of infantile colic in breast-fed infants. *Lancet* 2, 437–439, 1978.
10. Warner, J. O. Food allergy in fully breast-fed infants. *Clin. Allergy* 10, 133–136, 1980.
11. Evans, R. W., Allardyce, R. A., Fergusson, D. M., and Taylor, B. Maternal diet infantile colic in breast-fed infants. *Lancet* 1, 1340–1342, 1981.
12. Jarrett, E. E. Activation of IgE regulatory mechanisms by transmucosal absorption of antigen. *Lancet* 2, 223–225, 1977.
13. Juto, P., and Strannegard, O. T lymphocytes and blood eosinophils in early infancy in relation to heredity for allergy and type of feeding. *J. Aller. Clin. Immunol.* 64, 38–42, 1979.
14. Juto, P., and Bjorksten, B. Serum IgE in infants and influence of type of feeding. *Clin. Allergy* 10, 593–600, 1980.
15. Firer, M. A., Hosking, C. S., and Hill, D. J. Effect of antigen load on development of milk antibodies in infants allergic to milk. *Br. Med. J.* 283, 693–696, 1981.

16. Gerrard, J. W., and Shenassa, M. Food allergy: Two common types as seen in breast and formula-fed babies. *Ann. Allergy* 50, 375–379, 1983.

17. Illingworth, R. S. Evening colic in infants: A double-blind trial of dicyclomine hydrochloride. *Lancet* 2, 1119–20, 1959.

18. O'Donovan, J. C., and Bradstock, A. S. The failure of conventional drug therapy in the management of infantile colic. *Am. J. Dis. Child.* 133, 999–1001, 1979.

19. Brazelton, T. B. Crying in infancy. *Pediatrics* 29, 579–588, 1962.

20. Harris, M. J., Petts, V., and Penny, R. Cow's milk allergy as a cause of infantile colic: Immunofluorescent studies on jejunal mucosa. *Austral. Paediatr. J.* 13, 276–281, 1977.

21. Liebman, W. M. Infantile colic: Association with lactose and milk intolerance. *JAMA* 245, 723–733, 1981.

22. Goldman, A. S., Anderson, D. W., Sellers, W. A., Saperstein, S., Kniker, W. T., and Halpern, S. R. Milk allergy 1. Oral challenge with milk and isolated milk protein in allergic children. *Pediatrics* 32, 425–443, 1963.

23. Jakobsson, I., and Lindberg, T. Cow's milk proteins cause infantile colic in breast-fed infants: A double-blind crossover study. *Pediatrics* 71, 268–271, 1983.

24. Barr, R. G., Wooldridge, J. A., Hanley, J., Jajko, L., and Boisjoly, C. Formula change reduces crying behavior: Evidence for role of intestinal gas. (Abstr.) Presented at the APS-SPR meetings, May 2nd, 1984.

18

Offspring of High-Risk Allergic Families

Robert S. Zeiger
Kaiser Permanente Medical Center and University of California–San Diego, San Diego, California

I. INTRODUCTION

Prevention of allergic disease in infancy including food allergies depends on the ability to overcome the natural forces constantly working to sensitize humans to produce IgE antibody. The obstacles confronting any effective allergy prevention program are multiple and include heredity, environmental exposure, parental compliance and solvency, and viral infections. Prevention of IgE-mediated disorders could potentially be approached by selectively interfering with the major forces (genetic, cellular, and environmental) that, in concert, appear to be responsible for the ultimate phenotypic expression of atopy. Practically speaking, however, at the present time physicians interested in prevention of allergic diseases are limited to manipulating the modulating effect of the environment by reducing the allergenic load. To design or understand a potentially effective prevention program, one must appreciate various aspects of the development of allergic disease (1).

II. EFFECT OF GENETIC LOAD

The burden inflicted by genetic forces in the development of human allergies is huge, if not overwhelming. Prospective clinical studies of 2-4-year-old infants born to atopic parents have shown that the risk for allergy approaches 50-58% in the presence of unilateral allergic parentage and reaches 67-100% with bilateral allergic parentage (1). The genetic mechanisms regulating IgE sensitization include both allergen-nonspecific (basal IgE production and generalized IgE hyper-responsiveness) and allergen-specific factors (immune response and immune suppressor genes.)

Basal IgE production determined by serum IgE levels may be controlled by a two-allele system (a dominant allele [R] and a recessive allele [r]) in which low IgE level is inherited as an autosomal dominant trait and high IgE as autosomal recessive (2). In the general population the r allele is common, represented by its calculated frequency of 0.49 to 0.52 (3). The direct relationship of high maternal IgE levels to elevated newborn cord IgE (4) and the continued elevation of infant IgE when sequentially determined during childhood (5) attest to the strength of phenotypic expression of the (r) alleles for IgE production. Influencing the hereditary regulation of basal IgE production are both allergen-nonspecific generalized IgE hyperresponsiveness (linked to HLA-B8) and allergen-specific immune response and suppressor genes which are linked to several of the haplotypes in the HLA system.

III. DEVELOPMENT OF SENSITIZATION

The ultimate expression of allergic illness results from an intricate interrelationship between the "atopic" genetic constitution and the encountered environment. Environmental exposure to allergens potentially may occur as early as prenatally and as innocuously as through breast milk. The time of onset and variety of early solid feeding, the magnitude of inhalant and drug allergen exposure, and the critical effect of viral infection influence significantly the development of atopy.

A. Prenatal Sensitization

Nonspecific IgE produced by the fetus has been documented in humans as early as 11 weeks of gestation in fetal lung and liver and by 21 weeks in the spleen (6). IgE can be detected in amniotic fluid by 13 weeks (7), in infant cord blood by PRIST in from 13-82% of term pregnancies depending in part on atopic status of parents (5,8-10), maternal IgE (4,10), prenatal progesterone administration (4), and maternal helminth infection with microfiliaria (9).

Specific IgE sensitization has been documented to occur prenatally to such allergens as penicillin (11), wheat (12), milk (4,13), egg (8), and microfilariae (9). Nevertheless, specific prenatal sensitization to food allergens probably is a rare event, probably occurring in less than 0.1% of human newborns (5,14,15). Consistent with infrequent prenatal food sensitization, we have failed to demonstrate food-specific IgE by radioallergosorbent tests (RAST) in cord bloods from paired cord/4-month serum samples in 24 infants who possessed food-specific IgE at 4 months. In contrast, intrauterine infection with helminths, organisms capable of eliciting IgE responses, may induce specific microfilariae IgE in up to 25% of cord bloods in the human fetus (9).

The effect of maternal diet during late pregnancy on development of atopic manifestations in early infancy in 212 infants of atopic families was recently examined (Magnusson, K. K., Kjellman, N. I. M. and Johansson, S. G. O., submitted to European Academy of Allergology and Clinical Immunology June 1985). Mothers were randomized prenatally to a diet either avoiding cow's milk and egg, supplemented with Nutramigen and calcium (prophylaxis; n = 104) or to normal food (control; n = 108). Postnatally, infants in both groups were encouraged to breast feed and to supplement with Nutramigen until 3 months of age. No significant differences were found between prophylaxis or control infants, respectively, in mean birth weight (3546 vs. 3545 g), in incidence of positive skin tests (13 vs. 21%), or in atopic eczema or food allergy (5 vs. 7%). These findings are consistent with the infrequent occurrence of prenatal food sensitization and demonstrate that prenatal dietary avoidance cannot be expected to prevent atopy in infants of atopic families.

B. Postnatal Food Sensitization

1. Potential Adverse Effects of Breast Feeding

Adverse immunologic events have been attributed to breast feeding. The passage or transmission of dietary substances consumed by the mother through breast milk may potentially sensitize her offspring. As little as 1 part per billion of egg antigen within breast whey has been detected by P-K testing of recipient skin sensitized to human antiegg serum (16). Bovine milk protein has been identified in samples of maternal breast whey by passive cutaneous anaphylaxis (PCA) (9/9) (17) by Ouchterlony (48/67) (18) and by ELISA for casein (13/28) and B-lactoglobulin (5/28) (19). These observations point out the availability of maternally consumed dietary allergens in breast milk with the potential to sensitize at-risk offspring.

Human postnatal sensitization through breast milk of presumably exclusively breast-fed infants has been reported but never conclusively documented. Atopic manifestations as varied as atopic dermatitis (20-26), angioedema (26,27), rhinitis (24,26), and gastrointestinal tract allergy (24,26), have been described, in nondocumented exclusively breast-fed infants. The retrospective nature of these studies fails to rule out the possibility that some or all of these infants may have inadvertently been given the foodstuffs directly. Interestingly, three of four egg-skin test-positive "exclusively breast-fed" 4-month-old infants prospectively followed prenatally and postnatally, whose mothers "totally refrained" from egg consumption during the last trimester and during lactation, probably became sensitized to egg surreptitiously administered by grandparents (10). The concept that allergic sensitization may be promoted through passage of dietary allergens in breast milk is provocative, quite possibly real, though unproven, but merits consideration when implementing preventive measures to reduce allergic sensitization.

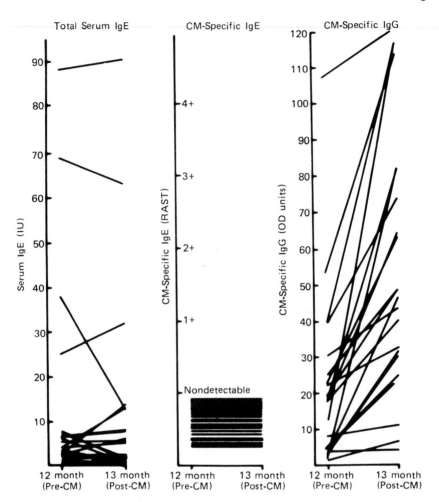

Figure 1 Effect of delayed cow's milk (CM) ingestion on immunologic responses to CM. Twelve-month-old prophylactic infants on milk avoidance and without specific CM IgE were challenged with the ad lib introduction of CM at 12 months. Paired total serum IgE, specific IgE (RAST), and CM-specific IgG were determined at 12 and 13 months.

Studies have warned of the potential risk of allergic sensitization in the breast-fed allergy-prone infant in which inadvertent, infrequent, and small quantities of foodstuffs (e.g., cow's milk) are ingested (28). Others have postulated that small quantities or delayed introduction of food allergens such as cow's milk potentially could increase later sensitization in humans as has been documented in animal models (29). Notwithstanding, we determined the effect of delayed cow's milk ingestion for one year on clinical and immunologic parameters in infants of allergic parents following a strict food prophylaxis (avoidance) regimen (see Sec. IV). First, only 11 of 267 (4%) of prophylactic infants demonstrated specific IgE to cow's milk (CM) at one year compared to 9/57 (16%) formula-fed atopic children followed by Juto and Bjorksten (30). Interestingly, most of these 11 infants consumed milk against protocol advice as documented by concomitant elevated serum cow's milk IgG determined by ELISA. Secondly, 25 prophylactic infants, with absent cow's milk IgE at 12 months, were fed ad lib whole cow's milk from 12 to 13 months, yet did not demonstrate significant increase in specific CM IgE or total serum IgE despite significant increases in CM-specific IgG ELISA (Fig. 1). Only one of these infants, a hyper-IgE responder, developed specific CM IgE by two years. An additional 125 prophylactic infants similarly tested failed to invoke a specific CM IgE response 1 month following deliberate CM ingestion. Such findings strongly suggest that delayed CM ingestion does not increase the risk of CM IgE or nonspecific sensitization in infants of allergic parents (31).

2. Effect of Cow's Milk Versus Breast Milk Feedings

Since the monumental and illuminating study of Grulee and Sanford (32) in 1936, which documented a seven fold reduction in the incidence of eczema in breast-fed compared to cow's milk-fed 9-month-old infants, many corroborating and contradictory studies have been published. To place these many conflicting studies in proper perspective, prospective infant feeding studies are critically summarized, divided into those evidencing benefit (Table 1) and those demonstrating a lack of effect (Table 2) and their design weaknesses are listed. None of these studies were randomized, creating bias in subject (family) recruitment which inherently confounds the studies' findings. For example, mothers who practice prolonged breast feeding generally delay introduction of solid foods, may utilize less day care assistance, and may smoke less. Delayed solid food feeding may in turn reduce eczema (33); decreased viral exposure may reduce the potential for respiratory illness, bronchiolitis, and infectious asthma as well as the potential for increased IgE sensitization (associated with viral infections) (34); abstinence from smoking would eliminate the stimulatory effect of cigarette smoke on IgE production (35) and asthma. Moreover, in some studies the control group consisted of families dropped from the breast-feeding groups due to noncompliance with the study protocol (36). We have noted that atopic parents specifically recruited and followed for an intervention study based on breast feeding and delayed solid food exposure, exhibited less maternal ($p = 0.007$) and paternal ($p = .001$) smoking, generated fewer low-birth-weight infants ($p = .042$), and significantly, introduced solid foods later than atopic parents not selected for or refusing recruitment. Such findings of noncompara-

Table 1 Prospective Nonrandomized Studies of Effect of Breast (B) vs. Cow's Milk (CM) Feeding on Development of Allergy: Studies Reporting Benefit of (B)

Study (yr)	B(n)/CM(n)	Interval (yr)	Eczema (E) allergy (A) outcome	Design weaknesses[a]
Grulee (1936) [32]	9749/1707	3/4	E:C = 7 X B	2,3,4,5,6
Matthew (1977) [36]	23/19	1	E:13% B vs 47% C[b]	1,2,3,5,7,8,9
Saarinen (1979) [38]	25/39	3	E:@3y↓B[b]	2,3,5,9
Ziering (1979) [57]	25/25	2	A:B = 34%, C = 65%	1,2,3,5,9
Chandra (1979) [39]	37/37	3	E:11% B vs 59% C[c]	2,3,5,9,10
Juto (1980) [30]	46/22	1	A:@ 3 & 6 mo ↓B[b]	1,2,3,4,5,9
Gruskay (1982) [40]	48/201	14	A:B ↓46%@14y	2,3,5,6
Businco (1983) [8]	34/41	2	A:B = 18%, C = 37%	1,2,3,5,9

[a]Design weaknesses: 1 = late solids in B; 2 = not randomized; 3 = no blinding; 4 = unselected sample; 5 = compliance not documented; 6 = lack immunology; 7 = environmental control in B; 8 = dropout rate high; 9 = small (n); 10 = B < 4 mo.
[b]$p < .05$.
[c]$p < 10^{-3}$.

Table 2 Prospective Nonrandomized Studies of Effect of Breast (B) vs. Cow's Milk (CM) Feeding on Development of Allergy: Studies Nonsupportive of Benefit of (B)

Study (yr)	B(n)/CM(n)	Interval (yr)	Outcome[a]	Design weaknesses[b]
Kaufman (1972) [41]	38/54	2	E > 50% B + CM	1,2,3,5,8,9
Halpern (1973) [42]	193/349	0.5-7	A = 16%B + CM	1,2,3,4,5,6,9
Kaufman (1976) [43]	38/56	2	E = 32%B; 23%CM	1,2,3,5,8,9
Hide (1981) [44]	204/62	1	A = 45%B, 53%CM E = 10%B, 13%CM	1,2,3,5,6,7,9
Gordon (1982) [45]	112/85	2	N.S.	1,2,3,5,9
Van Asperen (1984) [46][c]	54/25	1 1/3	E = 52%B, 40%CM	2,3,5,8,9
Van Asperen (1984) [46][d]	19/60	1 1/3	E = 58%B, 45%CM	2,3,5,8

[a]E = eczema, A = allergies.
[b]1 = Early solids; 2 = nonrandomized; 3 = no blinding; 4 = unselected; 5 = undocumented compliance; 6 = lack immunology; 7 = dropout rate high; 8 = (n) small; 9 = B < 3 months.
[c]Breast only for 2 months.
[d]Breast only for 4 months.

tiveness of control and experimental groups, added to the design flaws listed in Table 1 (8,30,32,36-40) and Table 2 (41-46), greatly weaken the impact of the findings of these studies.

Two common factors apparent in those studies which suggested that breast feeding reduced allergic disease were prolonged breast feeding (>4 months and preferably 6 months) and delayed solid food introduction. Relative importance of each factor could not be resolved by these studies (see Sec. III.B.4). Immunologic parameters which were associated with breast feeding and delayed solid feeding included significantly reduced serum IgE levels at ages less than 4 months (38) and by one year (39). In addition, infants with reduced T cells at one month post partum demonstrated higher serum IgE levels and peripheral eosinophilia when fed cow's rather than breast milk (47).

Great weaknesses in design are also found in the studies denying benefit of breast feeding on allergic sensitization (41-46). Common to all but one of the negative studies listed in Table 2 was the rather brief period of breast feeding (<3 months and frequently <6 weeks) and early introduction of solid feeding (41-45).

3. Effect of Soy Feeding on Allergic Sensitization

Three prospective randomized studies have examined the potential beneficial role of soy versus cow's milk feeding on development of allergies in infancy (48-50). Although, Johnstone and Dutton appeared to demonstrate a significant reduction in asthma (in those <3 years of age) and perennial allergic rhinitis (in those <6 years of age) in soy versus cow's milk feeding regimens, no differences were evidenced for eczema development (just the manifestation most expected to benefit from dietary avoidance) or hay fever (48). Confounding this study and possibly responsible for the benefits seen, was the concurrent delayed introduction of solid foods to the soy group. Moreover, immunologic parameters were never documented.

Two subsequent studies failed to confirm the above findings. Specifically, a methodologically strong clinical and immunological investigation of infants of bilaterally allergic parents failed to demonstrate any protective effect of soy versus cow's milk feeding on the development of allergy in the first 3 years of life. The incidence of atopy was greater than 60% in infants by three years in both the soy and cow's milk fed groups, a particularly high occurrence. These findings are not unexpected, since infant sensitization to soybean protein has been documented to cause anaphylaxis (51) and asthma (52). Additionally, IgE antibodies to soy occur commonly (67%) in children with IgE antibodies to milk (53). Present evidence therefore cannot support the use of soybean formulas for the purpose of preventing food-induced IgE-mediated disorders.

4. Effect of Early Solid Feeding on Allergic Sensitization

To minimize allergenic load, delayed solid food feedings to atopic-prone infants has been recommended for decades. Interestingly, half of the studies in Table 1 which noted a reduction in allergy in breast-fed infants added solid foods later in the breast than cow's milk fed groups. In an attempt to evaluate the effect of dietary patterns on development of eczema by 2 (33) and asthma by 4 years (54), an unselected birth cohort of 1262 infants were prospectively studied by Fergusson et al. Infants of atopic parents developed two and half times the incidence of eczema when fed solid foods during the first four months compared to infants not given solid foods during this interval. A direct relationship was noted between number of solid foods introduced during the first four months and the incidence of eczema. The authors argued that breast feeding did not exert any significant effect on the rates of eczema and that the benefits of sole breast feeding derived from the absence of solid food introduction. Kajosarri and Saarinen, however, noted that eczema developed by one year in only 14% of atopic-prone infants exclusively breast fed for 6 months compared to 35% ($p < .01$) in a similar group of breast-fed infants in which solid foods were added at 3 months (55). In contrast to findings for eczema, Fergusson et al. (54) found no evidence to indicate that either breast feeding or patterns of solid feeding practices significantly affected development of asthma by 4 years in the same cohort of infants. This latter finding is consistent with most studies implicating viral infections rather than foods in the causation of asthma in early childhood (0–3 years).

IV. EFFECT OF STRICT POSTNATAL DIETARY AVOIDANCE

Over the past 5 years we have studied the effect of a rather comprehensive dietary avoidance regimen (Table 3) on the development of atopy in infants of immunologically confirmed atopic parents, of whom 50% are bilaterally allergic. The objective of this dietary regimen is to avoid highly allergenic foods; particularly milk, egg, peanut, nuts, soy, corn, and fish during the first 12–36 months of life of infants at high risk of developing atopy. Nutramigen, owing to its low potential for sensitization, is the sole formula utilized. To reduce the potential or real possibility of food sensitization through exposure to allergenic food peptides in breast milk, mothers totally restrict their consumption of milk, egg, and peanut during lactation, while taking supplemental calcium (total 1500 mg daily). Environmental avoidance of allergens was also stressed and evaluated by home visits by a trained environmental nurse.

Infants are then formally evaluated at 4 months, 1 year, and yearly thereafter by physical exam, nasal cytology, Multitest skin tests, RASTs, and serum IgE levels (PRIST) for the possible development of allergic sensitization. Given the idealized prophylaxis regimen just described several critical issues arise: (a) natural history of allergic disease in the infants and (b) compliance of parents. The outcome of the first 2-3 years of 200 maternal-infant pairs who voluntarily consented to adhere to the prophylaxis regimen will now be discussed.

A. Development of Atopy

Eczema was diagnosed by a blinded physician utilizing standard criteria. Food allergy was defined by reproducible cutaneous (eczema, hives, or rash), respiratory (cough, wheezing, rhinitis), or gastrointestinal (heavy vomiting) symptoms upon food ingestion. Reactions were confirmed by food challenge. Asthma was diagnosed by auscultatory findings of wheezing and/or response to bronchodilators. Criteria for the diagnosis of allergic rhinitis included characteristic nasal symptoms with positive IgE sensitization and nasal eosinophilia.

Despite this strict avoidance protocol regimen, food allergy developed in 14%, eczema in 12%, infectious asthma in 24%, and allergic rhinitis in 7% of the prophylaxis infants by 36 months (Table 4). Peak onset of both eczema and food allergy occurred within the first 12 months and declined thereafter. The onset of infectious asthma was somewhat later in infancy, rather evenly distributed between 12 and 36 months. In contrast, allergic rhinitis was rare before 2 years.

Eczema was typically mild, sporadic, and associated with positive specific IgE in 19/23 (83%) of infants. Improvements in eczema generally accompanied withdrawal of the incriminating food with flaring evident on re-exposure. Double-blind food challenge of infants with historical food-induced worsening of eczema and positive food-specific IgE were characteristically positive (56).

Table 3 Dietary Avoidance Regimen

A. Infant
    Prolonged breast feeding (>4 months)
    Nutramigen supplementation
    Delayed solid food introduction
        6-12 months (vegetables, rice, meat, fruit)
        12-18 months (milk, wheat, corn, citrus, soy)
        24 months (egg)
        36 months (peanut, fish)
B. Maternal elimination (milk, egg, peanut)
    Last trimester
    Lactation

Table 4 Development of Atopic Conditions in Prophylaxis Infants

		Onset incidence (%)			
Age (mo)	No. of infants	Eczema	Food allergy	Infectious asthma	Allergic rhinitis
4	197	3.0	3.0	0.5	0
12	185	5.9	7.0	6.0	0.5
24	170	3.5	2.9	9.4	1.2
36	140	0	0.7	7.9	5.6
Cumulative (%)		12.4	13.6	23.8	7.3

Egg was the major food trigger of eczema with milk second in frequency, an order corresponding with frequency of specific food IgE (Table 5). Onset of food-specific IgE peaked at 1 year and declined thereafter (Table 6). Nutramigen was well tolerated; only 1 infant developed gastrointestinal symptoms on repeated challenge to the Nutramigen formula containing sucrose. This infant was able to tolerate Nutramigen with corn syrup solids and absent sucrose.

Of 14 infants with a historical adverse food reaction and possessing specific food IgE, 13 (93%) experienced a positive food challenge to the incriminated food during double-blind challenge. In contrast, only 1 of 11 (9%) infants with a positive historical adverse reaction and negative food-specific IgE experienced a positive food challenge. There existed a significant association of elevated serum IgE, positive food-specific IgE, and atopic disease with positive food challenges compared to negative food challenges (56). Most interestingly 4 breast-fed

Table 5 Onset of Food-Specific IgE in Prophylaxis Infants

		Onset of food-specific IgE (n)						
Age (mo)	No. of infants	Egg	Milk	Peanut	Soy	Wheat	Corn	Cod
4	197	6	2	0	0	0	0	0
12	185	17	9	5	1	1	2	1
24	170	1	1	2	6	3	1	1
36	140	1	0	1	1	0	1	0
Cumulative		25	12	8	8	4	4	2

Table 6 Development of IgE Sensitization in Prophylaxis Infants

Age (mo)	No. of infants	Onset incidence (%)	
		Food-specific IgE	Inhalant-specific IgE
4	197	4.1	0.5
12	185	11.8	1.1
24	170	1.8	5.9
36	140	2.1	8.5
Cumulative (%)		19.8	16.0

asymptomatic infants with demonstrable specific food IgE by skin test and RAST (milk, egg, or peanut) developed allergic symptoms (rash, gastrointestinal, and/or respiratory) on their initial exposure to these foods which occurred during double-blind food challenge. Such findings are consistent with the recent reporting of 8 infants with immediate hypersensitivity reactions during their first known exposure to milk, egg, or peanut (26). Whether sensitization occurred through breast feeding or inadvertent direct exposure remain impossible to determine.

Episodes of wheezing occurred during respiratory illnesses except in 3 infants during blinded food challenges. Persistent or recurrent IgE mediated asthma was not seen in any infant up to 36 months. Twenty-one of the 36 infants (56%) with wheezing experienced a single episode. In contrast to infants with eczema, those with infectious asthma evidenced both a significantly lower incidence of specific IgE to foods ($p < 0.0001$) and lower frequency of increased total serum IgE at 4 months ($p < 0.05$) but not in cord blood. While four of the infants experienced both eczema and asthma, the majority of infants with asthma within the first 3 years have yet to develop specific IgE. Such findings confirm that asthma in infancy even in an atopic-prone population typically does not involve food or inhalant but rather viral triggering.

The distribution of onset of inhalant specific IgE can be seen to be later in infancy than with food-specific IgE (Table 6). Interestingly, onset of inhalant-specific IgE appears as new food-specific IgE begins to wane. Inhalant-specific IgE was most frequently associated with allergic rhinitis.

B. Compliance

As noted above, despite a prophylaxis regimen, available professionals providing nutritional and environmental guidance, frequent and personal follow-up, atopic sensitization and allergic disease developed in these prospectively followed infants at risk for atopy. The two most obvious factors responsible for the above findings are parental noncompliance and genetic penetrance.

Previous studies have established that ingestion of foodstuffs in infancy will induce brisk immune responses. Quantitation of the immunologic responses to such common allergenic foods as milk and egg; therefore, can serve as an objective assay of dietary compliance (Fig. 2). We have been able to develop a sensitive ELISA for cow's milk (CM)-specific IgG and now are attempting to establish one for egg-specific IgG. The pattern of IgG response to cow's milk in paired samples from cord through 2 years in prophylaxis infants has revealed that at 4 and 9 months CM IgG is barely detectable signifying excellent avoidance and therefore compliance (in the range of 90%). However, by one year about 30% of the infants had significant CM IgG indicating ingestion of CM and break in compliance. CM was deliberately introduced at 12 months leading to significant

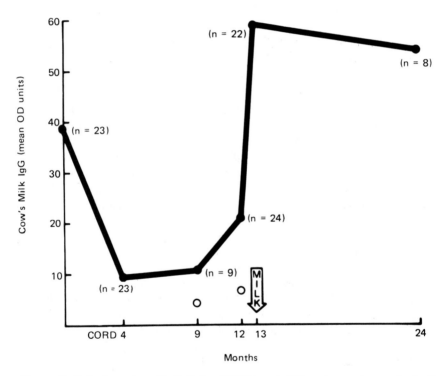

Figure 2 Paired cow's milk IgG by ELISA at different ages in prophylactic group infants. Ad lib whole cow's milk was added at 12 months.

CM IgG by 13 months (Fig. 2). Using this assay we could demonstrate that 20/57 (35%) infants with elevated 1-year CM IgG (>10 OD units) compared to only 10/108 (9%) with low CM IgG developed food allergy and/or specific food IgE (p = 0.00014). These findings suggest strongly that parental breaks in dietary protocol may be responsible for a segment of the sensitized infants. Of the 10 infants with low CM IgG, egg rather than milk was the usual sensitizing food. Future assay of egg-specific IgG should help to determine the compliance in this group of sensitized infants.

V. SUMMARY

The desire to alter the natural incidence of atopic illness has piqued physicians' imaginations for decades. Specifically, the phenotypic expression of IgE-mediated disorders, which appears regulated by multiple genetic factors and modulated by environmental experiences (allergen exposure, infection, smoking), has been a target for prevention medicine since the 1920s when dietary intervention was espoused in infancy. Such intervention to be successful must overcome many risk factors which in concert markedly increase the risk for atopic disease development (Table 7). During the past 60 years, much controversy has emerged from multiple clinical studies designed to evaluate the effect of dietary and other environmental exclusions on the subsequent manifestation of atopy. A randomized prospective study of allergy prophylaxis during infancy is mandatory to determine definitely the benefits and feasibility of such a regimen as well as its long-term effects on the development of atopy. From our recent findings which demonstrate the development of atopy in infants entered in a strict prophylaxis protocol, it becomes apparent that monumental obstacles confront preventive efforts to overcome the strength of the allergic constitution. Within the very near future, results from our prospective, prenatally randomized allergy prophylaxis study should be available for critical scrutiny of the effectiveness and feasibility of allergy prevention during infancy.

Table 7 Risk Factors in Atopy Development

Parental atopy
Early solid foods
Nonbreast feeding
Season of birth
Cord IgE
Infant IgE
Infant-specific IgE
↓ Infant T cells

ACKNOWLEDGMENTS

Supported in part by Kaiser Permanente research funds, NICHHD contract No. 1-HD-0-2832, Mead Johnson and Company, Marion Laboratories, and Lincoln Diagnostics. We thank Susette Craddock for expert assistance and preparation of the manuscript. Susan Heller, PNP, provided the excellent clinical follow-up of the infants.

REFERENCES

1. Schatz, M., Zeiger, R. S., Mellon, M., and Porreco, R. The course and management of asthma and allergic disease during pregnancy. In: *Allergy: Principles and Practice,* Middleton, E., Jr., Reed, C. E., and Ellis, E. F. (eds.). C. V. Mosby, St. Louis, 1983.
2. Marsh, D. G., Bias, W. B., and Ishizaka, K. Genetic control of basal serum IgE level and its effect on specific reaginic sensitivity. *Proc. Natl. Acad. Sci. USA* 71, 3588, 1974.
3. Rao, D. C. Lalovel, J. M., Morton, N. E., and Gerrard, J. W. Immunoglobulin E revisited. *Am. J. Hum. Genet.* 32, 620, 1980.
4. Michel, F. B., Bousquet, J., Greillier, P., Robinet-Levy, M., and Coulomb, Y. Comparison of cord blood immunoglobulin E concentrations and maternal allergy for the prediction of atopic disease in infancy. *J. Allergy Clin. Immunol.* 65, 422, 1980.
5. Kjellman, N. M., and Croner, S. Cord blood IgE determination for allergy prediction—a follow-up to seven years of age in 1,651 children. *Ann. Allergy* 53, 167, 1984.
6. Miller, D. L., Hirvonen, T., and Gitlin, D. Synthesis of IgE by the human conceptus, *J. Allergy Clin. Immunol.* 52, 182, 1973.
7. Singer, A. D., Hobel, C. J., and Heiner, D. C. Evidence for secretory IgE in utero. *J. Allergy Clin. Immunol.* 53, 94, 1974.
8. Businco, L., Marchetti, F., Pelligrini, G., and Berlini, R. Predictive value of cord blood IgE levels in "at-risk" newborn babies and influence of type of feeding. *Clin. Allergy* 13, 503, 1983.
9. Weil, G. J., Hussain, R., Kumaraswami, V., Tripathy, S. P., Phillips, K. S., and Ottesen, E. A. Prenatal allergic sensitization to helminth antigens in offspring of parasite-infected mothers. *J. Clin. Invest.* 71, 1124, 1983.
10. Hamburger, R. N., Heller, S., Mellon, M., O'Connor, R. D., and Zeiger, R. S. Current status of the clinical and immunologic consequences of a prototype allergic disease prevention program. *Ann. Allergy* 51, 281, 1983.
11. Levin, S., Altman, Y., and Sela, M. Penicillin and dinitrophenyl antibodies in newborns and mothers detected with chemically modified bacteriophage. *Pediatr. Res.* 5, 87, 1971.
12. Kaufman, H. S. Allergy in the newborn: Skin test reactions confirmed by the Prausnitz-Kustner test at birth. *Clin. Allergy* 1, 363, 1971.

13. Delepesse, M., Sarfati, M., Lang, G., and Sehon, A. H. Prenatal and neonatal synthesis of IgE. *Monogr. Allergy* 18, 83, 1983.

14. Kjellman, N. I. M., and Johansson, S. G. O. IgE and atopic allergy in newborn and infants with a family history of atopic disease. *Acta. Paediatr. Scand.* 65, 495, 1976.

15. Croner, S., Kjellman, N. I., Eriksson, B., and Roth, A. IgE screening in 1701 newborn infants and the development of atopic disease during infancy. *Arch. Dis. Child.* 57, 364, 1982.

16. Donnally, H. H. The question of elimination of foreign protein (egg white) in woman's milk. *J. Immunol.* 19, 15, 1930.

17. Gamo, I., Yabuuchi, H., Nishida, M., et al.: Studies on prophylaxis of cow's milk allergy by digestive enzymes. *Acta Paediatr. Japonica* 8, 1, 1966.

18. Jakobsson, I., and Lindberg, T. Cow's milk as the cause of infantile colic in breast-fed infants. *Lancet* 2, 437, 1978.

19. Stuart, C. A., Twiselton, R., Nicholas, M. F., and Hide, D. W. Passage of cow's milk protein in breast milk. *Clin. Allergy* 14, 533, 1984.

20. Shannon, W. R. Demonstration of food proteins in human breast milk by anaphylactic experiments on guinea pigs. *Am. J. Dis. Child.* 22, 223, 1921.

21. Talbot, F. B. Eczema in childhood. *Med. Clin. North Am.* 1, 985, 1918.

22. O'Keefe, E. S. The relation of food to infantile eczema. *Boston Med. Surg. J.* 183, 569, 1920.

23. Ratner, B., Jackson, H. C., and Gruehl, H. L. Transmission of protein hypersensitivities from mother to offspring. V. Active sensitization in utero. *J. Immunol.* 14, 303, 1927.

24. Gerrard, J. W. Allergy in breast-fed babies to ingredients in breast milk. *Ann. Allergy* 42, 69, 1979.

25. Warner, J. O. Food allergy in fully breast-fed infants. *Clin. Allergy* 10, 133, 1980.

26. Van Asperen, P. P., Kemp, A. S., and Mellis, C. M. Immediate food hypersensitivity reactions on the first known exposure to the food. *Arch. Dis. Child.* 58, 253, 1983.

27. Lyon, G. M. Allergy in an infant of three weeks. *Am. J. Dis. Child.* 36, 1012, 1928.

28. Kaplan, M. S., and Solli, N. J. Immunoglobulin E to cow's milk protein in breast fed atopic children. *J. Allergy Clin. Immunol.* 64, 122, 1979.

29. Jarrett, E. E., and Hall, E. Selective suppression of IgE antibody responsiveness by maternal influence. *Nature* 280, 145, 1979.

30. Juto, P., and Bjorksten, B. Serum IgE in infants and influence of type of feeding. *Clin. Allergy* 10, 593, 1980.

31. Mellon, M., Heller, S., O'Connor, R. D., Hamburger, R. N., and Zeiger, R. S. No increase in cow's milk (CM) sensitization after delayed CM ingestion in infancy. *J. Allergy Clin. Immunol.* 71, 40, 1983.

32. Grulee, C. G., and Sanford, H. N. The influence of breast and artificial feeding on infantile eczema. *J. Pediatr.* 9, 223, 1936.

33. Fergusson, D. M., Horwood, L. J., Beautrias, A. L., Shannon, G. T., and Taylor, B. Eczema and infant diet. *Clin. Allergy* 11, 325, 1981.

34. Frick, O. L., German, D. F., and Mills, J. Development of allergy in children. I. Association with virus infections. *J. Allergy Clin. Immunol.* 63, 228, 1979.

35. Kjellman, N. I. M. Effect on parental smoking on IgE levels in children. *Lancet* 1, 993, 1981.

36. Matthew, D. J., Taylor, B., Norman, A. P., and Turner, M. W. Prevention of eczema. *Lancet* 1, 321, 1977.

37. Orgel, H. A., Hamburger, R. N., Bazaral, M., et al.: Development of IgE and allergy in infancy. *J. Allergy Clin. Immunol.* 56, 296, 1975.

38. Saarinen, U. M., Backman, A., Kajossari, M., and Simes, M. Prolonged breast-feeding as prophylaxis for atopic disease. *Lancet* 2, 163, 1979.

39. Chandra, R. K. Prospective studies of the effect of breast feeding on incidence of infection and allergy. *Acta Paediatr. Scand.* 68, 691, 1979.

40. Gruskay, F. L. Comparison of breast, cow, and soy feedings in the prevention of onset of allergic disease' A 15-year prospective study. *Clin. Pediatr.* 21, 486, 1982.

41. Kaufman, H. S. Diet and heredity in infantile atopic dermatitis. *Arch. Dermatol.* 105, 400, 1972.

42. Halpern, S. R., Sellars, W. A., Johnson, R. B., Anderson, D. W., Saperstein, S., and Reisch, J. S. Development of childhood allergy in infants fed breast, soy or cow milk. *J. Allergy Clin. Immunol.* 51, 139, 1973.

43. Kaufman, H. S., and Frick, O. L. The development of allergy in infants of allergic parents: A prospective study concerning the role of heredity. *Ann. Allergy* 37, 410, 1976.

44. Hide, D. W., and Guyer, B. M. Clinical manifestations of allergy related to breast and cow's milk feeding. *Arch. Dis. Child.* 56, 172, 1981.

45. Gordon, R. R., Ward, A. M., Noble, D. A., and Allen, R. Immunoglobulin E and the eczema-asthma syndrome in early childhood. *Lancet* 1, 72, 1982.

46. Van Asperen, P. P., Kemp, A. S., and Mellis, C. M. Relationship of diet in the development of atopy in infancy. *Clin. Allergy* 14, 525, 1984.

47. Juto, P., Moller, C., Engberg, S., and Bjorksten, B. Influence of type of feeding on lymphocyte function and development of infantile allergy. *Clin. Allergy* 12, 409, 1982.

48. Johnston, D. E., and Dutton, A. M. Dietary prophylaxis of allergic diseases in children. *N. Engl. J. Med.* 274, 715, 1966.

49. Brown, E. B., Josephson, B. M., Levine, H. S., and Rosen, M. A prospective study of allergy in a pediatric population. *Am. J. Dis. Child.* 117, 693, 1969.

50. Kjellman, N. I., and Johansson, S. G. Soy versus cow's milk in infants with a biparental history of atopic disease: development of atopic disease and immunoglobulins from birth to 4 years of age. *Clin. Allergy* 9, 347, 1979.

51. Mortimer, E. R. Anaphylaxis following ingestion of soybean. *J. Pediatr.* 58, 90, 1961.

52. Peters, G. A. Bronchial asthma due to soybean allergy. *Ann. Allergy* 23, 1970, 1965.

53. Dannaeus, A., Johansson, S. G. O., Foucard, T., and Ohman, S. Clinical and immunological aspects of food allergy in childhood. 1. Estimation of IgG, IgA, and IgE antibodies to food antigens in children with food allergy and atopic dermatitis. *Acta Paediatr. Scand.* 66, 31, 1977.

54. Fergusson, D. M., Horwood, L. J., and Shannon, F. T. Asthma and infant diet. *Arch. Dis. Child.* 58, 48, 1983.

55. Kajosaari, M., and Saarinen, U. M. Prophylaxis of atopic disease by six months' total solid food elimination. *Arch. Paediatr. Scan.* 72, 411, 1983.

56. Mellon, M., Heller, S., O'Connor, R. N., Hamburger, R., Zeiger, R. Double blind food challenges (FC) in a prospective allergy prevention program for high risk infants. *J. Allergy Clin. Immunol.* 75, Part II, 296, 1985.

57. Ziering, R., O'Connor, R., Mellon, M., and Hamburger, R. University of California in San Diego Prophylaxis of Allergy in Infancy Study: An Interim Report. *J. Allergy Clin. Immunol.* 63, 199, 1979.

19

Protein Hydrolysates in Cystic Fibrosis

John D. Lloyd-Still
Northwestern University Medical School and Children's Memorial Hospital, Chicago, Illinois

Alice E. Smith
Children's Memorial Hospital and University of Illinois, Chicago, Illinois

Kathy A. Powers
Children's Memorial Hospital, Chicago, Illinois

Hans U. Wessel
Northwestern University Medical School and Children's Memorial Hospital, Chicago, Illinois

I. INTRODUCTION

Studies on growth in cystic fibrosis (CF) performed in the 1960s (1) and 1970s (2) show similar patterns with the height and weight values between the 3rd and 10th percentiles. The growth spurt that occurred following diagnosis and initiation of therapy in patients under 2 years of age was followed later by a declining growth rate. Growth retardation was found to correlate significantly with severity of pulmonary involvement (1,2).

Because an improved prognosis has been reported in CF patients with normal fat absorption (3), CF patients have been nutritionally supplemented by a variety of means including oral, nasogastric, jejunostomy, and intravenous hyperalimentation regimens. Despite initial success, most of these treatments result in relapse unless the force feeding regimen is continued long term, and in practice most patients become noncompliant after a variable interval.

257

The advent of neonatal screening for CF has theoretically made it possible to initiate treatment before malnutrition occurs and growth is impaired. Farrell et al. (4) compared 19 consecutively diagnosed CF infants treated with Pregestimil with a retrospective group treated with pancreatic enzymes, and concluded that normalization of weight and height could readily be achieved in infants with cystic fibrosis.

Since 1975, Pregestimil was the prescribed formula for all infants newly diagnosed with CF and pancreatic insufficiency in our CF Center. Growth (height and weight) records were available on 52 infants diagnosed under 1 year of age and treated with Pregestimil (another 96 patients with CF diagnosed after infancy or treated before Pregestimil was available were excluded). Eighteen children presented with meconium ileus (13 required surgery, 5 responded to gastrografin enemas); another 24 were diagnosed under 6 months of age, and 10 were diagnosed between 6 and 12 months of age. The growth data was compared to previous studies (1,2).

II. METHODS

Growth records for the first 36 months of life were analyzed for median, mean ± 1 S.D., and range of height and weight at birth, 3,6,9,12,18,24,30, and 36 months. These values were compared with published data (2,5) on CF children by plotting the results on the National Center for Health Statistics growth charts (6). Weight and height records were also expressed as standard scores or standard deviations from norms for age and sex compared with previous data (2). Results were calculated and plotted for the total of 52 infants, as well as for a subgroup of 18 CF infants with meconium ileus.

The relationship of caloric intake and specific nutrient composition has been studied in 64 of our CF patients aged between 0.3 and 18 years to determine if such detailed knowledge could predict clinical status (7). Source data included anthropometrics (age, height, weight, percentile of height and weight), dietary parameters (%RDA for calories, protein, iron, calcium, percent of total calories as protein, fat, carbohydrate, fat/kg), Shwachman score, and lung function data (% of predicted forced expiratory volume [FEV], midmaximim expiratory flow rate [MMEF] 25-75, and maximum expiratory flow rate [V_{max}] 75) which was available in 35 patients. Dietary data was derived from 72 hour dietary records supplied by parents (8).

III. RESULTS

The median values for height, weight, and sex are shown in Figures 1 and 2, which also includes the data from Sproul and Huang (1) and the 1982 CF Foundation patient data base registry (5). Patients with meconium ileus had better

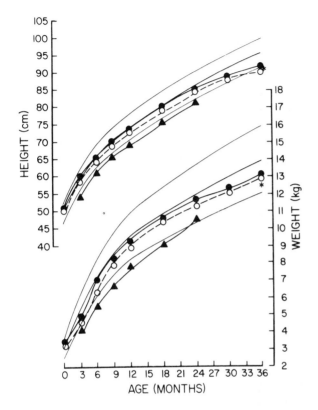

Figure 1 Height and weight percentiles (National Center for Health Statistics, Ref. 6) for girls, comparing data from ▲ Sproul et al., 1964 (1), ○ total CF group (n = 52), ● meconium ileus (n = 18), and * the 1982 CF Registry (5).

growth than the total group, and had values close to the 50th percentile after 9 months of age. Four patients died at a mean age of 7.5 months (range 6-9 months).

The weight and height growth expressed as standard scores or standard deviation for norms for age and sex are shown in Figures 3 and 4. Figure 4 shows an improvement compared to the data of Berry et al. (2). Meconium ileus patients again fared better than the total group. However, despite initial improvement there appears to be a fall off in height growth between 2 and 3 years. No patient continued on Pregestimil past 18 months of age.

Nutritional analysis on 64 of our CF patients (7) showed that the caloric intake averaged 95 ± 31% of RDA; range of 42-206%. Protein intake averaged 214 ± 70% of RDA; range of 85-380%. Other constituents were greater than 100% of

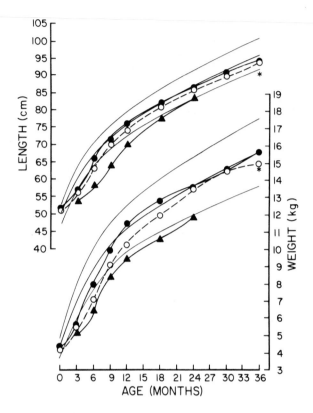

Figure 2 Height and weight percentiles (National Center for Health Statistics, Ref. 6) for boys, comparing data from ▲ Sproul et al., 1964 (1), ○ total CF group (n = 52), ● meconium ileus (n = 18), and * the 1982 CF Registry (5).

RDA in all patients. Linear regressions and multiple stepwise regressions revealed no significant correlations between any individual dietary parameter and age, height, weight, percentile of weight or height, Shwachman score, and pulmonary parameters. No dietary parameters predicted either Shwachman score, percentile of weight, or lung function. Of all parameters, Shwachman score correlated best with percentile of weight (r = .495), percentile FEV (r = .451), %MMEF25-75 (r = .442), %VMax 75 (r = .377), age (r < .368), weight (r < .333), and height (r < .305) in that order. All other correlation coefficients were < .230.

IV. DISCUSSION

There are three major factors which could affect growth in CF: (a) prenatal and genetic influences, (b) nutritional disturbances (especially pancreatic insuffici-

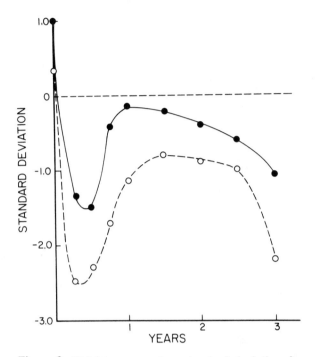

Figure 3 Height expressed as standard deviation from the norm (0.0) for age and sex for ○ the total CF group (n = 52) and ● meconium ileus (n = 18).

ency), and (c) pulmonary disease. The stature of CF parents is within the normal range (1), but there is some evidence that the birth weight in CF infants is 250 g below the norm allowing for gestational age (9,10). Birth weight in meconium ileus is increased (11), as is confirmed in our patients, and is thought to be secondary to the obstructed meconium.

Our findings show several changes from previous studies. First, there is still a high (7.7%) mortality in infants with CF treated with modern nutritional management. Four infants succumbed to progressive lung disease, despite being diagnosed soon after birth with early institution of pancreatic enzymes and predigested formula. Major psychosocial problems were present in all families which made management more difficult. These infants pursued a similar course to others reported in the literature (12). Thus, in our opinion, it is an oversimplification to state that normalization of weight and height could be readily achieved in all infants with cystic fibrosis (4).

However, the impressive growth patterns in the 18 infants with meconium ileus support the contention of Farrell et al. (4) that early institution of nutritional therapy is conducive to improved growth in these infants. These findings are even more remarkable when compared to previous studies (11,13) showing a

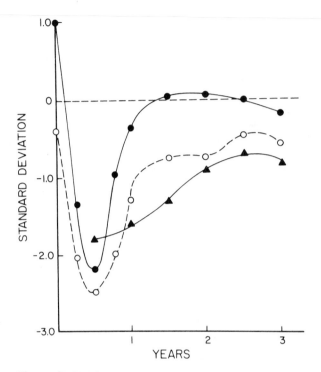

Figure 4 Weight expressed as standard deviation from the norm (0.0) for age and sex for ○ the total CF group (n = 52) and ● meconium ileus (n = 18), compared with data from ▲ Berry et al., 1975 (2).

mortality between 40 and 60% for meconium ileus. Other factors responsible for these improved results include the use of gastrografin enemas (5 out of 18 patients), a shorter period of hospitalization (mean of 12 days), the use of total parenteral nutrition (9 out of 18 patients), and the diagnosis of CF during initial hospitalization (17 out of 18 patients). Patients with meconium ileus received Pregestimil significantly longer (average duration 9.7 months ± 3.6) than patients without meconium ileus (mean 6.7 months ± 2.9) (p<.01), and the growth records were higher at all age periods after 6 months (Figures 1 and 2).

Despite emphasizing nutritional supplementation in all our CF patients, the growth patterns of our older patients are similar to the CF Foundation patient registry (5). This implies that despite a successful initial response to nutritional therapy, the disease progresses relentlessly. Contrasting findings in survival figures have recently been reported from Boston and Toronto where major changes in nutritional practices are evident (14).

In our experience (7), detailed dietary intake analysis provided important information about dietary composition, but had no predicted value with regard to the clinical status of CF patients as determined by Shwachman score, lung function, or percentile of weight. Our data indicated that the Shwachman score and percentile of weight decreased progressively with age, whereas dietary intake parameters did not change appreciably. These findings suggested that dietary manipulations have in all probability only limited effects on deterioration of pulmonary status which ultimately determines outcome in cystic fibrosis. Only prospective studies will show whether the improved nutritional parameters demonstrated in our infants treated with Pregestimil result in increased long-term survival.

REFERENCES

1. Sproul, A., and Huang, N. Growth patterns in children with cystic fibrosis. *J. Pediatr.* 65, 664-676, 1964.
2. Berry, H. K., Kellogg, F. W., Hunt, M. M., Ingberg, R. L., Richter, L., and Gutjaar, C. Dietary supplement and nutrition in children with cystic fibrosis. *Am. J. Dis. Child.* 129, 165-171, 1975.
3. Corey, M., Gaskin, K., Durie, P., Levison, H., and Forstner, G. Improved prognosis in CF patients with normal fat absorption. *J. Pediatr. Gastroenterol. Nutr.* 3, S99-S105, 1984.
4. Farrell, P., Sondel, S., Palta, M., and Mischler, E. Prevention of growth retardation in infants with cystic fibrosis. In: *Proceedings 9th International Cystic Fibrosis Congress,* Brighton, England, 1984, John Wiley & Sons, New York, 1984, p. 391.
5. Cystic Fibrosis Patient Registry 1982 Data Base. Cystic Fibrosis Foundation, Rockville, Maryland.
6. Hamill, P. V. V., Drizd, T. A., Johnson, C. L., Reed, R. B., Roche, A. F., and Moore, W. M. Physical growth: National Center for Health Statistics percentiles. *Am. J. Clin. Nutr.* 32, 607-629, 1979.
7. Smith, A. E., Wessel, H. U., and Lloyd-Still, J. D. The relationship of caloric intake and dietary composition to severity of clinical status in cystic fibrosis. *Proceedings 9th International Cystic Fibrosis Congress,* Brighton, England, 1984, John Wiley & Sons, New York, 1984, p. 318.
8. Smith, A. E., and Lloyd-Still, J. D. Value of computerized dietary analysis in pediatric nutrition: An analysis of 147 patients. *J. Pediatr.* 103, 820-824, 1983.
9. Boyer, P. H. Low birth weight in fibrocystic disease of the pancreas. *Pediatrics* 76, 778-784, 1955.
10. Hsia, D. Y. Y. Birth weight in cystic fibrosis of the pancreas. *Ann. Hum. Genet.* 23, 289-299, 1959.
11. Holsclaw, D. S., Eckstein, H. B., and Nixon, H. H. Meconium ileus. *Am. J. Dis. Child.* 109, 101-113, 1965.

12. Lloyd-Still, J. D., Khaw, K. T., and Shwachman, H. Severe respiratory disease in infants with cystic fibrosis. *Pediatrics* 53, 678-682, 1974.
13. Gurwitz, D., Corey, M., Francis, P. W. J., Crozier, D. N., and Levison, H. Perspectives in cystic fibrosis. *Pediatr. Clin. North Am.* 26, 603-615, 1979.
14. Corey, M., McLaughlin, F. J., Williams, M., and Levison, H. A comparison of CF clinic populations in Toronto and Boston. *Cystic Fibrosis Club Abstracts, 26th Annual Meeting,* Anaheim, CA, 1985, Vol. 26, p. 67.

APPENDIX

Infant Formula and Enteral Products to Meet Nutritional Needs

Nancy Moses
North Shore University Hospital, Manhasset, New York

Given the special and diverse needs for the nutritional management of sick infants, children, and adults, many infant formulas and enteral nutritional supplements have been developed. These commercially available formulas vary considerably in their composition and cost. It is therefore necessary for physicians and nutritionists to review the various components of the enteral products prior to selecting the appropriate dietary treatment for a particular medical problem. This appendix is an up-to-date tabular review of the infant formulas and enteral products used in current medical practice.

The infant formulas listed in Tables 1-3 are categorized according to the type and form of protein source (milk-based; soy-based; casein hydrolysates). The formulas and dietary supplements listed in Table 4 are designed for the dietary management of specific metabolic problems of infancy. Information regarding special premature formulas are reported in Chapter 16 of this book (Table 3, p. 218).

The formulas listed in Tables 5-10 are nutritional supplements developed for use in children, adolescent, and adult populations. These formulas are categorized according to type and form of protein, formula osmolality, and lactose content. Table 11 lists formulas for special metabolic situations such as pulmonary, hepatic, and renal diseases. Modular nutritional supplements of protein, carbohydrate, and fat sources are listed in Table 12.

The data on the nutrient composition of all listed products were obtained from product information distributed by the respective manufacturers. This information is presented in the tables on the basis of a volume of 1 liter.

In addition to formula composition, another factor that should be considered in selecting a nutritional supplement is cost. Therefore, the tables include the estimated cost of these products based on either the retail or wholesale market price.

In summary, there are numerous infant formulas and nutritional supplements that are commercially available for the dietary management of various medical problems. The information provided by these tables should assist health professionals in selecting the appropriate enteral formulation for their patients of any age group.

Table 1   Human Milk and Milk-Based Infant Formulas[a]

	Human milk[b]	Enfamil	Similac	SMA
Nutrient source				
Protein	Whey, casein	Whey, casein (nonfat cow's milk)	Whey, casein (nonfat cow's milk)	Nonfat cow's milk, demineralized
g/liter	11	15	15	15
Fat	Human	Coconut oil, soy oil	Soy oil, coconut oil	Oleo, coconut, oleoic, and soy oil
g/liter	45	38	36	36
Carbohydrate	Lactose	Lactose	Lactose	Lactose
g/liter	68	69	72	72
Caloric content				
Calories/L	750	670	676	670
% Protein calories	7	9	9	9
% Fat calories	55	50	48	48
% Carbohydrate calories	38	41	43	43
Nutrient analysis (amount per liter)				
Vitamin A IU	1898	2083	2000	2642
Vitamin D IU	22	416	400	444

Table 1 (continued)

	Human milk[b]	Enfamil	Similac	SMA
Nutrient analysis (continued)				
Vitamin E IU	1.8	21	20	9.5
Vitamin C mg	43	54	55	58
Thiamin mg	0.16	0.52	0.7	0.7
Riboflavin mg	0.36	1.0	1.0	1.05
Niacin mg	1.47	8.3	7	10
Vitamin B_6 mg	0.1	0.4	0.4	0.4
Vitamin B_{12} μg	0.3	1.6	1.5	1.1
Folic acid μg	52	104	100	53
Vitamin K μg	15	57	55	58
Pantothenic acid mg	1.84	3.1	3.0	2.1
Calcium mg	340	458	510	420
Phosphorus mg	140	312	390	330
Magnesium mg	40	52	41	53
Zinc mg	4	5.2	5	3.7
Iron mg	0.5	1.0[c]	1.5[d]	12.6
Copper mg	0.4	0.6	0.6	0.5
Sodium mg(mEq)	160 (7)	185 (8)	230 (10)	150 (7)
Potassium mg(mEq)	510 (13)	729 (19)	800 (21)	560 (14)
Chloride mg(mEq)	390 (11)	416 (12)	500 (14)	370 (10)
Cost/liter	0	$2.04[e]	$2.04[e]	
Cost/1000 kcal	0	$3.04	$3.04	
Producer	Mother	Mead Johnson	Ross	Wyeth
Form	Ready-to-use liquid	Concentrate, ready-to-use liquid, powder	Concentrate, ready-to-use liquid, powder	Concentrate, ready-to-use, liquid, powder

[a]Composition based on normal recommended dilution.
[b]Data on human milk from S. J. Fomon, *Infant Nutrition,* 2nd ed., Saunders, Philadelphia, 1974, p. 362, and I. Macy, H. Kelly, and R. Sloan, *The Composition of Milks*, National Academy of Sciences, Washington, D.C., 1953.
[c]Enfamil with Iron contains 12.5 mg/liter iron.
[d]Similac with Iron contains 12 mg/liter iron.
[e]Costs based on customer price of one case of ready-to-use liquid formula in a pharmacy in Great Neck, New York.

Table 2 Soy-Based Infant Formulas

	Prosobee	Isomil[a]	Nursoy	Advance	Soyalac	I-Soyalac
Nutrient source						
Protein	Soy protein isolate, L-methionine	Soy protein isolate, L-methionine, taurine, L-carnitine	Soy protein isolate, L-methionine	Nonfat milk, soy protein isolate, taurine	Soybean solids, L-methionine	Soybean protein isolate, L-methionine
g/liter	20	18	21	20	21	21
Fat	Coconut oil, soy oil	Soy oil, coconut oil	Oleo, coconut oils	Soy oil, corn oil	Soy oil	Soy oil
g/liter	36	37	36	27	37	37
Carbohydrate	Corn syrup solids	Corn syrup, sucrose	Sucrose	Corn syrup	Corn syrup, sucrose	Sucrose, tapioca dextrins
g/liter	69	68	69	55	66	66
Caloric content						
Calories/liter	667	676	670	540	680	680
% Protein calories	12	11	12	15	12	12
% Fat calories	48	49	48	45	49	49
% Carbohydrate calories	40	40	40	40	39	39
Nutrient analysis (amount per liter)						
Vitamin A IU	2083	2000	2604	2000	2100	2100
Vitamin D IU	417	400	417	400	420	420
Vitamin E IU	21	20	9	20	16	16
Vitamin C mg	54	55	57	50	63	63

	Mead Johnson	Ross Laboratories	Wyeth	Ross	Loma Linda	Loma Linda
Thiamin mg	0.5	0.4	0.7	0.75	0.53	0.53
Riboflavin mg	0.6	0.6	1.0	0.90	0.63	0.63
Niacin mg	8	9.0	9.5[b]	10	8.5	8.5
Vitamin B_6 mg	0.42	0.4	0.4	0.6	0.4	0.4
Vitamin B_{12} μg	2.1	3.0	2.1	2.5	2.1	2.1
Folic acid μg	104	100	52	100	106	106
Vitamin K μg	104	100	104	55	53	53
Pantothenic acid mg	3.1	5.0	3.1	4.0	3.2	3.2
Calcium mg	625	700	635	510	630	630
Phosphorus mg	495	500	445	390	420	420
Magnesium mg	73	50	68	64	74	74
Zinc mg	0.8	5.0	3.6	5.0	5.3	5.3
Iron mg	12.5	12.0	12.5	12.0	13.0	13.0
Copper mg	0.6	0.5	0.5	0.6	0.5	0.5
Sodium mg(mEq)	243 (11)	320 (10)	207 (9)	230 (10)	350 (15)	350 (15)
Potassium mg(mEq)	824 (21)	950 (24)	741 (19)	900 (23)	740 (19)	740 (19)
Chloride mg(mEq)	542 (15)	430 (12)	370 (10)	520 (14)	390 (11)	390 (11)
Cost/liter	$2.04	$2.04	$1.66	$1.86	$2.12	$2.12
Cost/1000 kcal	$3.06	$3.06	$2.48	$3.44	$3.12	$3.12
Producer	Mead Johnson	Ross Laboratories	Wyeth	Ross	Loma Linda	Loma Linda
Form	Concentrate, ready-to-use liquid, powder	Concentrate, ready-to-use liquid	Concentrate, ready-to-use liquid	Ready-to-use liquid	Concentrate, ready-to-use liquid, powder	Concentrate, ready-to-use liquid

[a] Isomil SF has the same composition as Isomil excluding sucrose.
[b] Niacin mg equivalents.

Table 3 Protein Hydrolysate Infant Formulas

	Nutramigen	Pregestimil
Nutrient source		
Protein	Casein hydroly-sate	Casein hydrolysate
g/liter	22	19
Fat	Corn oil	Corn oil, medium-chain triglycerides
g/liter	26	27
Carbohydrate	Sucrose, modified tapioca starch	Corn syrup solids, modified tapioca starch
g/liter	88	91
Caloric content		
Calories/liter	640	640
% Protein calories	13	11
% Fat calories	35	35
% Carbohydrate calories	52	54
Nutrient analysis (amount per liter)		
Vitamin A IU	1667	2083
Vitamin D IU	417	417
Vitamin E IU	10	16
Vitamin C mg	54	54
Thiamin mg	0.5	0.5
Riboflavin mg	0.6	0.6
Niacin mg	8	8
Vitamin B_6 mg	0.4	0.4
Vitamin B_{12} μg	2.1	2.1
Folic acid μg	104	104
Vitamin K μg	104	104
Pantothenic acid mg	3.1	3.1
Calcium mg	625	625
Phosphorus mg	469	417
Magnesium mg	73	73
Zinc mg	4.2	4.2
Iron mg	12.5	12.5
Copper mg	0.6	0.6
Sodium mg(mEq)	312 (14)	312 (14)
Potassium mg(mEq)	677 (17)	729 (19)
Chloride mg(mEq)	469 (13)	573 (16)
Cost/liter	$2.90	$3.24
Cost/1000 kcal	$4.53	$5.06
Producer	Mead Johnson	Mead Johnson
Form	Powder	Powder

Table 4 Special Infant Formulas

	Portagen	Lofenalac	RCF	Product 3232 A[a]	MSUD Diet Powder[b]	Product 3200 AB[c]	Product 3200 K[d]
Nutrient source							
Protein	Sodium caseinate	Casein hydrolysate	Soy protein isolate, L-methionine, taurine, L-carnitine	Casein hydrolysate	Free amino acids[e]	Casein hydrolysate[f]	Soy protein isolate
g/liter	24	22	20	19	12	22	21
Fat	MCT oil (86%), corn oil (14%)	Corn oil	Soy oil, coconut oil	MCT oil, corn oil	Corn oil	Corn oil	Corn oil, coconut oil
g/liter	32	26	36	28	28	27	37
Carbohydrate	Corn syrup solids, sucrose	Corn syrup solids, modified tapioca starch	—	Modified tapioca starch	Corn syrup solids, modified tapioca starch	Corn syrup solids, modified tapioca starch	Corn syrup solids
g/liter	78	88	0	91	88	88	67
Caloric content							
Calories/liter	667	667	405	650	667	667	667
% Protein calories	14	13	20	11	14	13	12
% Fat calories	40	35	80	36	39	36	49
% Carbohydrate calories	46	52	—	53	47	51	39

Table 4 (continued)

Nutrient analysis (amount per liter)	Portagen	Lofenalac	RCF	Product 3232 A[a]	MSUD Diet Powder[b]	Product 3200 AB[c]	Product 3200 K[d]
Vitamin A IU	5208	1667	2000	2500	1667	1667	1667
Vitamin D IU	521	417	400	500	417	417	417
Vitamin E IU	21	10	20	25	10	10	10
Vitamin C mg	54	54	55	78	54	54	54
Thiamin mg	1.0	0.5	0.4	0.5	0.5	0.5	0.5
Riboflavin mg	1.2	0.6	0.6	0.6	0.6	0.6	0.6
Niacin mg	13.5	8.3	9.0	8.3	8.3	8.3	8.3
Vitamin B_6 mg	1.4	0.4	0.4	0.4	0.42	0.42	0.42
Vitamin B_{12} μg	4.2	2.1	3.0	2.1	2.1	2.1	2.1
Folic acid μg	104	104	100	104	104	104	104
Vitamin K μg	104	104	100	125	104	104	104
Pantothenic acid mg	7.0	3.1	5.0	3.1	3.1	3.1	3.1
Calcium mg	625	625	700	625	687	687	573
Phosphorus mg	469	469	500	417	375	469	417

Magnesium mg	135	73	50	73	73	73	52
Zinc mg	6.2	4.2	5.0	4.2	4.2	4.2	5.2
Iron mg	12.5	12.5	1.5	12.5	12.5	12.5	12.5
Copper mg	1.0	0.6	0.5	0.6	0.6	0.6	0.6
Sodium mg(mEq)	312 (14)	312 (14)	320 (14)	286 (12)	260 (11)	312 (14)	260 (11)
Potassium mg(mEq)	833 (21)	677 (17)	770 (20)	729 (19)	687 (18)	677 (17)	573 (15)
Chloride mg(mEq)	573 (16)	469 (13)	590 (16)	573 (16)	521 (14)	469 (13)	417 (12)
Cost/liter^g	$2.38	$4.65	$1.90				
Cost/1000 kcal	$3.57	$6.97	$4.69				
Producer	Mead Johnson	Mead Johnson	Ross Laboratories	Mead Johnson	Mead Johnson	Mead Johnson	Mead Johnson
Form	Powder	Powder	Concentrated liquid	Powder	Powder	Powder	Powder

[a]Mono- and disaccharide-free diet powder; nutrient composition in normal dilution of 20 kcal/oz with 81 g powder and 59 g carbohydrate.
[b]Maple syrup urine disease.
[c]Low phenylalanine and tyrosine formula powder for use in the dietary management of hereditary tyrosinemia.
[d]Soy protein isolate formula powder without added methionine for the dietary management of infants with homocystinuria.
[e]Protein is incomplete with inadequate amounts of leucine, isoleucine, and valine for normal growth.
[f]Protein is incomplete with inadequate amounts of phenylalanine for normal growth.
[g]Cost based on price of one case formula purchased by hospital in Great Neck, New York.

Table 5 Blenderized, Whole Protein Nutritional Supplements

	Vitaneed	Ccmpleat-B	Compleat Modified
Nutrient source			
Protein	Beef puree, sodium and calcium caseinates	Beef puree, nonfat milk	Beef puree, calcium caseinate
g/liter	35	43	43
Fat	Beef puree, partially hydrogenated soy oil	Beef puree, corn oil	Beef puree, corn oil
g/liter	40	43	37
Carbohydrate	Maltodextrin, green bean, peach, carrot puree	Hydrolyzed cereal solids, fruit and vegetable purees, nonfat milk	Hydrolyzed cereal solids
g/liter	125	128	140
mOsm/kg H_2O	310	405	300
Caloric content			
Calories/cc	1.0	1.07	1.07
Total calorie:N ratio	179:1	156:1	156:1
Nonprotein calorie:N ratio	154:1	131:1	131:1
% Protein calories	14	16	16
% Fat calories	36	36	30
% Carbohydrate calories	50	48	54
Nutrient analysis (amount per liter)			
Vitamin A IU	2500	3332	3332
Vitamin D IU	200	268	268
Vitamin E IU	30	20	20
Vitamin C mg	150	60	60
Thiamin mg	1.5	1.5	1.5
Riboflavin mg	1.7	1.7	1.7
Niacin mg	20	13	13
Vitamin B_6 mg	2.0	2.0	2.0
Vitamin B_{12} μg	6.0	4.0	4.0
Folic acid μg	200	280	280
Vitamin K μg	150	68	68
Pantothenic acid mg	5	7	7

Table 5 (continued)

	Vitaneed	Compleat-B	Compleat Modified
Calcium mg	500	680	680
Phosphorus mg	500	1320	920
Magnesium mg	200	268	268
Sodium mg(mEq)	500 (22)	1280 (56)	680 (30)
Potassium mg(mEq)	1250 (32)	1400 (36)	1400 (36)
Chloride mg(mEq)	850 (24)	880 (24)	480 (14)
Zinc mg	15	10	10
Copper mg	1.0	1.3	1.3
Iron mg	9.0	12.0	12.0
Lactose (g)	0	26.1	0
Standard require-ments (cc)[a]	2400	1800	1800
Cost/liter	$3.86	$6.08	$7.68
Cost/standard req.	$9.26	$10.22	$12.92
Cost/1000 kcal	$3.86	$5.68	$7.18
Producer	Biosearch	Sandoz Nutrition	Sandoz Nutrition
Form	Ready-to-use liquid	Ready-to-use liquid	Ready-to-use liquid

[a]Standard requirements represent the highest recommended level of intake for any age group (excluding pregnant and lactating women) proposed in the 1980 Recommended Dietary Allowances.

Table 6 Hypertonic, Lactose-Containing Nutritional Supplements

	Meritene Liquid	Meritene Powder[b]	Sustacal Powder[d]	Carnation Instant Breakfast[f]
Nutrient source				
Protein	Skim milk, sodium caseinate	Nonfat dry milk, calcium caseinate	Nonfat milk	Nonfat milk, soy protein, Na caseinate
g/liter	58	65	75.9	62
Fat	Corn oil	Milk fat	Milk fat	Milk fat
g/liter	32	32	34.1	33
Carbohydrate	Corn syrup solids	Sucrose, corn syrup solids, fructose	Sucrose, corn syrup solids	Sucrose, corn syrup solids
g/liter	110	113	178	146
mOsm/kg H_2O	505	690	1010	g
Caloric content				
Calories/cc	1.0	1.0[c]	1.33[e]	1:1
Total calorie:N ratio	108:1	96:1	106:1	114:1
Nonprotein calorie:N ratio	78:1	71:1	80:1	89:1
% Protein calories	24	26	23	22
% Fat calories	30	29	23	26
% Carbohydrate calories	46	45	54	52
Nutrient analysis (amount per liter)				
Vitamin A IU	4000	4545	6185	5208
Vitamin D IU	320	364	493	417
Vitamin E IU	24	27	37	15
Vitamin C mg	72	54.5	74	108
Thiamin mg	1.8	1.4	1.9	1.7

	Sandoz (Doyle) Ready-to-use	Sandoz (Doyle) Powder	Mead Johnson Powder	Carnation Powder
Riboflavin mg	2.1	2.5	2.2	2.3
Niacin mg	16	18	26	22
Vitamin B_6 mg	2.4	1.8	2.6	2.3
Vitamin B_{12} μg	4.8	6.5	7.4	3.1
Folic acid μg	320	364	493	417
Vitamin K μg	—	73		NA
Pantothenic acid mg	8	9.1	13.0	7.3
Calcium mg	1200	2073	2148	1696
Phosphorus mg	1200	1818	1778	1608
Magnesium mg	320	364	500	479
Sodium mg(mEq)	880 (38)	1018 (44)	1222 (53)	1008 (44)
Potassium mg(mEq)	1600 (41)	2655 (68)	3370 (86)	2962 (76)
Chloride mg(mEq)	1600 (44)	2073 (58)	1778 (49)	g
Zinc mg	12	13.5	18.5	13.7
Copper mg	1.6	1.8	2.6	2.0
Iron mg	14.4	16.4	22.2	15.9
Lactose (g)	56.7	97.5	85.8	84.0
Standard requirements (cc)[a]	1250	1100	850	1400
Cost/liter	$3.46	$2.67	$2.88	$1.83
Cost/standard req.	$4.32	$3.34	$2.45	$2.56
Cost/1000 kcal	$3.46	$2.67	$2.17	$1.66
Producer	Sandoz (Doyle)	Sandoz (Doyle)	Mead Johnson	Carnation
Form	Ready-to-use	Powder	Powder	Powder

[a]Data on human milk from S. J. Fomon, *Infant Nutrition*, 2nd ed., Saunders, Philadelphia, 1974, p. 362, and I. Macy, H. Kelly, and R. Sloan, *The Composition of Milks*, National Academy of Sciences, Washington, D.C., 1953.
[b]With added whole milk.
[c]Standard dilution.
[d]With added whole milk, vanilla flavor.
[e]40 cal/oz dilution.
[f]With added whole milk.
[g]Information not found.

Table 7 Hypertonic, Lactose-Free, Whole Protein Nutritional Supplements

	Sustacal Liquid	Ensure Liquid	Travasorb Liquid	Precision High Nitrogen	Precision Low Residue	Citrotein
Nutrient source Protein	Calcium and sodium caseinate, soy protein isolate	Sodium and calcium caseinates, soy protein isolate	Sodium and calcium caseinate, soy protein isolate	Egg white solids	Egg white solids	Egg white solids
g/liter	61	37	36	44	46.3	40.8
Fat	Partially hydrogenated soy oil	Corn oil	Corn oil, partially hydrogenated soy oil	Medium chain triglycerides, partially hydrogenated soybean oil	Medium-chain triglycerides, partially hydrogenated soybean oil	Partially hydrogenated soybean oil
g/liter	23	37	36	1.3	1.6	1.6
Carbohydrate	Sucrose, corn syrup	Hydrolyzed corn starch, sucrose	Sucrose, corn syrup solids	Maltodextrins, sucrose	Maltodextrins, sucrose	Sucrose, maltodextrins
g/liter	140	143	142	217	249	120.7
mOsm/kg H_2O	620, 700[b]	450	450	557	525	480-515[d]
Caloric content Calories/cc	1.0	1.06	1.06	1.05[c]	1.11[c]	0.66[c]
Total calorie:N ratio	102:1	169:1	174:1	150:1	268:1	101:1
Nonprotein calorie:N ratio	79:1	153:1	155:1	125:1	243:1	76:1

% Protein calories	24	14	14	17	9	25
% Fat calories	21	31.5	31.5	1	1	2
% Carbohydrate calories	55	54.5	54.5	82	90	73
Nutrient analysis (amount per liter)						
Vitamin A IU	4700	2500	2637	1750	2917	5164
Vitamin D IU	370	200	211	140	235	415
Vitamin E IU	29	22.8	31.6	10.5	17.5	31
Vitamin C mg	56	152	160	31.5	52.5	233
Thiamin mg	1.4	1.5	1.6	0.8	1.3	3.1
Riboflavin mg	1.7	1.7	1.8	0.9	1.5	3.5
Niacin mg	20	20	21	7	12	42
Vitamin B_6 mg	2.0	2.0	2.1	1.1	1.8	4.3
Vitamin B_{12} μg	5.6	6.0	6.3	2.1	3.5	12.4
Folic acid μg	370	200	211	140	235	815
Vitamin K μg	230	36	1013	35	58	—
Pantothenic acid mg	9.8	5.0	5.3	3.5	5.8	20.6
Calcium mg	1010	520	527	350	585	1048
Phosphorus mg	930	520	527	350	585	1048
Magnesium mg	380	200	211	140	234	415
Sodium mg(mEq)	940 (41)	800 (35)	738 (32)	980 (43)	700 (30)	699 (30)
Potassium mg(mEq)	2100 (54)	1480 (38)	1266 (32)	910 (23)	875 (22)	699 (18)
Chloride mg(mEq)	1570 (44)	1360 (38)	1055 (29)	1190 (33)	1121 (31)	932 (26)
Zinc mg	14.1	15.0	15.8	5.25	8.8	15.5

Table 7 (continued)

	Sustacal Liquid	Ensure Liquid	Travasorb Liquid	Precision High Nitrogen	Precision Low Residue	Citrotein
Copper mg	2.0 m	1.0	1.1	0.7	1.16	2.06
Iron mg	16.9	9.0	9.5	6.3	10.5	37.3
Lactose (g)	0	0	0	0	0	0
Standard requirements (cc)	1290	2300	2275	3430	2050	1145
Cost/liter	$3.89	$3.24		$9.93	$4.67	$3.54
Cost/standard req.	$5.02	$7.48		$34.07	$9.57	$4.05
Cost/1000 kcal	$3.89	$3.06		$10.43	$5.18	$5.00
Producer	Mead Johnson	Ross Laboratories	Travenol Laboratories	Sandoz (Doyle)	Sandoz (Doyle)	Sandoz Nutrition (Doyle)
Form	Ready-to-use liquid	Ready-to-use liquid, powder	Ready-to-use liquid	Powder	Powder	Powder

aStandard requirement represents the highest recommended absolute level of intake for any age group (except pregnant and lactating women) proposed in the 1980 Recommended Dietary Allowances.
bApplies to chocolate flavor only.
cStandard dilution.
dVaries with flavors.

Table 8 Isotonic, Lactose-Free, Whole Protein Nutritional Supplements

	Isocal	Osmolite	Precision Isotonic	Travabsorb MCT	RENU	Entri-Pak with Entrition	Osmolite HN
Nutrient source							
Protein	Calcium and Na caseinate, soy protein isolate	Na and Ca caseinates, soy protein isolates	Egg white solids, sodium caseinate	Lactalbumin, potassium caseinate	Calcium and sodium caseinate	Sodium and calcium caseinates	Sodium and calcium caseinate, soy protein isolate
g/liter	34	37	30	49	35	35	44
Fat	Soy oil blend (80%), medium-chain triglycerides (20%)	Medium-chain triglycerides (50%), corn oil (40%), soy oil blend (10%)	Partially hydrogenated soybean oil	Medium-chain triglycerides (80%), sunflower oil (20%)	Soy oil	Corn oil	Medium-chain triglycerides (50%), corn oil (40%), soy oil (10%)
g/liter	44	38	31.2	33	40	35	36
Carbohydrate	Maltodextrin	Hydrolyzed corn starch	Maltodextrin, sucrose	Corn syrup solids	Maltodextrin, sucrose	Maltodextrin	Hydrolyzed corn starch, sucrose
g/liter	133	143	150	123	125	136	139
mOsm/kg H$_2$O	300	300	300	250	300	300	310
Caloric content							
Calories/cc	1.06	1.06	1.0	1.0[b]	1.0	1.0	1.06
Total calorie:N ratio	192:1	178:1	208:1	125:1	179:1	178:1	150:1
Nonprotein calorie:N ratio	167:1	153:1	183:1	100:1	154:1	154:1	125:1
% Protein calories	13	14	12	20	14	14	17
% Fat calories	37	31.4	28	29	36	31.5	30
% Carbohydrate calories	50	54.6	60	51	50	54.5	53

Table 8 (continued)

Nutrient analysis (amount per liter)	Isocal	Osmolite	Precision Isotonic	Travabsorb MCT	RENU	Entri-Pak with Entrition	Osmolite HN
Vitamin A IU	2600	2604	3332	2500	2500	2500	3750
Vitamin D IU	210	208	268	200	200	200	300
Vitamin E IU	40	24	20	30	30	30	34
Vitamin C mg	159	158	60	150	150	150	137
Thiamin mg	2.0	1.58	1.5	1.5	1.5	1.9	1.7
Riboflavin mg	2.3	1.8	1.7	1.7	1.7	1.7	1.9
Niacin mg	26	21	13	20	20	20	22
Vitamin B_6 mg	2.6	2.1	2.0	2.0	2.0	2.0	2.3
Vitamin B_{12} µg	7.9	6.2	4.0	6.0	6.0	6.0	7.1
Folic acid µg	210	208	268	200	200	200	458
Vitamin K µg	132	37	67	75	150	100	54
Pantothenic acid mg	13.2	5.2	6.8	5.0	5	10	11
Calcium mg	630	542	680	500	500	500	750
Phosphorus mg	530	542	680	500	500	500	750
Magnesium mg	210	208	268	200	200	200	300

	Mead Johnson	Ross Laboratories	Sandoz Nutrition (Doyle)	Travenol Laboratories	Biosearch	Biosearch	Ross Laboratories
Sodium mg(mEq)	530 (23)	542 (24)	800 (35)	350 (15)	500 (22)	700 (31)	917 (40)
Potassium mg(mEq)	1320 (34)	1000 (26)	1000 (26)	1740 (45)	1252 (32)	1200 (30.7)	1542 (40)
Chloride mg(mEq)	1060 (29)	833 (23)	1080 (31)	1215 (34)	852 (24)	1000 (28)	1417 (39)
Zinc mg	10.6	15.4	10	15	15	7.5	17
Copper mg	1.1	1.04	1.3	1.0	1.0	1.0	1.5
Iron mg	9.5	9.2	12	9.0	9.0	9.0	13.7
Lactose (g)	0	0	0	0	0	0	0
Standard requirements (cc)[a]	2300	2200	1800	2400	2400	2400	1600
Cost/liter	$4.02	$2.25	$8.40		$3.66	$4.95	$2.53
Cost/standard req.	$9.26	$4.95	$15.12		$8.79	$11.88	$4.05
Cost/1000 kcal	$3.79	$2.12	$8.40		$3.66	$4.95	$2.39
Producer	Mead Johnson	Ross Laboratories	Sandoz Nutrition (Doyle)	Travenol Laboratories	Biosearch	Biosearch	Ross Laboratories
Form	Liquid	Liquid	Powder	Powder	Liquid, ready-to-use liquid	Ready to deliver	Ready-to-use liquid

[a]Data on human milk from S. J. Fomon, *Infant Nutrition*, 2nd ed., Saunders, Philadelphia, 1974, p. 362, and I. Macy, H. Kelly, and R. Sloan, *The Composition of Milks*, National Academy of Sciences, Washington, D.C., 1953.
[b]Standard dilution.

Table 9 Hypertonic, High Calorie, High Nitrogen, Whole Protein Nutritional Supplements

	Sustacal HC	Ensure Plus	Magnacal	Ensure HN	Isotein HN	Sustagen	Ensure Plus HN	Two Cal HN
Nutrient source								
Protein	Calcium and sodium caseinate	Sodium and calcium caseinates, soy protein isolates	Sodium and calcium caseinates	Sodium and calcium caseinates, soy protein isolates	Delactosed lactalbumin, Na and Ca caseinates	Nonfat milk, powdered whole milk, Ca caseinate	Sodium and calcium caseinates, soy protein isolates	Sodium and calcium caseinates, soy protein isolates
g/liter	61	54	70	44	69	111	63	82
Fat	Corn oil	Corn oil	Soy oil	Corn oil	Soy oil; medium-chain triglycerides (25%)	Milk fat	Corn oil	Corn oil, medium-chain triglycerides
g/liter	58	53	80	35	34	17	49	90
Carbohydrate	Corn syrup solids, sucrose	Hydrolyzed corn starch, sucrose	Maltodextrin, sucrose	Hydrolyzed corn starch, sucrose	Maltodextrin, fructose	Corn syrup solids, dextrose, lactose	Hydrolyzed corn starch, and sucrose	Hydrolyzed corn starch, sucrose
g/liter	190	197	250	139	158	312	197	214
mOsm/kg H_2O	650	600	590	470	300	1100	650	750
Caloric content								
Calories/cc	1.50	1.50	2.0	1.06	1.2	1.85	1.5	2.0
Total calorie:N ratio	160:1	171:1	179:1	150:1	110:1	102:1	150:1	150:1
Nonprotein calorie:N ratio	134:1	146:1	154:1	79:1	85:1	77:1	124:1	127:1
% Protein calories	16	15	14	17	23	24	17	17
% Fat calories	34	32	36	30	25	8	30	40
% Carbohydrate calories	50	53	50	53	52	68	53	43

Nutrient analysis (amount per liter)								
Vitamin A IU	4200	3708	5000	3750	2856	5208	5208	5208
Vitamin D IU	340	292	400	300	230	417	417	417
Vitamin E IU	25	32	60	34	17	47	47	47
Vitamin C mg	76	158	300	137	51	312	250	187
Thiamin mg	1.9	2.6	3.0	1.7	1.3	4.0	3.1	2.5
Riboflavin mg	2.1	2.7	3.4	1.9	1.5	4.5	3.5	2.8
Niacin mg	25	31	40	22	11	52	42	33
Vitamin B$_6$ mg	2.5	3.1	4	2.3	1.7	5.2	4.2	3.3
Vitamin B$_{12}$ μg	7.6	9.4	12	7.1	3.4	15.6	12.5	10.0
Folic acid μg	510	312	400	458	240	417	833	667
Vitamin K μg	210	54	300	54	58	260	75	75
Pantothenic acid mg	13	8	10	11	5.8	26	21	17
Calcium mg	850	625	1000	750	583	3333	1042	1042
Phosphorus mg	850	625	1000	750	583	2500	1042	1042
Magnesium mg	340	312	400	300	230	417	417	417
Sodium mg(mEq)	850 (36)	1725 (75)	1000 (44)	917 (40)	617 (27)	1250 (54)	1167 (51)	1042 (45)
Potassium mg(mEq)	1480 (38)	2292 (59)	1250 (32)	1542 (40)	1097 (28)	3333 (85)	1792 (46)	2292 (59)
Chloride mg(mEq)	1270 (36)	1958 (54)	950 (27)	1417 (39)	960 (27)	2812 (78)	1583 (44)	1542 (43)
Zinc mg	13	23	30	17	8.6	21	15.8	24
Copper mg	1.7	1.6	2.0	1.5	1.1	2.1	2.1	2.1
Iron mg	15	14:1	18	13.7	10.3	18.7	18.7	18.7
Lactose (g)	0	0	0	0	0	113	0	0
Standard requirements (cc)[a]	1400	1920	1200	1600	2060	960	1150	1150
Cost/liter	$4.51	$4.22	$6.02	$1.79	$5.48	$7.73	$3.73	$3.47
Cost/standard req.	$6.31	$8.10	$7.22	$2.86	$11.29	$7.42	$4.29	$3.99

Table 9 (continued)

	Sustacal HC	Ensure Plus	Magnacal	High Nitrogen Ensure HN	Isotein HN	Sustagen	Ensure Plus HN	Two Cal HN
Cost/1000 kcal	$3.01	$2.81	$3.01	$1.69	$6.57	$4.24	$2.49	$1.73
Producer	Mead Johnson	Ross Laboratories	Biosearch	Ross Laboratories	Sandoz Nutrition (Doyle)	Mead Johnson	Ross Laboratories	Ross Laboratories
Form	Ready-to-use liquid	Ready-to-use liquid	Ready-to-use liquid	Ready-to-use liquid	Powder	Powder	Ready-to-use liquid	Ready-to-use liquid

[a]Data on human milk from S. J. Fomon, *Infant Nutrition*, 2nd ed., Saunders, Philadelphia, 1974, p. 362, and I. Macy, H. Kelly, and R. Sloan, *The Composition of Milks*, National Academy of Sciences, Washington, D.C., 1953.

Table 10 Hypertonic, Protein Hydrolysate, and Free Amino Acid Nutritional Supplements

	Criticare HN	Vital HN	Travasorb STD	Travasorb STD	Vivonex STD	Vivonex HN	Vivonex T.E.N.
Nutrient source							
Protein	Hydrolyzed casein and free amino acids	Partially hydrolyzed whey, meat, and soy, free amino acids	Enzymatically hydrolyzed lactalbumin	Enzymatically hydrolyzed lactalbumin	Free amino acids	Free amino acids	Free amino acids
g/liter	38	42	30	45	21	44	38
Fat	Safflower oil	Safflower oil; medium-chain triglycerides (45%)	Medium-chain triglycerides (60%), sunflower oil (40%)	Medium-chain triglycerides (60%), sunflower oil (40%)	Safflower oil	Safflower oil	Safflower oil
g/liter	3	11	13	13	1.5	0.9	2.8
Carbohydrate	Maltodextrin, modified corn starch	Hydrolyzed corn starch, sucrose	Glucose oligo-saccharides, sucrose	Glucose oligo-saccharides	Glucose oligo-saccharides	Glucose	Maltodextrin
g/liter	222	185	190	175	231	210	206
mOsm/kg H_2O	650	460	560	560	550	810	630
Caloric content							
Calories/cc	1.06	1.0	1.0	1.0	1.0	1.0	1.0
Total calorie:N ratio	173:1	150:1	208:1	138:1	306:1	150:1	175:1
Nonprotein calorie:N ratio	148:1	125:1	183:1	113:1	281:1	123:1	149:1

Table 10 (continued)

	Criticare HN	Vital HN	Travasorb STD	Travasorb STD	Vivonex STD	Vivonex HN	Vivonex T.E.N.
% Protein calories	14	17	12	18	8	18	15
% Fat calories	3	9	12	12	1	1	3
% Carbohydrate calories	83	74	76	70	91	81	82
Nutrient analysis (amount per liter)							
Vitamin A IU	2600	3333	2500	2500	2778	1667	2500
Vitamin D IU	210	267	200	200	222	133	200
Vitamin E IU	40	30	15	15	17	10	15
Vitamin C mg	159	60	45	45	33	20	60
Thiamin mg	2.0	1.0	0.8	0.8	0.8	0.5	1.5
Riboflavin mg	2.3	1.1	0.9	0.9	0.9	0.6	1.7
Niacin mg	26	13	10	10	11	7	20
Vitamin B_6 mg	2.6	1.5	1.0	1.0	1.1	0.7	2.0
Vitamin B_{12} µg	7.9	4.0	3.0	3.0	3.3	2.0	6.0
Folic acid µg	210	267	200	200	222	133	400
Vitamin K µg	132	47	75	75	37	22	22
Pantothenic acid mg	13.2	6.7	5	5	6	3.3	10

	Mead Johnson	Ross Laboratories	Travenol Laboratories	Travenol Laboratories	Norwich Eaton	Norwich Eaton	Norwich Eaton
Calcium mg	530	667	500	500	556	333	500
Phosphorus mg	530	667	500	500	556	333	500
Magnesium mg	210	267	200	200	222	133	200
Sodium mg(mEq)	630 (27)	467 (20)	920 (40)	920 (40)	468 (20)	529 (23)	460 (20)
Potassium mg(mEq)	1320 (34)	1333 (34)	1170 (30)	1170 (30)	1172 (30)	1173 (30)	782 (20)
Chloride mg(mEq)	1060 (29)	900 (25)	1500 (42)	1365 (38)	722 (20.4)	815 (23)	819 (23)
Zinc mg	10.6	10	7.5	7.5	8.3	5.0	10
Copper mg	1.1	1.3	1.0	1.0	1.1	0.7	1.0
Iron mg	9.5	12	9.0	9.0	10	6.0	9.0
Lactose (g)	0	0	0	0	0	0	0
Standard requirements (cc)[a]	2260	1800	2400	2400	2160	3600	2400
Cost/liter	$12.50	$7.67			$5.20	$9.97	
Cost/standard req.	$28.25	$13.79			$11.23	$35.88	
Cost/1000 kcal	$11.79	$7.67			$5.20	$9.97	
Producer	Mead Johnson	Ross Laboratories	Travenol Laboratories	Travenol Laboratories	Norwich Eaton	Norwich Eaton	Norwich Eaton
Form	Ready-to-use liquid	Powder	Powder	Powder	Powder	Powder	Powder

[a]Data on human milk from S. J. Fomon, *Infant Nutrition*, 2nd ed., Saunders, Philadelphia, 1974, p. 362, and I. Macy, H. Kelly, and R. Sloan, *The Composition of Milks*, National Academy of Sciences, Washington, D.C., 1953.

Table 11 Nutritional Supplements for Special Metabolic Problems

	Traumacal	Stresstein	Traum-Aid HBC	Lonalac	Portagen
Nutrient source					
Protein	Calcium and sodium caseinates	Free amino acids	Free amino acids	Casein	Sodium caseinate
g/liter	83[a]	69[b]	56[c]	53	35
Fat	Soybean oil (70%), medium-chain triglycerides (30%)	Medium-chain triglycerides, soybean oil	Partially hydrogenated soybean oil, medium-chain triglycerides, monodiglycerides	Coconut oil	Medium-chain triglycerides (86%), corn oil (14%)
g/liter	68	27	12	55	48
Carbohydrate	Corn syrup, sucrose	Maltodextrin	Maltodextrins	Lactose	Corn syrup solids
g/liter	142	171	166	74	115
mOsm/kg H_2O	490	910	675		320
Caloric content					
Calories/cc	1.5	1.2[d]	1.0	1.0[d]	1.0
Total calorie:N ratio	116:1	109:1	132:1	118:1	178:1
Nonprotein calorie:N ratio	90:1	84:1	102:1	93:1	153:1
% Protein calories	22	23	22	21	14
% Fat calories	40	20	11	49	41
% Carbohydrate calories	38	57	67	30	45
Nutrient analysis (amount per liter)					
Vitamin A IU	2500	2499	1667	1500	7812

	Enrich	Pulmocare	Ross SLD	Travabsorb Renal	Amin-Aid	Travabsorb Hepatic	Hepatic-Aid II
	Sodium and calcium caseinates	Sodium and calcium caseinates	Egg white solids	Crystalline L-amino acids	Crystalline L-amino acids	Crystalline L-amino acids	Crystalline L-amino acids
	39	62	38	23	19	29	44
	Corn oil	Corn oil	—	Medium-chain triglycerides oil (70%), sunflower oil (30%)	Soybean oil, mono- and diglyceride	Medium-chain triglycerides oil (70%), sunflower oil (30%)	Soybean oil, mono- and diglycerides
	37	91	0.5	18	46	14	36
	Hydrolyzed corn starch, sucrose, soy poly-saccharide	Hydrolyzed corn starch, sucrose	Sucrose, hydro-lyzed corn starch	Clucose oligo-saccharides, sucrose	Maltodextrin, sucrose	Glucose oligo-saccharides, sucrose	Maltodextrin, sucrose
	160	104	140	271	366	209	169
	480	490		590	850	690	560
	1.1	1.5	0.72	1.4	1.9	1.1	1.2
	181:1	149:1	118:1	364:1	643:1	232:1	167:1
	156:1	124:1	93:1	339:1	618:1	207:1	142:1
	14	17	21	7	4	11	15
	29	55	1	12	21	12	28
	57	28	78	81	75	77	57
	3542	5208	4274				

Table 11 (continued)

	Traumacal	Stresstein	Traum-Aid HBC	Lonalac	Portagen
Vitamin D IU	200	201	133	—	781
Vitamin E IU	38	15	20	—	31
Vitamin C mg	148	30	33	—	81
Thiamin mg	1.9	0.8	0.5	0.6	1.6
Riboflavin mg	2.2	0.8	0.6	2.7	1.9
Niacin mg	25	10	7.0	1.2	21
Vitamin B_6 mg	2.5	1.1	0.7	—	2.1
Vitamin B_{12} μg	7.5	3.0	2.0	—	6.2
Folic acid μg	200	210	133	—	156
Vitamin K μg	127	36	50	—	156
Pantothenic acid mg	12.7	5.1	3.3	—	10
Calcium mg	750	510	400	1760	937
Phosphorus mg	750	510	400	1562	703
Magnesium mg	200	201	133	141	208
Sodium mg(mEq)	1180 (51)	660 (29)	533 (23)	40 (2)	469 (20)
Potassium mg(mEq)	1390 (36)	1110 (28)	1167 (30)	1958 (50)	1250 (32)
Chloride mg(mEq)	1600 (45)	990 (28)	833 (24)	781 (22)	859 (24)
Zinc mg	14.8	7.5	6.7	—	9.4
Copper mg	1.5	1.0	0.7	—	1.6
Iron mg	8.9	9.0	6.0	—	18.7
Lactose (g)	0	0		74	0
Standard requirements (cc)[a]	2000	2400	3000	N/A	2560
Cost/liter	$5.42	$16.49			$3.57
Cost/standard req.	$10.83	$40.30		N/A	$9.14
Cost/1000 kcal	$3.61	$13.99			$3.57
Producer	Mead Johnson	Sandoz Nutrition	American McGaw	Mead Johnson	Mead Johnson
Form	Ready-to-use liquid	Powder	Powder	Powder	Powder

[a]22.5% of protein provided by branched chain amino acids.
[b]44% branched chain amino acids.
[c]Branched chain amino acids 36% of the total amino acids and 60% of total essential amino acids by weight.
[d]Standard dilution.
[e]Water-soluble vitamins only.

Enrich	Pulmocare	Ross SLD	Travabsorb Renal	Amin-Aid	Travabsorb Hepatic	Hepatic-Aid II
283	417	342				
31	47	38				
125	250	77				
1.6	3.1	2.0				
1.8	3.5	2.2				
21	42	26				
2.1	4.2	2.6				
6.2	12.5	7.7				
417	833	513				
50	75	31				
10	21	13				
708	1042	855				
708	1042	855				
283	417	342				
833 (36)	1292 (56)	855 (37)		322(14)	437 (19)	322 (14)
1542 (40)	1875 (48)	855 (22)		<195(<5)	1131 (29)	<195 (<5)
1417 (39)	1667 (46)	1026 (28)				
15.8	23.3	20				
1.4	2.1	1.7				
12.9	18.7	15.4				
0	0	0				
1700	1150	1400	2100[e]		2100[e]	
$3.55	$4.14	$2.93	$13.71	$22.06	$26.49	$40.85
$6.03	$4.76	$4.11	N/A	N/A	N/A	N/A
$3.23	$2.76	$4.09	$9.80	$11.61	$24.08	$34.04
Ross Laboratories	Ross Laboratories	Ross Laboratories	Travenol Laboratories	American McGaw	Travenol Laboratories	American McGaw
Ready-to-use liquid	Ready-to-use liquid	Powder	Powder	Powder	Powder	Powder

Table 12 Modular Supplements for Oral and Tube Feedings

	Protein		Carbohydrate			Fat		
	Casec	Propac	Moducal	Sumacal	Polycose[a]	MCT oil	Microlipid	Lipomul Oral
Calories	4.0/g	4.0/g	3.8/cc	3.8/cc	3.8/cc	7.7/cc	4.5/cc	6.0/cc
Protein source	Calcium caseinate	Whey	—	—	—	—	—	—
g/1000 kcal	237.8	192.5	0	0	0	0	0	0
Carbohydrate source	—	—	Maltodextrin	Maltodextrin	Corn starch hydrolysate	—	—	—
g/1000 kcal	0	12.5	250	250	247	0	0	1.1
Fat source	—	—	—	—	—	Coconut oil	Safflower oil, polyglycerol	Corn oil
g/1000 kcal	5.4	20	0	0	0	120.5	111.1	109.9
Producer	Mead Johnson	Biosearch	Mead Johnson	Biosearch	Ross Laboratories	Mead Johnson	Biosearch	Upjohn
Form	Powder	Powder	Powder	Powder	Powder, liquid	Liquid	Liquid	Liquid
Cost/1000 kcal		$10.37	$2.06	$1.51	$2.07	$2.62	$3.36	

[a]Use powder form for comparison.

INDEX